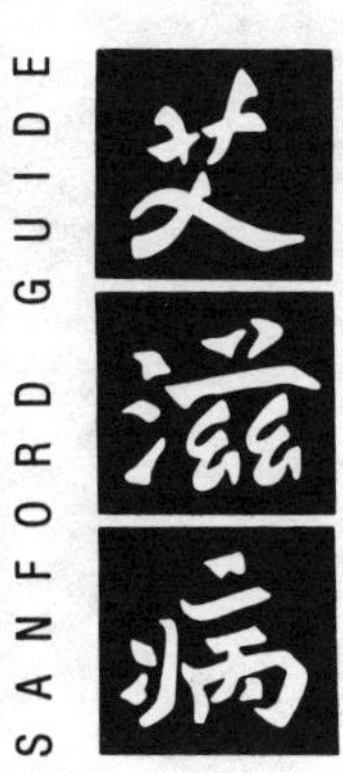

Seventh Edition

THE SANFORD

GUIDE TO HIV/AIDS THERAPY

Merle A. Sande, MD

David N. Gilbert, MD

Robert C. Moellering, Jr, MD

1998

THE SANFORD GUIDE TO HIV/AIDS THERAPY 1998
(7TH EDITION)

EDITORIAL BOARD

Merle A. Sande, M.D.
University of Utah School of Medicine
Salt Lake City, Utah

David N. Gilbert, M.D.
Providence Portland Medical Center
Oregon Health Sciences University
Portland, Oregon

Robert C. Moellering, Jr., M.D.
Beth Israel Deaconess Medical Center
Harvard Medical School
Boston, Massachusetts

The Sanford Guide to HIV/AIDS Therapy is published annually by:

ANTIMICROBIAL THERAPY, INC.
P.O. Box 70
Hyde Park, VT 05655 USA

PUBLISHER'S NOTE

You, the user, should know that the SANFORD GUIDES are not prepared for any single pharmaceutical company or distributor. Though it is distributed by multiple companies in the health care field, the SANFORD GUIDES have been independently prepared and published since their inception in 1969. The SANFORD GUIDES are not subject to any form of approval prior to publication. Decisions regarding content are solely those of the editors.

Our thanks to the Editorial Board, Carolyn Wickwire for her continued dedication to preparation of this complex manuscript, Gateway Graphics for printing and oversight of production, and Delaware Valley Bindery for finishing of this edition of the SANFORD GUIDE.

Printed in the United States of America

ISBN 0-933775-35-0

— TABLE OF CONTENTS —

TABLE 1
ASSESSMENT OF HIV INFECTION RISKS AND RECOMMENDATIONS FOR HIV TESTING

I. General

HIV risk assessment is an essential component of primary care for all patients. In talking to patients, avoid medical jargon (e.g., "intercourse"), vague terms ("sexually active"), group designations ("homosexual"), or judgmental terms ("promiscuous"). Learn the language and terminology understood and used by patients. Question responses to the depth necessary to elicit risky behavior and to define extent of risk of acquisition and transmission.

II. Specific Behaviors Associated With HIV Transmission

    A. Sexual Behaviors [The role of antiretroviral drugs for post-sexual exposure is currently being considered but data are lacking *(NEJM 336:1097, 1997)*]

        1. Sexual Partner(s)
- HIV-infected partners
- Partners who are at risk but have not been HIV tested [risk of HIV often underappreciated by partners; example, 15.7% crack cocaine smokers HIV+ vs 5.2% in non-smokers, women > men (sex for money or drugs) *(NEJM 331:1422, 1994)*]
- Multiple partners
- Presence of mucosal ulceration or other STD in either partner *(CID 23:449, 1996)*

        2. Sexual Practices

          a. High infection risk
- Unprotected anal receptive intercourse
- Unprotected vaginal receptive intercourse

          b. Infection risk documented
- Unprotected oral receptive intercourse *(AnIM 125:257, 1996)*
- Unprotected anal insertive intercourse
- Unprotected vaginal insertive intercourse (risk may be higher during menses)
- Unprotected oral insertive intercourse

          c. Lower infection risk
- Any of the above with latex/vinyl condom (vaginal or penile) protection. However, very few studies have been done to assess effectiveness of condoms in preventing HIV transmission. Based on contraceptive efficacy (97%) and defect rate (0.04%), effectiveness calculated as 8–27%/year *(J Sex Marital Therapy 15:5, 1989)*. In 343 HIV-neg. women partners of HIV+ men, seroconversion for those who used condoms with every encounter was 1.1/100 person years while for those who used condoms intermittently or not at all, rate was 7.2/100 person years *(J AIDS 6:497, 1993)*. In Thailand, aggressive condom campaign reduced seroprevalence from 7.2 to 3.8% in military conscripts.
- Cunnilingus, especially with rubber dam, microwaveable plastic food wrap or other water-impervious barrier
- Circumcision ↓ risk to male *(CID 23:449, 1996)*

          d. Safer
- Deep kissing
- Protected sex with HIV test negative partner
- Mutual monogamy
- Mutual masturbation
- Masturbation or massage

          e. Safest
- Abstinence

        3. Conditions That Facilitate HIV Sexual Transmission *(CID 23:449, 1996; NEJM 336:1072, 1997)*

Male-to-Female Transmission	Relative Risk Reported
(a) Oral contraceptives	2.5– 4.5
(b) Gonococcal cervicitis	1.8– 4.5
(c) Candida vaginitis	3.3– 3.6
(d) Genital ulcers	2.0– 4.0
(e) Vitamin A deficiency	2.6–12.9
(f) CD4 count <200	6.1–17.6
Female-to-Male Transmission	
(a) Lack of circumcision	5.4–8.2
(b) Genital ulcers	2.6–4.7
(c) Sex during menses	3.4
Titers of viral DNA in vaginal secretions increased *(JID 175:57, 1997)*	
(a) With low CD4 count	9.6 (<200 vs >500)
(b) Vitamin A deficiency	2.6
(c) Presence of cervical mucopus	2.1
(d) Acute primary HIV infection	↑
Titers of viral DNA in semen (ejaculate) *(JID 172:1469, 1995)*	
(a) Gonococcal urethritis	3.2
(b) Acute primary HIV infection	↑ *(NEJM 333:1783, 1995)*

    B. Injection (intravenous or "skin popping") Drug Use (IDU) or Smoking Crack Cocaine. Assess injectable anabolic steroid use! Assess sexual behaviors in all drug users! Infection rates in crack cocaine-smoking women are as high as in men who had sex with men (41% vs 43%).

        Drug Use Practices:

        1. Riskiest
- Sharing uncleaned needles, syringes, other paraphernalia (works), especially in "shooting galleries". HIV DNA found on 85% of needles/syringes and ⅓–⅔ cottons, cookers, wash waters from shooting galleries *(J AIDS 11:301, 1996)*.
- Practicing "registering," "booting" or "back loading"

2. Less risky
   - Sharing cleaned needles, syringes, works. (Household bleach is effective, especially after washing and when contact time is greater than 5 minutes. It is important to rinse with water after bleach use)
   - Drug paraphernalia used repeatedly but by single user
3. Least risky
   - Single use needles, syringes, works
   - Sterile needles, syringes, works (needle/syringe exchange appears effective and has not increased drug use)

C. Blood Product Infusion Recipient

Blood Product Risks:
1. Riskiest
   - Receipt of multiple units of blood products between 1978–1985
   - Receipt of blood products obtained from donors in countries where screening is unreliable or not done
2. Less risky
   - Receipt of heterologous blood products in U.S. after 1985 (risk per unit 1:450,000 to 1:660,000 units or 1:28,000 after an average of 5.4 units) *(NEJM 333:1721, 1995)*. [This is because of a window (about 20 days) between infection and seroconversion (18–27 donations/yr are in this window).] HIV p24 antigen testing of all blood products (instituted 3/96) reduces the "window" by 6 days and ↓ infectious donations by 25%/yr to 1:600,000-1:880,000 units *[MMWR 45(RR2):1, 1996]*. Rhogam and hepatitis B vaccine (serum-derived) have never been reported to transmit HIV-1.
   - Receipt of donor-selected blood products in U.S. after 1985 (but no safer than random donors)
3. Safest
   - Receipt of autologous blood products
   - Receipt of genetically engineered blood product substitutes

D. Perinatal Infection [A study on timing of HIV transmission from mother to child in Zaire estimated that 6% occur intrauterine, 18% intrapartum/early postpartum and 4% late postpartum (breast feeding) *(JID 174:722, 1996)*]
   1. General
      a. Routine perinatal screening recommended in U.S., especially in high prevalence areas/populations but should be offered to all
      b. ACTG 076, a placebo-controlled trial, demonstrated that zidovudine decreased transmission of HIV from mother to infant from 25.5% to 8.3% *(See Table 6, page 21) (NEJM 331:1173, 1994)*.
         - There has been no documentation of teratogenic effects related to zidovudine treatment *(NEJM 326:857, 1992)*
         - Several other studies have confirmed reduction to <10% but not 0% in clinical practice setting *(JAMA 275:1483, 1996; JID 174:1207, 1996)*
         - Studies in 3rd World examining ZDV rx just at time of birth in progress but complicated by ethical considerations for use of placebo control group *(NEJM 337:853, 1997)*
      c. Diagnosis of infection in neonates remains problematic
         - All newborns of HIV+ mothers carry maternal HIV antibodies, sometimes as long as 15 months
         - Although overall transmission rate in U.S. is 12–30%, only ½ of infected children are virus + by any test at birth
         - "Almost all" HIV-infected infants can now be diagnosed by 6 months of age by one or a combination of: culture, polymerase-chain reaction (PCR), serologic detection of p24 antigen or branched HIV DNA amplification assay *(JID 173:168, 1996) (see Table 2)*.
   2. Relative risk determinants
      a. Highest risk
         - Newborn of HIV+ mother who has delivered a previously infected child (risk 37–65%)
         - Maternal plasma HIV-1 RNA level: 15/20 transmitters >50,000 copies/ml, 0/63 transmitted with <20,000 copies/ml *(JAMA 275:599, 1996)*.
         - Low CD4 count *(JID 175:567, 1997)*
         - Premature rupture of membranes: >4 hrs transmission rate 25% vs 14% <4 hrs *(NEJM 334:1617, 1996)*
      b. At risk
         - Newborn of HIV+ mother (risk varies 15–60%)
           - ·· No evidence delivery method (C-section) alters risk
         - Newborn of mother with unrecognized risk in partners
         - Breast-fed newborn of HIV+ mother
      c. Lowest risk
         - Mother with negative HIV test

E. Occupational Exposure *(See Table 7, page 33) (AJM 102:S5B, 1997; NEJM 337:1485, 1997; CDC Guidelines, MMWR 45:470, 1996; AnIM 125:497, 1996)*

Relative Risk Determinants:
1. Riskiest [risk may be decreased by glove use, which removes > 50% blood from exposure site in some studies but HIV-size microbes can pass through ⅓ of latex gloves tested *(J All Clin Imm 97:575, 1996)*. With double-glove use, blood-hand contacts ↓ from 71 to 32/100 procedures *(Abst. 412, 2nd CRV, 1995)*]
   - Deep parenteral inoculation (RR 16.8) via hollow needle of blood from source with high-titer viremia; seroconversion or advanced HIV disease (RR 7.8)
   - Parenteral inoculation of materials containing high titer virus in research laboratory setting
   - Failure to use ZDV after inoculation (RR 0.1 when used)

   2. Less risky
- Small volume exposure via non-hollow needle
- Mucosal exposure/non-intact skin exposure [risk is too low to be quantified in prospective studies; not zero but estimated to be at least a log (90%) lower than needlestick risk. Risk may be increased if large volume or prolonged contact occurs]

   3. Risk not identified
- Cutaneous contact (intact skin)
- Exposure to urine, saliva, sweat, tears

F. Donor Organ or Tissue Transplantation

   1. Test potential donors for HIV [(note "window" between infection and seroconversion *(C.2 above)*]
   2. Assess donors for risk factors
   3. Evaluate risk/benefits
- Risk following artificial insemination with semen from HIV+ donor is 3.5% *(JAMA 273:854, 1995; Lancet 351:728, 1998)*. HIV testing recommended but **not legally required** (FDA considering regulation 1997).

III. Recommendations for HIV Testing

A. HIV pre-test counseling should be provided to **all persons at risk** and HIV testing recommended. Use pre-test counseling to encourage reduction of risk for acquisition and/or transmission (*Examples:* "What do you expect your test results to be? Why? What will you do if you are HIV+? Is there anything different you will do if you are HIV–?").

B. "At Risk" Persons May Include:
   1. All persons (men and women) with identified risk behaviors
   2. All persons with sexually transmitted diseases
   3. All persons with conditions associated with HIV infection *(see Table 1, pages 2–4)*
   4. All persons with tuberculosis [among patients seen in TB clinics in 1988–1989, 3.4% (range 0–46%) were HIV+ *(J Inf Dis 165:87, 1992)*]
   5. Pregnant women in areas of high prevalence. Some authorities recommend testing all pregnant women (controversial).
   6. Women of childbearing age in areas of high prevalence
   7. All patients, age 15–54 years, in-patient or out-patient, receiving care in institutions where HIV prevalence is ≥ 1% or AIDS diagnosis rate is ≥ 1.0 per 1000 discharges *[MMWR 42:(RR-2), 1993 (Jan. 15)]*. Such screening would involve only 593 of the 5558 U.S. Acute Care Hospitals and 12% of all patients but would detect 68% of HIV+ patients hospitalized for conditions other than symptomatic HIV disease *(NEJM 327:445, 1992)*. Recent studies in high-prevalence areas have shown 5% HIV+ (women > men) between ages 60–79 *(Arch Int Med 155:184, 1995)*. This raises questions about the 54-year upper age cutoff. For guidelines regarding the conduct of blinded HIV serosurveys in hospitals, contact Seroepidemiology Branch, Mail Stop E-46, CDC, Atlanta, GA 30333.
   8. Patients with unexplained lymphadenopathy, fever, weight loss

C. Post-Test Counseling: Provide test results preferably in person, assess mental status, review risk reduction/third-party risks *(see II.A,B above)*, provide follow-up referral.

FIGURE 1

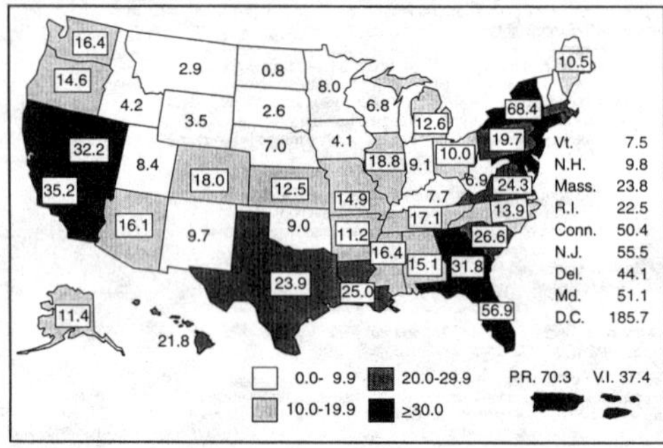

From MMWR 45:316, 1996
By 1997, 573,800 persons ≥13 yrs of age with AIDS had been reported to CDC in the United States. For the first time since the beginning of the epidemic, death rates from AIDS have declined (13% ↓ 1995 → 1996) *(MMWR 46:165, 1997)*

TABLE 2

LABORATORY TESTS COMMONLY USED IN THE DIAGNOSIS AND MANAGEMENT OF INFECTION WITH HIV-1, HIV-2, HTLV-1, AND HTLV-2

An outline of available tests followed by specific comments:

1. HIV-1 and HIV-2 antibody tests
   A. Serum antibody detection
      (1) ELISA ± Western blot
      (2) Rapid detection methods
      (3) Home test kits
   B. Detection of HIV-1 and HTLV-1 and -2 antibody in other body fluids
      (1) Antibody in saliva
      (2) Antibody in urine
2. HIV-2 antibody tests
3. HTLV-1 antibody tests
4. HTLV-2 antibody tests
5. Detection/quantitation of HIV
   A. HIV p24 antigen
   B. Qualitative PCR: Circulating cells or plasma
   C. Quantitative plasma viral "burdens"
6. Guide to logarithmic change
7. CD4/CD8 T-lymphocyte counts
   A. CD4 T-lymphocytes
   B. CD8 T-lymphocytes
8. Categories of laboratory resistance of HIV
   A. Genotypic resistance
   B. Phenotypic resistance

Test	Primary Purpose(s)	Sensitivity %	Specificity %	Comment
1. HIV-1 antibody tests (*Ln 348:176, 1996; Med Lett 39:81, 1997*)				
A. Detection of antibody in serum or plasma				
(1) Enzyme immunoassay (EIA) followed by Western blot for confirmation. Current assay detects antibodies to both HIV-1 and HIV-2.				False-pos. EIA in multiparous women, post-influenza or Hep B vaccination, post-multiple blood transfusions, and pts with autoimmune disease. Uncommon with present assay.
	For all high-risk groups (*Table 1*); becomes positive approx. 2 mos. post-disease acquisition in majority; 6 mos. after infection, 95% pts antibody-positive (*AJM 102: 117, 1997*)	99.9	99.9	False-neg. EIA in blood donors is 1 per 500,000 units (*NEJM 334:1685, 1996*). Causes: (1) window between acquisition and antibody response (2–6 mos.), (2) pts with agammaglobulinemia, (3) disease due to genetic variant HIV. Current licensed serologic test detects HIV subtypes (also called clades) A–H; **may not detect subtype O** or HIV-2. Test kits that will detect subtype O and HIV-2 are in final stages of evaluation. Positive Western blot requires detection of antibodies to at least 2 of the following HIV antigens: p24, Gp41, Gp120, Gp160. General ref.: Metcalf et al., Chapter 11 in AIDS: BIOLOGY, DIAGNOSIS, TREATMENT AND PREVENTION. DeVita et al., Eds., Lippincott-Raven, 1997.
(2) Rapid detection methods: Results available in 30 minutes or less				
Examples: Single use diagnostic system (SUDS)	When quick answer needed, e.g., test blood of source pt in occupational exposure. Pts who may not comply with return visit: ER, STD clinics	99.9	99.6	High temperature and inadequate centrifugation can cause false-positives. Need to confirm positive test with standard serology. Cost: approx. $9/test. *Refs.: AnIM 125:471 & 509, 1996; J Clin Micro 33:2899, 1995.*
(3) Home test kits, e.g., Home Access	Encourage individuals at risk to determine their antibody status. Convenient. Anonymity maintained.	100	99.95	Better described as home specimen collection systems. Patient pricks fingertip and blood spotted on filter paper. Positives confirmed with standard antibody. Counseling included. Takes 3–7 days. Cost: $35–50. *Ref.: Arch Int Med 157:309, 1997.*
B. Detection of HIV-1 antibody in other body fluids				
(1) Antibody in saliva (OraSure) (*Ref.: JAMA 277:254, 1997*)	Major advantage is avoidance of need for a needlestick. Easy to use; collected by health care worker	99.9	99.9	Test pad placed between cheek and gum for 2–5 mins. Collects oral mucosal transudate containing IgG antibody. Lab does EIA test for antibody; positives undergo Western blot confirmation. Cost: $99 for 3-test kit. Takes 3 days.
(2) Antibody in urine (Sentinel or Calypte): HIV-1 Urine ELISA)	Rapid—results in 2.5 hrs. Like rapid tests, could be used on source blood if occupational exposure or in ERs, STD clinics	98.7	99.1	Non-invasive and rapid turnaround time attractive but lower sensitivity is a concern. Positives confirmed with serum antibody test. Cost: individual test ?; 192-test kit $816.

TABLE 2 (2)

Test	Primary Purpose(s)	Sensitivity %	Specificity %	Comment
2. HIV-2 antibody tests—62 pts with HIV-2 infections in U.S. as of 6/95; most are immigrants from West Africa. *See serum assay for HIV-1/HIV-2, above*				
3. HTLV-1: Detection of antibody Human T-lymphocyte virus-1	1. Screen all donated blood and blood components 2. Test pts with compatible illness: (a) Adult T-cell lymphoma (b) Tropical spastic hemiparesis (myelopathy)	>98	>98 *(see Comment)*	Infection endemic in SW Japan, Caribbean, Melanesia and parts of Africa. Risk factors similar to HIV. Infection is lifelong. Specificity good but transient false-positives in 2–5% of blood donors who had received influenza vaccine in last 4 months *(MMWR 42:173, 1993).*
4. HTLV-2: Detection of antibody Human T-lymphocyte virus-2	Thus far, an investigative tool in that there is no definite association with any disease process. Donated blood is NOT screened.			Based on antibody studies, infection with HTLV-2 is endemic in Native Americans and injection drug users.

Test	Current Use	% Positive	Advantages	Disadvantages	Comment
5. Detection/quantitation of HIV					
A. HIV-1 p24 antigen (Assumes acid pretreatment to dissoci-ate immune complexes)	• Diagnosis of acute HIV syndrome (anti-body not detectable for ≥2 months) • Used to screen all donated blood [MMWR 45(RR-2), 1996]	% positive depends on method/stage of disease, e.g., in acute retroviral syn.: 100%; if CD4 200–500, 45–70%; if CD4 <200, 75–100%	Detection of infection before antibody appears (up to first 55 days)	Not as good as quant. nucleic acid methods as measure of effectiveness of therapy; a new test couples p24 to an ELISA with quanti-tation similar to DNA PCR methods (AIDS 11:F47, 1997).	In newborns at risk, HIV PCR (if available) preferable to p24 antigen (JID 173:68, 1996)
B. Qualitative PCR: circulating cells or plasma	Can use in early disease instead of p24 antigen, e.g., acute HIV, newborns; also to resolve indeterminate Western blots. Can use circulating cells or plasma	>99% for HIV variants from U.S. and Europe (subtype B). May fail to detect African HIV-1 variants (JID 174:244, 1996)	In meta-analysis, 97% sen-sitivity & 98% specificity with 1.9% false-pos. and 3.0% false-neg. (AnIM 114:803, 1996).	Not generally available; qualitative; expensive	Trend is to use quantitative PCR methods. Hard to interpret meta-analysis data due to rapid changes in PCR methods and implementation of quality assur-ance procedures.
C. Quantitative measurement of plasma "viral burdens" (Lancet 347:71, 1996)	• Clinical uses for viral burdens: (1) Deci-sions to initiate antiretroviral rx (Table 5). (2) Prognosis. Levels of ≥100,000 viral RNA equivalents per ml plasma = poor prognosis (AnIM 122:573, 1995). (3) Monitor response to antiretroviral rx. (Nature Medicine 2:625, 1996). (4) Pre-dict likelihood of transmission of HIV from mother to fetus. (5) Diagnosis of infection in newborn (JID 173:68, 1996).	Depending on stage of dis-ease & sensitivity of specific method: 86–>98%	At least 3 competing methods. Test availability varies with locale. Ability to accurately quantitate lower levels of viremia (<500 viral RNA equivalents/ml) being developed rapidly. Changes in viral burden of ≤0.3 log may be just technical variation; changes ≥0.5 log reflect real changes in viral burden. Recommend using same test for individual patient follow-up because of discrepancies between the 3 different techniques. These tests should NOT be used for dx of HIV infection; false-positive rate of 2–3% at low titers ~500 copies/ml range) has been anecdotally reported.		

TABLE 2 (3)

Test	Current Use	% Positive	Advantages	Disadvantages	Comment
5. Detection/quantitation of HIV, Quantitative measurement of plasma "viral burdens" *(continued)* (1) Due to assay differences, use same assay repeatedly for a given patient (2) For given assay, need change of ≥0.5 log for significant change	• Current methods: (1) Couples reverse transcription (RT) to a DNA PCR amplification (RT-PCR) (2) Amplification of RNA of HIV; a nucleic acid sequence-based amplification (NASBA)	>98	Lower limit of sensitivity approx. 40 copies/ml (ultrasensitive)	**Preferred anticoagulant[1]:** ACD/EDTA	For information, call Hoffman-La Roche (800-526-1247). Values roughly 2x higher than bDNA. RT-PCR is less efficient than bDNA at quantitation of subtypes A, E, F, G, O *(J Clin Micro 36:716, 1998)*.
	(3) Identification of HIV RNA, then signal amplification by DNA branched-chain technique (referred to as bDNA)	>98	Lower limit of sensitivity 40–80 copies/ml (volume-dependent)	ACD/EDTA/HEP	For information, call Organon Tecknika (919-620-2680)
		>98	Lower limit of sensitivity approx. 50 copies/ml	EDTA	For information, call Chiron (800-522-8378)

6. A guide to logarithmic changes; for a person starting with 100,000 copies of HIV-RNA:

Log Drop	n-Fold Change	Copies of HIV RNA Remaining
0.3	2-fold	50,000
0.5	3-fold	33,000
1.0	10-fold	10,000
1.5	30-fold	3,300
2.0	100-fold	1,000

7. CD4/CD8 antigen T-lymphocyte counts (CD=cluster differentiation)—*Revised CDC Guidelines on Methods now available in MMWR 46(No. RR-2):1–29, 1997*

Test	Current Use	% Positive	Advantages	Disadvantages	Comment
A. CD4 T-lymphocyte count (T-helper lymphocyte)	(1) Assess magnitude of injury to host immune system; (2) Changes used to monitor effectiveness of antiretroviral rx. Normals: CD4 500–1400/mm³. CD8 180–865/mm³; CD4/CD8 ratio 1.1–3.5; (3) Initiation of prophylaxis vs opportunistic infections *(Table 9)*	Not applicable	Generally available. Rate of ↓ in CD4 count correlates with HIV disease progression *(NEJM 334:426, 1996)*; changes in CD8 counts may/may not parallel CD4 count changes.	Test must be done ≤2 days after blood collection. Counts influenced by man variables: time of day, time of year, lab doing test, intercurrent infection *(CID 21:1121, 1995)*. Cost varies from $60–$150. Viral "burden" appears a better measure of prognosis and response to therapy.	Fluoresceinated monoclonal antibodies are added to pt blood & the % fluorescent cells counted in cell sorter. CD4 count calculated as: WBC x % lymphocytes x % CD4 cells. To avoid influence of change in WBC, can use % of CD4 (≥29% = CD4 count of >500; 14–28% = CD4 200–499; <14% = CD4 <200/mm³)
	NOTE: FDA approved an immunologic assay method for CD4 counts (called TRAX CD4) (5/95). Valid on blood stored for ≤5 days. Cost approx. $20/test. Other similar tests, not requiring flow cytometry, under evaluation *(J AIDS 10:522, 1995)*.				
B. CD8 T-lymphocyte count (T-suppressor/cytotoxic lymphocyte)	Often measured in parallel with CD4, even though role in disease process less well defined—*see Comment*	Not applicable			3–4 wks following infection, both CD4 & CD8 counts ↑ but CD8 is greater with inversion of normal CD4/CD8 ratio. CD8 cells believed to play a role in control of viral replication in many cells including CD4 cells *(Science 271: 324, 1996)*.

[1] **ACD** = acid citrate dextran; **EDTA** = ethylenediaminetetraacetic acid; **HEP** = heparin

8. Categories of Laboratory Resistance of HIV

A. Genotypic resistance
   1. Definition
      a. Changes in nucleotide sequence of virus
      b. Single, or more often multiple, gene mutations predict resistance of anti-HIV drugs
   2. Several methods under evaluation
      a. Point mutation assays
      b. Gene sequencing
      c. Analysis of gene chip nucleotide arrays

   3. Advantages
      a. Can be done fairly rapidly
      b. Technically less demanding than phenotypic assays
   4. Disadvantages
      a. Inability to predict mutational interactions; interpretation complex
      b. Genotype does not equal phenotype
   5. Reported mutations: NOTE—multiple mutations may be present.

Drug	Location of Mutations [mutant codon(s)]
Resistance to Nucleoside Analogs Reverse Transcriptase Inhibitors (RTI):	
Didanosine (Videx, ddI)	$74 \pm$ (65, 75, 184)
Lamivudine (Epivir, 3TC)	184
Stavudine (Zerit, d4T)	50, 75
Zalcitabine (HIVID, ddC)	$65 \pm$ (69, 74, 75, 184)
Zidovudine (Retrovir, ZDV)	$215 \pm$ (41, 67, 70, 210, 219)
Resistance to Non-Nucleoside RTIs:	
Delavirdine (Rescriptor)	103 or $181 \pm$ (236)
Nevirapine (Viramune)	103 or $181 \pm$ (98, 106, 108, 188, 190)
Resistance to Protease Inhibitors (JAMA 277:145, 1997):	
Indinavir (Crixivan)	82 or $46 \pm$ (10, 20, 24, 54, 63, 64, 84, 90)
Nelfinavir (Viracept)	$30 \pm$ (35, 36, 46, 71, 77, 84, 88)
Ritonavir (Norvir)	82 or $84 \pm$ (10, 20, 36, 46, 54, 63, 71, 90)
Saquinavir (Invirase)	48 or $90 \pm$ (10, 54, 63, 71, 90)

B. Phenotypic resistance
   1. Definition:
      a. Response of HIV in laboratory after incubation with antiviral agent(s)
      b. Analogous to testing susceptibility of bacteria to antibiotics
   2. Two methods in development
      a. Compare susceptibility of control sensitive virus to susceptibility of patient's virus (VIRCO)
      b. Determine in vitro inhibitory concentration$_{90}$ (IC_{90}) of test drug against patient's virus (VIROLOGIC)
   3. Advantage: "Readouts" similar to testing of bacteria
   4. Disadvantages:
      a. 2–3 weeks required
      b. Expensive

C. REMEMBER: NOT ALL CLINICAL FAILURE IS DUE TO DRUG RESISTANCE.

TABLE 3A
1993 REVISED CDC HIV CLASSIFICATION SYSTEM AND EXPANDED AIDS SURVEILLANCE DEFINITION FOR ADOLESCENTS AND ADULTS
(MMWR 41:RR-17, Dec. 18, 1992)

The revised system emphasizes the importance of CD4 lymphocyte testing in clinical management of HIV infected persons. The system is based on 3 ranges of CD4 counts and 3 clinical categories giving a matrix of 9 exclusive categories. This system is less valuable in clinical decision analysis in 1997 because of availability of measures of viral RNA.

CRITERIA FOR HIV INFECTION: Persons 13 years or older with repeatedly (2 or more) reactive screening tests (ELISA) + specific antibodies identified by a supplemental test, e.g., Western blot ["reactive" pattern = + vs any two of p24, gp41, or gp120/160 (MMWR 40:681, 1991)]. Other specific methods of diagnosis of HIV-1 include virus isolation, antigen detection, and detection of HIV genetic material by PCR or branched DNA assay (bDNA).

CLASSIFICATION SYSTEM				Clinical Category A	Clinical Category B	Clinical Category C

	CLINICAL CATEGORY			Asymptomatic HIV infection
				Persistent generalized lymphadenopathy
				  (PGL)[1]
				Acute (primary) HIV illness
					Symptomatic, not A or C conditions.
					Examples include but not limited to:
					  Bacillary angiomatosis
					  Candidiasis, vulvovaginal: persist-
					    ent >1 month, poorly
					    responsive to rx
					  Candidiasis, oropharyngeal
					  Cervical dysplasia, severe, or
					    carcinoma in situ
					  Constitutional sx, e.g., fever
					    (38.5°) or diarrhea > 1 month
						Candidiasis: esophageal, trachea, bronchi
						Coccidioidomycosis, extrapulmonary
						Cryptococcosis, extrapulmonary
						† Cervical cancer, invasive
						Cryptosporidiosis, chronic intestinal (> 1 month)
						CMV retinitis, or CMV in other than liver, spleen, nodes
						HIV encephalopathy
						Herpes simplex with mucocutaneous ulcer > 1 month,
						  bronchitis, pneumonia
						Histoplasmosis: disseminated, extrapulmonary
						Isosporiasis, chronic, > 1 month
						Kaposi's sarcoma
						Lymphoma: Burkitt's, immunoblastic, primary in brain
						M. avium or M. kansasii, extrapulmonary
						M. tuberculosis, †pulmonary or extrapulmonary
						Pneumocystis carinii pneumonia
						† Pneumonia, recurrent (≥ 2 episodes in 1 year)
						Progressive multifocal leukoencephalopathy
						Salmonella bacteremia, recurrent
						Toxoplasmosis, cerebral
						Wasting syndrome due to HIV

CD4 Cell§ Category	**A**	**B**	**C**			
(1) ≥ 500/mm³	A1	B1	C1			
(2) 200–499/mm³	A2	B2	C2			
(3) < 200/mm³	A3	B3	C3			

* See table for clinical definitions. Shaded area indicates expansion of AIDS surveillance definition. Cats. A3, B3 and C require reporting as AIDS.

§ There is a diurnal variation in CD4 counts averaging 60/mm³ higher in the afternoon in HIV+ individuals. Blood for sequential CD4 counts should be drawn at about the same time of day each time (J AIDS 3:144, 1990). The equivalence between CD4 counts and CD4 % of total lymphocytes is ≥500 = ≥29%, 200–499 = 14–28%, <200 = <14%.

The above must be attributed to HIV infection or have a clinical course or management complicated by HIV.

[1] Nodes in 2 or more extrainguinal sites, at least 1 cm in diameter for ≥ 3 months

* These are the 1987 CDC case definitions (MMWR 36:15, 1987). The 1993 CDC Expanded Surveillance Case Definition includes all conditions contained in the 1987 definition (above) plus persons with documented HIV infection and any of the following: (1) CD4 T-lymphocyte count < 200/mm³ (or CD4 < 14%), (2) pulmonary tuberculosis,† (3) recurrent pneumonia† (≥ 2 episodes within 1 year) or (4) invasive cervical carcinoma.† There are no CDC definitions utilizing viral load available to date.

TABLE 3B: "PERFORMANCE STATUS" (KARNOFSKY SCALE)

Criteria of Performance Status (PS)		
Able to carry on normal activity; no special care is needed	100	Normal; no complaints; no evidence of disease
	90	Able to carry on normal activity; minor signs or symptoms of disease
	80	Normal activity with effort; some signs or symptoms of disease
Unable to work; able to live at home and care for most personal needs; a varying amount of assistance is needed	70	Cares for self; unable to carry on normal activity or to do active work
	60	Requires occasional assistance but is able to care for most needs
	50	Requires considerable assistance and frequent medical care
Unable to care for self; requires equivalent of institutional or hospital care; disease may be progressing rapidly	40	Disabled; requires special care and assistance
	30	Severely disabled; hospitalization is indicated although death not imminent
	20	Very sick; hospitalization necessary; active supportive treatment is necessary
	10	Moribund, fatal processes progressing rapidly
	0	Dead

TABLE 3C: RESISTANCE TO INFECTION AND LONG-TERM NON-PROGRESSORS *(Reference: NEJM 332:201, 209, 288, 1995)*

Certain persons have apparent resistance to HIV infection. These include prostitutes from various parts of Africa who have had multiple sexual exposure to infected semen and persons who have received infusions of infected blood products without apparent progressive HIV infection. Potential explanations include:

- A deletion mutation (delta 32) of the macrophage trophic CCR5 chemokine receptor which is necessary for the HIV fusion process by which the virus gains entry into these early target cells appears nearly complete protection from HIV infection *(Science 273:1797, 1856, 1996)*. This mutation allele is found in up to 20% of Caucasian descendants from northern European countries, of which 1–2% are homozygous for the mutation, 3–6% in southern European countries and essentially 0 in the black descendants from Africa *(Nature Med 3:338, 1997)*. To date <10 persons worldwide infected with HIV have been found to be homozygous for the delta 32 CCR5 mutation *(Nature Med 3:252, 1997)*.
- Early data also suggest that a mutation in another chemokine receptor CCR2 and in a B-chemokine product (SCYA1) may also play a role in protection.
- Several individuals were accidentally infused with blood products contaminated with an HIV-1 variant that was defective in the "nef" gene. These individuals were infected with the virus but did not develop progressive infection, suggesting a non-virulent virus. In SIV (simian virus) the nef gene is necessary for development of immunodeficiency.

Approximately 5% of HIV+ individuals have shown little or no progression of clinical disease or ↓ in CD4 counts over 10–15 years. HIV can be isolated by culture but viral RNA levels are usually low. Several explanations are possible:

- Many of these persons have high CD8 cell counts
- Up to ½ are heterozygous for the CCR5 mutation and have been shown to have lower viral RNA copies/ml of plasma and higher CD4 cell counts compared to CCR5 wild type at the same time period after infection. In vitro, cells from the heterozygous are more difficult than cells without the mutation to infect with HIV-1 *(AnIM 127:882, 1997; J AIDS & Human Retrov 16:10, 1997)*. Heterozygosity for CCR5 Δ32 mutation also substantially reduces progression of disease in children but does not appear to protect from HIV transmission from mother to child *(JAMA 279:277, 1998)*. Mutations in CCR2, SCYA1 and other chemokines and receptors may also play a role in slowing infection of macrophages and CD4 lymphocytes, thus slowing progression of disease.

TABLE 3D: GENETIC DIVERSITY OF HIV *(JAMA 275:210, 1996)*

- Genetic variation of HIV is extremely high with rapid turnover of HIV virions (10^{10} virions/day) *(Science 271:1582, 1996)*.
- 9 subtypes (also termed clades or genotypes) of HIV-1 have been classified.
- Geographic distribution of subtypes varies:

HIV-1 Subtype	Country		HIV-1 Subtype	Country
A	Central Africa		F	Brazil, Romania, Zaire
B	South American (including Brazil, U.S., Europe, Thailand		G	Zaire, Gabon, Taiwan
C	Brazil, India, southern Africa, China		H	Zaire, Gabon
D	Central Africa		O	Cameroon, Gabon (may not be detected with standard EIA, *see Table 2*)
E	Thailand, Central African Republic, China			

HIV-1 subtype O is almost as close to HIV-2 as it is to HIV-1 *(Lancet 343:1376, 1994)*
- Preliminary in vitro studies suggest subtype E may grow more efficiently in Langerhans cells from genital mucosa, which would favor heterosexual transmission *(Science 271:1291, 1996)*.
- Infections with subtypes other than B, i.e., E, D or A, have been introduced into the U.S. by individuals infected abroad *(Lancet 346:1198, 1995)*.

FIGURE 2

COURSE OF HIV INFECTION AND DISEASE IN ADULTS: CLINICAL DECISION POINTS

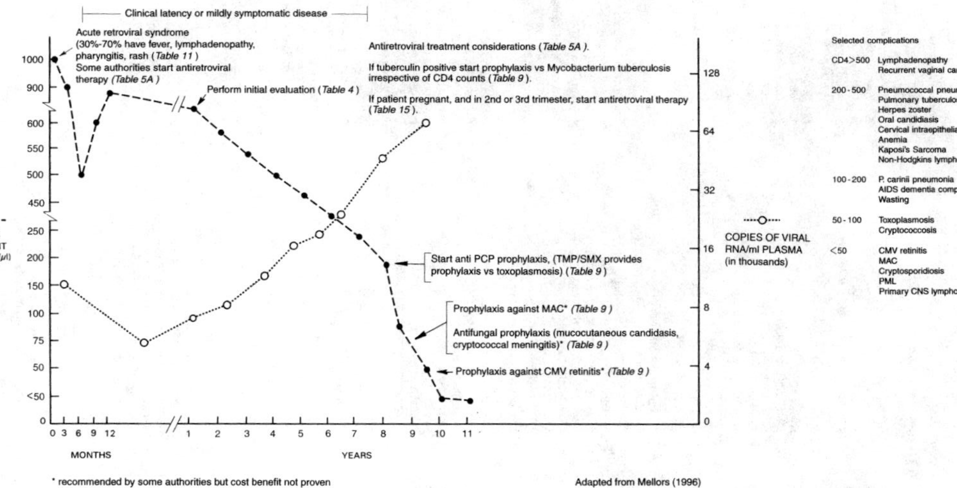

* recommended by some authorities but cost benefit not proven

Adapted from Mellors (1996)

TABLE 4

INITIAL EVALUATION OF THE HIV-INFECTED ADULT PATIENT
[JAMA 269:1144, 1993; CID 21(Suppl. 1):S12, 1995]

I. History

    A. General health status
        1. General well-being
        2. Constitutional symptoms
        3. History of infectious diseases: childhood infections, infections in adult life, previous physician visits, hospitalizations (where, when)
        4. Immunization history

    B. Drug history
        1. Medications and dosages
            A. Prescription
            B. Non-prescription
            C. Alternative therapies *(see Table 26)*
        2. "Recreational" drug use *(See Table 1, page 2) (see AJM 101:435, 1996, for review)*
            A. Intravenous/injection; crack cocaine
            B. Other
            C. Partners at risk
        3. Smoking history
        4. Alcohol history

    C. Sexual history
        1. Sexual practices *(See Table 1, page 2)*
        2. Sexually transmitted diseases
        3. Obstetrical/gynecologic history
        4. Contraceptive use
        5. Partners at risk

    D. Risks for opportunistic infections
        1. Travel history
        2. Geographic location of current/prior residence, e.g., southwestern, mideastern USA
        3. Occupational history, e.g., poultry workers
        4. Avocational activities
        5. Tuberculosis status: history of BCG vaccination, family members with and/or treated for tuberculosis, contacts (close) with patients with known tuberculosis, results of previous tuberculin tests and/or chest x-rays if known
        6. Pets, e.g., cats–Bartonella henselae; fish–M. marinum. Cat ownership not associated with toxoplasma antibody seroconversion *(JAMA 269:76, 1993)*

    E. Past history of viral hepatitis, to include type if known

II. Comprehensive Physical Examination

    A. Document weight and height
    B. Careful funduscopic and oral examination
    C. Dermatologic examination, to include back, buttocks, and extremities, hands, feet
    D. Exam of all lymph node areas: postoccipital, preauricular, cervical, submental, supra-clavicular, axillary, epitrochlear, inguinal (measure and record size if palpable, record as negative if not palpable)
    E. Rectal/genital examination, to include pelvic exam with Pap smear in women, inspection for perianal/genital Herpes simplex. Pap smears should be repeated every 12 months.
    F. Assess mental status for evidence of dementia.

III. Laboratory Evaluation

    A. Baseline
        1. Complete blood count with differential
        2. Renal function tests: BUN, creatinine
        3. Liver function tests: serum bilirubin, aspartate aminotransferase (AST, SGOT), alanine aminotransferase (ALT, SGPT), alkaline phosphatase

    B. HIV staging
        1. CD4 count
        2. Quantitative measurement of plasma HIV *(Table 2)*—"viral load" or plasma "viral burden"

    C. Additional studies
        1. PPD Intermediate (5TU),[1] *see Table 12, page 78*
        2. Chest x-ray
        3. VDRL or RPR (tests for syphilis)
        4. IgG antibody to toxoplasmosis
        5. Hepatitis B surface antigen (HBsAg), antibody to Hep B surface Ag (anti-HBsAg), antibody to Hep C
        6. CMV antibody, IgG

IV. Initial Health Care Maintenance

    A. HIV risk reduction education *(see Table 1)*
    B. Drug rehabilitation/safer needle use/needle exchange *(AJM 101:435, 1996)*
    C. Smoking cessation (smoking ↑ risk of thrush, hairy leukoplakia, bacterial pneumonia)
    D. Partner notification
    E. Reproductive counseling
    F. Psychosocial support
    G. Immunizations *(see Table 22)*. Immunizations have been shown to transiently ↑ HIV viral load, clinical significance uncertain *(AIDS Clin Care 8:11, 1996; NEJM 334:1222, 1996)*.
        1. Pneumococcal vaccine *(JID 174:1191, 1996)*
        2. Influenza vaccine (annually)
        3. Hepatitis B vaccine, if sexually active or sharing needles
    H. Preventive dentistry
    I. If CD4 count <100 cells/mm^3, baseline ophthalmologic evaluation

V. Primary Care of Patients Infected With HIV:

Multiple studies have now demonstrated that physicians and other health care givers who care for large numbers of HIV-infected persons and who make delivery of this care a major focus of their practice, training and continuing education have better outcomes *(see IDSA position statement, CID 26:275, 1998)*.

---

[1] Use of anergy testing with PPD testing is not recommended as a routine procedure *[MMWR 46(RR-15):1–10, 1997]*

TABLE 5A

ANTIRETROVIRAL THERAPY IN ADULTS 1998-9 *(See Table 2, pages 7 & 8, for tests of viral RNA)*

1997 and 1998 have continued to bring enormous changes to the care of the HIV-infected individual. With increased experience in clinical practice, a reduction in cost and a better understanding of the meaning of quantitative measures of viral RNA *(see Table 2)* and increased experience of utilizing **Highly Active Antiretroviral Therapy (HAART)**, clinicians have gained valuable lessons in managing this increasingly complex disease. In early 1998, the CDC reported a 45% reduction in mortality rate from AIDS compared to 1996, a reduction attributed to better antiretroviral therapy management. However, less optimistic reports revealed that in clinical practice, up to 53% of patients were "failing" HAART combination therapy (protease inhibitors used were indinavir or ritonavir) with the reappearance of viral vRNA after rx for 1 year *(Deeks, ICAAC 1997)*. The failure rates were highest in patients who had been on antiretroviral drugs before (antiretroviral experienced), especially when a protease inhibitor was added without changing the NRTI drugs at the same time, had advanced disease (CD4 count <200 and higher viral load), and had evidence of non-compliance with the therapy.

The following concepts are emerging that guide therapy in 1998-9:

- **The lower the vRNA levels can be driven the longer the therapeutic effect will last!** Initial results from the INCAS study *(ICAAC 1997)* demonstrated that rx that achieved a nadir vRNA level of 1000 copies/ml of plasma failed after 100 days, when the levels reached <500 copies/ml relapse of viral RNA occurred after 200 days, but if plasma vRNA copies were driven to <25 copies/ml (as measured by the ultrasensitive assay), relapse did not occur. Relapses were associated with appearance of resistant phenotype subpopulations. Thus, it appears that maintaining the viral load below the mutation rate for resistant genes is critical to maintenance of complete suppression of viral activity and termination of CD4 cell destruction.

- **Achieving the maximum therapeutic response is most successful in patients not previously treated (antiretroviral naive).** Therefore, initiating rx with less than an optimal regimen may result in generation of resistant subpopulations and a less than maximally effective response for the second cycle.

- **Monotherapy is clearly less optimal than triple combination therapy (HAART).** Use of double therapy (2 RTIs) may be effective in very early disease (500–5,000 copies vRNA/ml and CD4 <500) but is usually less effective than 2 NRTIs and a PI (or NNRTI).

- **Unfortunately, in some patients even with HAART rx one may not be able to drive the vRNA to undetectable (<500 copies/ml)** especially when initial viral load is high (>100,000 copies/ml). If the viral load has dropped by 2–3 logs and is stable at that point, most clinicians would follow and change rx only if the load rises by >1–2 log (with several determinations). Others have found ↑ CD4 (>100/mm³) on HAART without complete suppression of plasma RNA (>500 copies/ml) for up to 1 yr and recommend continuing rx as long as CD4 count stays up *(Lancet 351:723, 1998)*.

- **The definition of failure of a regimen** has not been completely validated *(JAMA 277:1962, 1997)* but is generally considered as:
  (1) Failure to achieve an undetectable vRNA or at least a >1 log decline after 4 weeks of rx
  (2) Return of vRNA to detectable by current techniques (>500 copies/ml of plasma) while on rx
  (3) Reproducible 3-fold ↑ (or 1–2 logs) from nadir of plasma vRNA copies while on rx
  (4) Persistent significant decline in CD4 cells with or without progression of clinical symptoms
  (5) Intolerance or toxicity of the therapy resulting in inconsistent dosing or intolerable side-effects

- **When changing rx because of clinical or virological failure, all 3 drugs (2 RTIs and the PI or NNRTI) should be changed** if possible, because the emergence of resistant viruses is likely (similar to the management of resistant tuberculosis). Cross-resistance among protease inhibitors is a particularly vexing problem. After indinavir or ritonavir failure, salvage rx with protease inhibitor-containing regimens is difficult and if a response occurs it usually appears to be short-lived *(ICAAC Abst. I-205, 1997)*. One report suggests that better responses may occur with indinavir or ritonavir after saquinavir or nelfinavir failures *(ICAAC Abst. I-204, 1997)*; however, another report found only limited activity *(ICAAC Abst. LB5, 1997)*. It seems obvious that once a protease inhibitor has been tried and failed, the next protease inhibitor is destined to be less effective.

- **If failure is the result of drug toxicity (bone marrow suppression, neuropathy or pancreatitis) without virological relapse, one can change the offending drug alone (ZDV, ddl or ddC).**

- **If CD4 counts are allowed to reach low levels, <200/mm³ and especially <50/mm³, clones of CD4 cells (especially uncommitted clones) are apparently irreversibly destroyed**, thus if antiretroviral rx successfully suppresses viral activity, clonal expansion of CD4 cells will occur but the total repertoire that was initially present may not return *(Nature Med, May 1997)*. Recently, several patients with prolonged effective HAART (>1–2 yrs) have demonstrated continued immune reconstitution, suggesting continued clonal awakening over time. Nevertheless, the ability to respond to the many infectious and malignant challenges may be limited in the future.

- **Initiation of antiretroviral rx early in the course of the disease when viral load is still low (and near complete suppression can still be achieved) and before clonal depletion of CD4 cells has occurred** is emerging as the most rational approach, but if and only if the patient is willing and committed to adherence to the regimen. Most clinicians list lack of adherence as the most common cause for therapeutic failure.

- There are patients who have demonstrated return of vRNA to detectable or >3-fold rise from nadir who have not shown decline of CD4 cells or progression of clinical symptoms. Whether this reappearance of vRNA represents emergence of nonpathogenic viral subpopulations or defective virions is not currently known. Most experts recommend changing rx if this occurs if there are viable drug combinations that have not been used. If most options have been tried, it seems reasonable to maintain current rx until CD4 cell decline or clinical symptoms progress. Then try rearranging previously used drugs or seek clinical trials of new therapies in development.

1. **When should antiretroviral treatment be started?**
   The most important factor in answering this question is to find out if the patient is ready to comply with the difficult regimens since lack of compliance guarantees failure of the treatment and facilitates the emergence of resistant subpopulations of virus making it much more difficult to treat the patient later. It also creates the potential for spread of resistant viruses to others. Studies indicate that about ⅓ of patients are totally adherent, ⅓ partially adherent and ⅓ almost totally nonadherent to prescribed rx. 2 important factors affect adherence: (1) the number of pills and (2) ease of administration of the regimen, qd better than bid, which is better than tid; mixing bid with tid medications mixed with food and without food makes total adherence nearly impossible. Every effort should be made to come to an agreement or contract with the patient as to what he/she is capable or willing to comply with prior to initiating rx. Frequent follow-up with advice and encouragement to the patient is important to help maintain compliance and to detect non-compliance.

Situation 1: CD4 count <500/mm³	**Situation 2:** CD4 count >500/mm³	**Situation 3:** CD4 count >500/mm³
Viral burden >5000 copies/ml	Viral burden >500 copies/ml	Viral burden undetectable
Comment: Treatment indicated	Comment: Recommendations vary. Authors favor rx if pt compliant and committed.	Comment: Retest periodically No rx

2. **What drugs should be used for initial therapy?** *(Summary in Medical Letter 39:111, 1997)*
   There are currently 11 FDA-approved drugs available in the United States for use against HIV:

The **nucleoside reverse-transcriptase inhibitors (NRTI)**, which include:

Group A drugs:	Standard dosage:
Zidovudine (ZDV)—Retrovir	300 mg bid or 200 mg tid
Stavudine (d4T)—Zerit	40 mg bid for >60 kg, 30 mg bid for <60 kg
Group B drugs:	
Didanosine (ddI)—Videx	200 mg bid (empty stomach) for >60 kg, 125 mg bid for <60 kg. A single daily dose of 400 mg po looks promising *(IDSA Absts 210, 211, 1997)*
Zalcitabine (ddC)— HIVID	0.75 mg tid
Lamivudine (3TC)—Epivir	150 mg bid

The **non-nucleoside reverse-transcriptase inhibitors (NNRTI)**, which include:

Nevirapine—Viramune	200 mg qd x2 weeks, then 200 mg bid
Delavirdine—Rescriptor	400 mg tid

The **protease inhibitors (PI)**, which include:

Saquinavir—Invirase	600 mg q8h with meals
Saquinavir—Fortovase	1200 mg q8h with meals
Indinavir—Crixivan	800 mg q8h, empty stomach or with light meal [1200 mg bid looks promising *(IDSA Abst. 225, 1997)*]
Ritonavir—Norvir	300 mg q12h with food, then dose escalate over 2 wks to 600 mg bid
Nelfinavir—Viracept	750 mg q8h with food [1250 mg bid looks promising *(5th CRV, Abst. 373)*]
Ritonavir/saquinavir	Each drug taken 400 mg bid
Indinavir/ritonavir	Each 400 mg bid [also produces serum levels similar to each drug alone at tid—promising *(ICAAC Abst. A-57, 1997)*]

When using 2 NRTIs together, it is recommended that an A drug be combined with a B drug, not an A with an A or a B with a B drug *(Chapter by Flexner & Hendrix in AIDS, Ed.: DeVita, 1997)*. This prevents additive toxicities and possible antagonism of action. Some clinicians like to initiate a **double** NRTI combination (esp. ZDV + 3TC) without a PI or NNRTI in patients with <5000 vRNA copies/ml; this has given suppression to <500 copies in most patients (80%) for up to 1 year, while most of those with >5000 copies failed. **Most recommend initiating triple combinations:** combine 2 NRTIs (A+B) with either a PI or an NNRTI. Addition of the PI (indinavir) improved results of both clinical & virologic parameters in antiretroviral naive & experienced patients *(NEJM 337:725 & 734, 1997)*. Significant drug-drug interactions occur with PIs *(see Table 17)* (esp. with ritonavir). Drug tolerance and the ability of the patient to balance food intake and convenience (quality of life issues) are major considerations. Virologic failure after 1 yr in 50% of pts *(S. Deeks, ICAAC 1997)*. Factors: previous rx, late-stage disease, poor compliance, and drug toxicity.

3. **How should patients be monitored?**
   Most authorities recommend measurements of viral load after 1 month, then every 3–4 months and more frequently if non-compliance is suspected, CD4 counts drop, or clinical symptoms appear or progress. It is also recommended that viral load be quantified every time adjustments in drugs or dosages are made, at 2–4 weeks, and again at 8–12 weeks, in order to document drug effect.

TABLE 5A (3)

4. **What is appropriate when antiretroviral regimen fails?** *(as defined above)*
   Failure of rx may be due to many different reasons and it is important to attempt to identify the cause. As mentioned, most failures are probably due to lack of compliance with the complicated triple drug therapies. Patients may not recognize that they are non-compliant or may be embarrassed to admit it.
   - If non-adherence is likely responsible for the jump in viral RNA, one may initially reinstitute original regimen, especially if patient stopped all drugs at once (it has been shown that even after a year on rx when drugs are stopped simultaneously, the viral isolates will still be sensitive to all 3 drugs and patients will again respond to reinitiation of original rx).
   - However, if the patient took the drugs erratically or if he/she was compliant and broke through with a rise in vRNA, the virus may well be resistant to all drugs and a change in rx is warranted. It is recommended that all drugs be changed if possible, as outlined below.
   - One factor worth considering when patients fail is drug malabsorption or drug-drug interactions that ↓ effective plasma drug concentrations. In several studies, plasma indinavir concentrations correlated with therapeutic effect: mean trough concentrations were 0.133 mg/L in responders and 0.023 mg/L in non-responders. In addition, levels above the IC50 (concentration of drug required to inhibit 50% of viruses in vitro) were present 90% of the dosing interval for responders but only 58% for those who failed *(ICAAC Absts. A-15, A-19, & IDSA Abst. I-173, 1997)*. Others have found that trough concentrations do not predict failure *(5th CRV, Abst. 337)*. Use of plasma drug levels in instances when the cause of failure is not apparent may be of some value.
   - Detection of mutations that confer resistance (genotyping) and phenotypic tests for resistance to antiretroviral drugs are commercially available and hold promise for clinical decision-making, but to date they have not been validated with clinical or surrogate marker outcomes *(J AIDS & Human Retrov 15:356, 1997)*.

   Alternative regimens for pts who fail rx:
   (1) 2 different NRTIs + a different PI
   (2) 2 different NRTIs + dual PI therapy, e.g., saquinavir + ritonavir
   (3) Dual PI therapy + an NNRTI
   (4) 2 new NRTIs + an NNRTI

SUMMARY OF SUGGESTED TREATMENT OF HIV INFECTION *(see above for details)*

CLINICAL SETTING	VIRAL RNA PER ML OF PLASMA	PRIMARY RX	ALTERNATIVE RX	COMMENT
Normal CD4	Below detectable limit	None	None	Follow viral burden q6–12 months
Normal or low CD4	>5000 copies/ml	(a) ZDV 300 mg po bid + (b) 3TC 150 mg po bid + protease inhibitor (PI) (Indinavir 800 mg po q8h or ritonavir 300 mg po bid with 2-wk escalation to 600 mg bid with food or nelfinavir 750 mg po tid)	(a) d4T 40 mg po bid + (b) (ddl 200 mg po bid or 3TC 150 mg po bid) + PI (indinavir or ritonavir or nelfinavir)	Do not give concomitant ZDV and d4T (overlapping toxicity). Whenever regimen initiated check viral burden 2–4 weeks and 8–12 weeks later.
	>500 but <5000 copies/ml	Some would use 2 NRTIs (A+B) ± either a PI or an NNRTI [nevirapine (200 mg po qd x2 wks, then 200 mg po bid) or delavirdine (400 mg tid)] *(see Comments)*	Some would not treat with CD4 counts >500/mm³	The authors prefer the aggressive approach (3 drugs) if the pt is willing to comply with the complex regimen.
Normal or low CD4 and failure of initial regimen	>500 copies/ml	d4T + ddl + (ritonavir or indinavir or nelfinavir—a PI not previously used) or d4T + 3TC +(ritonavir or indinavir or nelfinavir)	(Ritonavir 400 mg po bid + saquinavir 400 mg po bid) + 2 NRTIs (A+B)	Whenever regimen changed, check viral burden at time of change, 2–4 weeks later, and 8–12 weeks later
Acute retroviral syndrome	Very high	ZDV + 3TC + PI x2 years minimum [undetectable virus at 10 months in 12 pts *(Intl Cong on AIDS, Vancouver, 7/96)*]	Hope is to ↓ viral setpoint and slow progression of disease *(JID 176:798, 1997)*	
Needlestick injury		2 NRTIs (A+B) x1 month (add PI for high-risk exposure)	*See Table 7, page 34* for discussion of options based on severity of exposure and stage of disease of source patient	
Pregnancy		ZDV last half of pregnancy + during delivery, then infant x6 wks	Experimental combination regimen	No breast feeding *(see Table 6)*

Abbreviations: **NRTI** = nucleoside reverse transcriptase inhibitor; **NNRTI** = non-nucleoside reverse transcriptase inhibitor; **PI** = protease inhibitor; **ZDV** = zidovudine; **3TC** = lamivudine; **d4T** = stavudine; **ddl** = didanosine; **A & B** refer to Group A & B drugs *(see page 14)*; **5th CRV** = 5th Conference on Retroviruses & Opportunistic Infections, 1998

TABLE 5B: ANTIVIRAL DRUGS AND SIDE-EFFECTS

Antiretroviral Drugs. *For detailed pharmacology: Chap. by Flexner & Hendrix in AIDS, Ed. DeVita, 1997.*

Nucleoside Reverse Transcriptase Inhibitors (NRTI) (FDA-approved)

DRUG NAME(S) GENERIC (TRADE)	DOSAGE/ROUTE/COST*	COMMENTS/ADVERSE EFFECTS
Didanosine (ddI) (Didanosine) (Videx)	≥60 kg body weight Tablets 200 mg q12h on empty stomach Powder 250 mg q12h on empty stomach <60 kg body weight Tablets 125 mg q12h on empty stomach Powder 167 mg q12h on empty stomach Chewable tablets (25, 50, 100, 150 mg) must be chewed or crushed thoroughly before swallowing. Buffered powder for oral solution (100, 167, 250 mg packets) to be dissolved in 4 oz water is available. New tablet formulations are 35% smaller & softer (easier to chew) than original tablets. (100 mg tablet $1.61, 250 mg powder $4.00) (Approx. **$193/month** for 400 mg/d)	**Adverse effects: Pancreatitis** 6% (0.35% fatal), ↑ amylase 10%. ↑ amylase can be of salivary origin esp. with xerostomia. No intervention necessary unless symptomatic. In pts with history of pancreatitis 8/27 (30%) developed pancreatitis, avoid or use with caution in alcoholics. Hyperglycemia, occasional diabetes mellitus. **Peripheral neuropathy** 20%, 12% required dose reduction. Hepatic: ↑ SGOT 13%, fatal liver failure in 0.2%, hepatomegaly with severe steatosis, hypertriglyceridemia. **Other:** GI—**diarrhea** 28%, abdominal pain 10%, nausea 6%; skin—rash 9%; CNS—headache 7%; fever 12%. Lab: anemia (<8.0 gm, 2%), leucopenia (<2000, 16%), thrombocytopenia (<50,000, 2%), ↑ uric acid 2%. Pregnancy—use only if clearly needed. Approved for children. Pts on Na⁺ restriction, buffered tablets each contain 265 mg Na⁺. **Note:** Drugs whose absorption requires gastric acidity and can be blocked by buffers in ddI, e.g., indinavir, dapsone, ketoconazole, fluoroquinolones, should be given 2 hours apart from ddI. In one study in Europe, once-a-day dosing appeared effective at interim analysis, but not yet recommended. May work: serum T½ is 1.6 hr, but intracellular T½ is 25–40 hrs *(IDSA Absts. 210, 211, 1997)*. **Hydroxyurea** (500 mg bid) has been shown to ↑ available concentration of nucleoside analogs, particularly ddI, and ↑ antiretroviral activity: In a Swiss HIV Cohort Study, d4T, ddI & hydroxyurea achieved a log 4.5 reduction in viral RNA and 54% (39/72) were undetectable at 12 wks vs 28% with d4T and ddI alone. The drug is inexpensive and no cross-resistance has been found. We await further trials.
Lamivudine (3TC) (Epivir)	150 mg bid po in combination with ZDV (200 mg tid or 300 mg bid po). Also, oral solution of 10 mg/ml. (150 mg tab $3.84) (Approx. **$230/month** + ZDV, $288/month) NOTE: Combination tablets available (150 mg 3TC + 300 mg ZDV) = Combivir $8.61 ea. (**$516/mo.**) Dose: 1 Combivir bid po.	**Adverse effects: Well tolerated**. Side-effects reported for combination ZDV + 3TC, most due to ZDV. Fatigue & headache 35%, malaise 27%, nasal symptoms 20%, fever 10%. GI: nausea 33%, diarrhea 18%, nausea/vomiting 12%, anorexia 10%, abdominal pain 9%. Neurol.: neuropathy 12%, dizziness 10%, insomnia 11%, depression 9%. Other: rash, hair loss, vasculitis, photophobia, paresthesias in arms. Lab: leucopenia 7%, anemia 3%. In **pediatric** trials: **pancreatitis** 15%.
Stavudine, d4T (Zerit)	≥60 kg: 40 mg bid po (40 mg tab $4.05) <60 kg: 30 mg bid po (30 mg tab $3.90) (Approx. **$253/month** for 40 mg bid). Oral solution available.	**Adverse effects: Peripheral neuropathy** (15–20%). GI: nausea/vomiting, abdominal pain, diarrhea, pancreatitis 1% with 6 deaths attributed to d4T. CNS: sleep disorders, mania. Skin: rash. Hepatic: ↑ AST, ALT.
Zalcitabine (Dideoxycytidine), ddC (HIVID)	0.75 mg po q8h Higher doses too toxic. (0.75 mg tablet $2.30) (Approx. **$200/month** for 0.75 mg q8h)	**Adverse effects:** Major clinical toxicity is **peripheral neuropathy** (22–35%) (numbness and paresthesias → severe continuous pain, slowly reversible when ddC discontinued, ↑ with diabetes mellitus). Other: GI—**oral ulcers** 13%, dysphagia 3%, abdominal pain 3%; skin—**rash** 8%; CNS—headache 9%, myalgia 5%. Hepatomegaly with severe steatosis. Lab: Anemia (<7.5 gm) 5%, leucopenia (<1500, 9%). Fertile women should not receive ddC unless on effective contraception. Safety in children <13 yrs not established. Irreversible ototoxicity has been reported *(Int J STD & AIDS 8:201, 1997)*.
Zidovudine (ZDV), formerly azidothymidine (AZT) (Retrovir)	300 mg po bid 100 mg tab (po) $1.60 300 mg tab (po) $4.80 200 mg IV $17.23 50 mg/tsp, 240 ml $38.23 (Approx. **$288/month** for 600 mg/d) NOTE: Combination tablets of ZDV (300 mg) + 3TC (150 mg) available. Dose: 1 tab bid	**Adverse effects:** Most are dose-dependent. On 600 mg/d: Major clinical toxicity is **hematologic**: anemia (<8 gm, 1%), granulocytopenia (<750, 1.8%). Macrocytosis expected with all dosage regimens. Anemia may respond to epoetin alfa if endogenous serum erythropoietin levels are ≤500 mU/ml. Other: GI—**nausea 50%**, xerostomia, hypertriglyceridemia, hepatomegaly with severe steatosis and severe lactic acid acidosis *(AIDS Clin Care 6:17, 1994)*, anorexia 20%, vomiting 17%; CNS—**headache** 62%, **malaise** 53% (headache, malaise at initiation of rx less frequent if dose 200 mg qd for 5–7 days, then 400 mg q12h for 5–7 days, then 200 mg q8h); pigmentation of nails, [myopathy (7/41 pts on ZDV >270 days, creatine kinase ↑ 2 months before clinical signs, biopsies show abnormal giant mitochondria, strength returns ~8 weeks after ZDV discontinued, *Quart J Med 86:5, 1993)*]. **Asthenia and insomnia common complaints.**

* From 1997 Red Book, Medical Economics Data. Price is average wholesale price (AWP)

NOTE: All dosage recommendations are for adults (unless otherwise indicated) and assume normal renal function.

DRUG NAME(S) GENERIC (TRADE)	DOSAGE/ROUTE/COST*	COMMENTS/ADVERSE EFFECTS
Non-Nucleoside Reverse Transcriptase Inhibitors (NNRTI)		
Delavirdine (Rescriptor)	400 mg po tid (mix 4 100 mg tablets in 3 oz. of water to produce slurry). (100 mg $0.62) (Approx. **$233/month**)	Adverse events of moderate or severe intensity reported in ≥2% of pts but **skin rash has occurred in 18% attributed to the drug;** can continue or restart drug in most cases. Other side-effects include headache, nausea, vomiting, diarrhea and ↑ in liver enzymes in <5% of pts. See *drug-drug interactions, Table 17.* Cross-resistant HIV strains develop with nevirapine.
Nevirapine (Viramune)	200 mg daily for 2 wks, followed by full dose of 200 mg 2x/day (may lower risk of rash). (200 mg $4.13)(**$248/month**)	**Adverse effects: Rash in 37% enrolled in trials;** grade 3 rash in 5.6%, 6.7% stopped nevirapine because of rash. Stevens-Johnson reported *(Lancet 351:567, 1998).* Rash resolves in 50% of pts within 2 wks of stopping rx and in 80% by 1 month. "Serious" rash occurred in 5% of children enrolled in ACTG 250 trial of nevirapine. Fever, nausea and headache can occur. ↑ gamma glutamyl transpeptidase (GGT) in 10% of 252 vs 2% of controls. Nevirapine has good CSF penetration.
Protease Inhibitors: Recommend use only in combination with 2 NRTI (A+B) drugs	**Comment:** There have been 15 case reports of spontaneous bleeding episodes in HIV+ pts with hemophilia being treated with protease inhibitors at the time of the event. It is unknown whether there is a causal relationship between protease inhibitors and bleeding episodes; however, FDA & manufacturers recommend monitoring hemophiliac pts for spontaneous bleeding episodes whenever protease inhibitors are being used in HIV rx. HIV+ hemophiliac pts currently on protease inhibitors **should not discontinue** their rx; consult with provider if they have concerns *(FDA, July 1996).* All may be associated with hyperglycemia and/or hyperlipidemia. 6/105 pts given PIs developed symptomatic diabetes mellitus *(ICAAC Abst. LB-8, 1997).* Central obesity, gynecomastia, and **"buffalo hump"** fatty distributions (so-called lipodystrophy) have been reported with all PIs as well as effective HAART in general *(5th CRV, Abst. 409).*
Indinavir sulfate (Crixivan)	800 mg po tid (capsules). Rx: Two 400 mg caps po tid with 12 oz. liquid, without food. (400 mg cap $2.50) [Approx. **$450/month** + NRTI drug(s)]. Also now 200 mg tabs. In combination with ZDV and 3TC, indinavir 1000 or 1200 mg **bid** was as effective as 800 mg q8h in ↓ viral load (70% had <500 copies/ml in bid while 50% had <500 copies in q8h group at 32 wks *(5th CRV, Abst. 374).*	**Adverse effects: Kidney stones** due to precipitation of indinavir in collecting system (2–3% on 2.4 gm/d but much higher in "hot climates" *(AIDS 14:296, 1997),* 12/174 (6.9%) developed nephrolithiasis within 4 mos. of starting indinavir, 5/8 who continued rx had a 2nd episode *(ICAAC Abst. 183, 1997).* A German study reported 19/158 (12%) sonographically confirmed stones while another 11% had flank pain alone *(ICAAC Abst. 184, 1997).* Prevent (minimize) by good hydration (≥48 oz. water/day) *(AAC 42:332, 1998).* ↑ **indirect bilirubin 10–15% (≥2.5 mg/dl) due to a drug-induced Gilbert's syndrome (of no clinical significance),** GI: nausea 12%, vomiting 4%, diarrhea 5%. Anemia/neutropenia (~5%) *(Abst 287, 3rd CRV, 1996).* Headache 6%. Hyperglycemia has been reported in 7/1000 pts 1–7 months after initiation of rx *(Ln 350:713, 1997).* Rarely severe allergic reactions with repeated exposure *(CID 26:523, 1998).* 10 pts receiving indinavir for 4 wks had ↑ in cholesterol from 145 to 172 mg/dl and triglycerides ↑ from 95 to 142 mg/dl *(IDSA Abst. 233, 1997).* **Drug interactions: see Table 17.** Indinavir effect on cytochrome P-450 enzymes could inhibit the metabolism of terfenadine, astemizole, cisapride, triazolam, midazolam; risk of cardiac arrhythmias; do not give indinavir concurrently with these drugs.
Nelfinavir (Viracept)	750 mg po tid with food. (250 mg $2.06) (Approx. **$557/mo.**) Oral solution available In combination with d4T and 3TC, nelfinavir 1250 mg **bid** was as effective as 750 mg **tid** in ↓ viral load (2–2.5 log) and ↑ CD4 (120 cells/mm³); however, duration of follow-up only 16 wks *(5th CRV, Abst. 373).*	**Adverse effects: GI: Mild to moderate diarrhea in 14–52%,** elevated LFTs, but early indications are that it may be better tolerated than the currently approved PIs. Toxicity profile in general similar to other PIs. Also has potential for bid dosing and is well absorbed with food. Resistance develops slowly and resistant strains have remained susceptible to other PIs. However, because the potential for HIV cross-resistance between nelfinavir and other PIs has not been fully explored, it is unknown what effect nelfinavir rx will have on the activity of coadministered or subsequently administered PIs. Less effect on hepatic metabolism of other drugs than ritonavir but similar to other PIs *(see Table 17).*
Ritonavir (RTV) (Norvir)	600 mg po bid (capsules and oral solution). Capsules must be kept in refrigerator, solution can be kept at room temperature. [Rx: start with 3 100 mg caps po with chocolate milk (or Ensure® or Advera®) bid day 1; 4 caps bid po days 2, 3; 5 caps bid day 5; then 6 caps bid po qd.] (100 mg cap $1.56) [Approx. **$668/month** + NRTI drug(s)] Take with food.	**Adverse effects:** Overall common (85–100% but only 12% withdrawals). **Drug interactions:** More than any other anti-HIV drug. *See Table 17 and review package insert.* **GI:** bitter aftertaste (↓ by taking with chocolate milk, Ensure® or Advera®), nausea [23%, ↓ by initial dose escalation (titration)) regimen], vomiting (13%), diarrhea (13%), **circumoral paresthesias (5–6%),** ↑ γGTT, ↑ **triglycerides;** ↑ **LFTs/CPK/uric acid;** other: lightheadedness (9–14%). Due to **drug-drug interactions,** the following drugs **should not** be co-administered with ritonavir: amiodarone, astemizole, bepridil, bupropion, cisapride, clozapine, encainide, flecainide, meperidine, piroxicam, propafenone, propoxyphene, quinidine, rifabutin, and terfenadine. Interaction with glipizide, glyburide and tolbutamide may explain ↑ hyperglycemia. Also avoid sedatives and hypnotics, e.g., diazepam and flurazepam.

NOTE: All dosage recommendations are for adults (unless otherwise indicated) and assume normal renal function.

TABLE 5B (3)

DRUG NAME(S) GENERIC (TRADE)	DOSAGE/ROUTE/COST*	COMMENTS/ADVERSE EFFECTS
Protease Inhibitors (continued)		
Saquinavir (SQV) (Invirase) (Fortovase for softgel tab)	600 mg po tid (capsules). Rx: Three 200 mg caps po tid with food—high fat preferred. (Hard capsule 200 mg $2.12; soft-gel 200 mg $1.06). Invirase—hard capsules 600 mg po tid with meals (**$572/month**). Fortovase—soft capsules 1200 mg po tid with meals (**$573/month**)	Oral bioavailability ~ 4%, take with food. **Adverse effects:** Overall 37%—mostly mild, <5% moderate. GI: diarrhea, abdominal discomfort, nausea; headache (*Ln 345:952, 1995*). **Soft gelatin capsule formulation shows ↑ absorption to 10–13%** (now approved). Saquinavir + ritonavir also in study and results look promising with ↓ doses (RTV 400 mg bid and SQV 400 mg bid), ↓ toxicity (↑ hepatic dysfunction in pts with underlying hepatitis) and impressive reduction in vRNA (>80% of pts to undetectable) with bid dosing.

TABLE 5C
FOUR NEW DRUGS AVAILABLE THROUGH TREATMENT INVESTIGATIONAL NEW DRUGS PROTOCOLS[1]

DRUG	Adefovir (Preveon)	Efavirenz (DMP-266; Sustiva)	Abacavir (1592-U89)	Amprenavir (141W94)
SOURCE	Gilead 800-GILEAD5	DuPont Merck 800-870-8899	Glaxo Wellcome 800-501-4672	Glaxo Wellcome 800-501-4677
CLASS	Nucleoside RT inhibitor	Non-nucleoside RT inhibitor	Nucleoside RT inhibitor	Protease inhibitor
USUAL DOSE	120 mg po qd	600 mg po qhs	300 mg po bid	1200 mg bid
SIDE EFFECTS	Renal failure, hepatitis, pancreatitis, nausea, cognitive deficiency	Dizziness, headache, rash, diarrhea	Nausea, hepatitis, headache, insomnia, weakness. 3% have hypersensitivity reaction which can be fatal on rechallenge	Nausea, vomiting, diarrhea, hepatitis, insomnia, rash, fatigue
COMMENTS	Activity vs HBV, CMV, HSV	Promising with either PI (indinavir) (90% had <400 copies/ml after 60 wks) or ZDV + 3TC (90% had <400 copies/ml after 24 wks). Resistance could be a problem (*5th CRV, Abst. 692*).	Good CNS penetration	
ENROLLMENT CRITERIA	CD4 <50; viral load >30,000; failure with 2 NRTIs + PI	CD4 <400; viral load (any); failure or intolerant of current therapy	CD4 <100; viral load ≥30,000	CD4 ≥50; viral load ≥5,000; ≤4 weeks NRTI & NNRTI, ≤1 week 3TC or PI

[1] Adapted from *The Hopkins HIV Report:* Charles Raines

NOTE: *All dosage recommendations are for adults (unless otherwise indicated) and assume normal renal function.*

TABLE 6A
HIV/AIDS IN WOMEN/PREGNANCY

I. General Aspects

    A. In 1996, women constituted the fastest growing segment of adults with AIDS in the U.S. *(AJM 101:316, 1996)*. In 1993–Oct. 1995, 18% (43,383) of reported cases of AIDS were in women. For women age 25–44 years, HIV disease is 4th leading cause of death, in blacks the number one cause of death (22%). Seroprevalence from 1984 through 1993 stable at 1.7/1000 (regional prevalences up to 3.1/1000 in Northeast) *(MMWR 44:81, 1995)*. *See Figure 1, page 4 (Table 1)*.

    B. In 1994, of women with AIDS, 41% IDU, 38% heterosexual contact with HIV+ partner or "at risk", 19% no specific exposure, 2% contaminated blood. 77% cases occurred in blacks and Hispanics (especially Puerto Ricans in the Northeast), rates 16 and 7x higher than in white women. Rates in Hispanic of Mexican and Central American origin in Texas and California are similar to rates in white women.

    C. Transmission of HIV from men to women occurs more readily than from women to men, with a 4-fold ↑ in one study. Factors reported associated with ↑ risk: genital ulcers, anal intercourse, partner with advanced disease, non-menstrual bleeding, increased number of sexual exposures, oral contraceptives. Factors **not** associated with increased risk: intercourse during menstruation, number of STDs, circumcision status of partners. Lesbians may be at risk for HIV if they inject drugs or have partners with high-risk behaviors.

    D. Risk after several years of unprotected sex with same infected partner is 10–45%.

    E. Despite these aspects, relatively less is written about women's issues. Only small numbers of women have been included in therapy trials.

II. Initial Assessment: *See Table 4*

III. Clinical Manifestations *(Adapted from Wofsy, C., AIDS File 5:2–5, 1993; J AIDS 9:361, 1995)* (Few clinical studies available to date)

    A. AIDS-defining diagnoses:
Compared to men, women are more likely to present with *(JAMA 272:1915, 1994)*:
- Oral thrush (58%)
- Bacterial pneumonia
- Progressive multifocal leukoencephalopathy

Men more likely to have: non-visceral KS, oral hairy leukoplakia, PCP, invasive HSV.

    B. Human papillomavirus:
- Infection prevalence not increased
- Disease incidence increased! Cervical intraepithelial neoplasia (CIN) 21% (odds ratio 4.9 greater in HIV+) *(J AIDS 9:361, 1995)*
- Aggressive course, with high rate of progression to cancer if immunosuppressed
- Pap smear recommended for HIV+ women. If initial Pap smear negative, repeat in 6 months. If both are negative, annual Pap smears adequate (CDC Guidelines). We recommend every 6 months for those with CD4 <200. Colposcopy recommended for any suspicious lesions. There are no contraindications to standard treatment modalities for CIN.

    C. Recurrent/refractory vaginal candidiasis
- May be early manifestation (CD4 may be >500)
- HIV diagnosis often missed because testing not offered

    D. Other conditions
- PID may be more severe, 7–17% require hospitalization
- Menstrual disorders (41% HIV+ women had menstrual abnormalities vs 24% in case controls) include irregular periods, heavier or scantier periods, early menopausal symptoms, ↑ in premenstrual symptoms
- Incidence of Kaposi's sarcoma is estimated to be 3% in HIV+ women *(AIDS Reader Nov.-Dec., p. 206, 1996)*.

IV. Natural History *(see also PID 15:891, 1996)*. Several studies suggest shortened survival in women even after race, age and risk behavior controlled. 2-year survival in women who received ZDV 33% vs 53% in men. Median survival after an AIDS-defining illness was 13.4 months in women vs 17 months in men. In recent study, HIV+ women at ↑ risk of death, but not rate of disease progression *(JAMA 272:1915, 1994)*. In 1996, it was shown that the rate of clinical progression was similar between men and women if they received comparable medical care *(AJM 101:316, 1996)*. In addition, antiretroviral rx is equally effective in men and women.

V. Family Planning. 85% of women with AIDS are in child-bearing years. Certain contraceptives may pose health hazards for HIV+ women *(from Zeeman B, Hirschhorn LR, p. 616, in HIV Infection, Libman H, Witzburg RA. 3rd Ed., Little Brown & Co.)*

Method of Contraception	Failure Rate	Risks
Sterilization	0.4	No HIV protection
Oral contraceptive	3	May ↑ disease progression; drug-drug interactions common
IUD	3	↑ risk of PID
Latex condom	12	—
Diaphragm cervical cap	18	Potential vaginal abrasions
Sponge	18–28	Potential vaginal abrasions
Nonoxynol-9	21	Failure rate, irritation of vaginal mucosa

VI. Treatment Issues

    A. Little clinical data available

TABLE 6A (2)

B. Theoretical issues
  - Baseline anemia (iron deficiency)
  - Low mean body weight compared to men

C. Menstrual dysfunction
  - Amenorrhea should be evaluated, start with pregnancy test
  - Premature menopause occurs frequently, consider hormone replacement therapy

D. Recommended treatment regimens currently identical for men and women

VII. HIV in Pregnancy: Care of the Mother

A. Antepartum Care
  - **All** pregnant women should be offered HIV testing and counselling **regardless** of risk factors *(MMWR 43:RR-11, 1994)*.
  - Quantitative measure of HIV RNA
  - Obtain CD4 count at outset and each trimester (some ↓ in normal pregnancy)
  - Screening tests (HBsAg, RPR, chlamydia) as in any pregnancy

B. Use of antiviral therapy *(MMWR 47:RR-2, 1998)*. Basic principle is to consider optimal care for the woman as if she were not pregnant. Therefore, choice of therapy is based on viral load, CD4 count and prior treatment. Pregnancy may lead to considerations about timing of therapy, dosing and choice of agents, but women should be offered standard aggressive antiviral therapy.
  1. Zidovudine therapy is the minimum standard of care. ACTG protocol 076 regimen reduced transmission from 25.5% to 8.3% among women who were: *(NEJM 331:1173, 1994)*
     - antiretroviral naive
     - CD4 count >200
     - >14 weeks gestation
     Regimen consists of:
     - zidovudine 100 mg po 5x/day initiated at week 14–36
     - zidovudine IV during labor: 2 mg/kg loading dose, then 1 mg/kg/hr
     - zidovudine syrup for infant (2 mg/kg q6h) beginning 8–12 hours after birth for 6 weeks
     Subsequent studies (ACTG 185) have shown that zidovudine is also effective in women with <200 CD4 cells. Oral zidovudine started at week 36 of pregnancy without zidovudine for infant reduced transmission from 18% to 9% (Bangkok Perinatal Study, *MMWR 47:151, 1998*).
  2. Combination therapy is preferred for women for whom antiretroviral therapy would normally be recommended (e.g., CD4 <500, vRNA >5,000–10,000). Triple drug regimens with 2 nucleosides and a potent protease inhibitor or nevirapine are preferred. However, the safety of antiretroviral agents in pregnancy is not fully established.
     - Women should understand and be actively involved in the decision.
     - Zidovudine should be included in all regimens unless there is significant intolerance or evidence of resistance. Stavudine is preferred substitute.
     - IV zidovudine should be given intrapartum and zidovudine syrup given to infant as in ACTG 076 protocol.
     - Efficacy for mother, safety, and placental passage should be considered in selecting *(Table 15)*.
     - When possible, consider deferring therapy until after 14 weeks gestation to minimize risk of teratogenicity.
     - If only 2 nucleosides are used, consider zidovudine and didanosine. 3TC-containing 2-drug regimens should be avoided so as not to select for resistance.

C. Specific situations
  1. For women pregnant and not on antiretroviral therapy, begin therapy after 14 weeks gestation.
  2. For women on antiretroviral therapy when pregnancy is diagnosed:
     - If greater than 14 weeks, continue therapy. Consider including zidovudine if not part of regimen.
     - If less than 14 weeks, 2 choices:
       (a) Stop all drugs until >14 weeks gestation, then reintroduce all drugs.
       (b) Consider continuing all drugs after discussing risks vs maternal benefit.
  3. For HIV-infected women in active labor who have had no prior therapy:
     - Administer intrapartum zidovudine and zidovudine syrup to infant for 6 weeks
     - After delivery, obtain viral load and CD4 count for mother and plan appropriate therapy.
     - Single-dose nevirapine (200 mg po at onset of labor) achieves therapeutic concentrations in mother and infant for several days. Trial underway to test if this further reduces transmission.
  4. For infants born to HIV-infected women who have received no antepartum or intrapartum therapy, consider administering zidovudine syrup for 6 weeks if it can be started within 24–48 hours. Observational study of more than 900 births in NY state showed zidovudine to infant within 48 hours reduced transmission from 30% to 10% *(Birkhead, 5th Conf. on Retroviruses, 1998)*.

D. PCP prophylaxis: Recommended for women with CD4 count <200 or on prophylaxis because PCP during pregnancy can be more severe, perhaps due to delayed diagnosis.
  - TMP/SMX may be used, although use in last trimester may be associated with ↑ bilirubin. Risk of kernicterus unknown but small.
  - Dapsone: no known adverse effects, although experience limited.
  - Aerosolized pentamidine. Little systemic absorption, although less effective in advanced disease. Effect of ventilation changes due to pregnancy on distribution is unknown.

TABLE 6B
HIV IN THE FETUS AND NEWBORN

GENERAL:

- From Jan. 1993–Oct. 1995, 43,383 (18%) of newly reported cases of AIDS in the U.S. were in women, 85% of whom are of child-bearing age. The estimated 80,000 HIV+ women in 1992 will leave 125,000–150,000 orphan children when they die in the 1990s *(Ped 90:482, 1992)*.

TABLE 6B (2)

- Seroprevalence studies 1989–1993 indicated that 1.7/1000 women who gave birth in the U.S. were HIV+. In inner-city hospitals, e.g., Boston City Hospital, the seroprevalence (1992) was >3%. There are an estimated 12,000 HIV-infected children in the U.S.
- Detection of HIV-infected women, prevention of pregnancy, decreasing transmission to the fetus/infant and early detection and treatment of infected infants and prevention of OIs are major goals *(see Table 6A)*. 24% of mothers with HIV+ infants had no recorded risk factors *(JID 171:689, 1995)*. Further, there has been no improvement in clinical recognition of perinatal HIV infection over the past 4 years.

TRANSMISSION:[1]

- Over 90% of HIV+ children in U.S. acquired their infection from their mothers perinatally: in utero, during delivery, or postpartum through breast feeding. Risk of transmission 13–40% *(MMWR 44/RR-7, July 7, 1995)*.

- Time of transmission:
    - •• In utero: HIV has been identified in fetal tissues as early as 8 weeks. Probably in the majority, in utero transmission occurs late in pregnancy *(Lancet 345:518, 1995)*.
    - •• Intrapartum: at least ½ of transmissions believed to occur through exposure to mother's blood, cervical secretions or amniotic fluid during delivery.
    - •• Postpartum acquisition is rare. Only documented cases acquired through breast feeding. Breast-fed infants have a 14–30% additional risk of becoming infected. In mothers seroconverting during lactation, the risk is 1/3 *(Lancet 342:1437, 1993)*.

- Factors affecting transmission:
    - •• Plasma level HIV-1 RNA. 1 study, >100,000/ml 75% probability of transmission, ≤100,000 3% *(PNAS 92:12100, 1995)*, 2nd, 15/20 transmitters vs 4/75 non-transmitters >50,000. <20,000 0/63 transmitted *(JAMA 275:599, 1996)*. 3rd, 2/19 with <70,000 (10,000, <2000) transmitted *(Lancet 347:899, 1996)*. However, transmission has been documented at all levels of plasma HIV RNA.
    - •• HIV-infected mothers who give birth more than 4 hours after rupture of fetal membranes are almost twice as likely to transmit the virus to their newborns than are mothers who deliver earlier *(NEJM 334:1617, 1996)*.
    - •• Stage of infection: risk is 3-fold higher in HIV+ women with CD4 <400/mm³ compared with women whose CD4 is >700/mm³.
    - •• Vitamin A deficiency ↑ maternofetal transmission (Vitamin A <0.7 µmol/L 32%, ≥1.4 µmol/L 7%) *(Lancet 343:1593, 1994)*.
    - •• Other maternal independent factors: illicit drug use during pregnancy and birth weight *(NEJM 334:1617, 1996)*.

- Prevention of transmission
    - •• Zidovudine or alternative regimen for prevention of HIV transmission from mother to infant, *see Table 6A, page 21 for details and recommendations*
    - •• Intrapartum: avoid prolonged rupture of membranes. No amniotomies. Avoid fetal scalp blood samples and scalp electrodes
    - •• Cesarean delivery ↓ transmission 20–50%, but in some studies no ↓ *(Ped IDJ 14:169, 1995)* (still controversial question, ongoing multicenter trial in Europe will provide answer; *Lancet 348:865, 1996)*. In U.S., Cesarean section is not offered as a means to ↓ mother-to-infant transmission, but should be done for obstetrical reasons.
    - •• Avoid breast feeding if safe, adequate bottle feeding is available *(Lancet 342:1437, 1993; JID 174:722, 1996)*.
    - •• Manual cleansing of the birth canal with chlorhexidine immediately before delivery had no impact on HIV transmission *(Lancet 347:1647, 1996)*.

DIAGNOSIS: *(See Table 6C, page 22)*

- "All" infants born to HIV-infected women have anti-HIV IgG since IgG crosses placenta at 30–32 weeks or later in gestation. "All" will be ELISA and Western blot positive, although only 15–30% actually infected.

- Detection of anti-HIV IgA or IgM in a child indicates infection. IgA seems to be a more sensitive assay. However, IgA is detected in only 50% of infected infants by age 3–6 months *(Lancet 348:865, 1996)*.

- In infants less than 18 months, diagnosis of HIV infection depends on viral culture or HIV DNA PCR. HIV DNA PCR is the preferred assay. Quantitative plasma RNA PCR (e.g., Amplicor) may be more sensitive and specific *(JID 175:707, 1997)* but further studies are needed. "Positive" is based on + results from 2 of the 3 methods or one method on 2 occasions. 30–50% infants + at birth, almost 100% by 3–6 months. HIV+ infants who do not have definitive virologic diagnosis should have ELISA and Western blot repeated every 3 months (until age 1 year), then at 18 and 24 months of age *(JAMA 275:1342, 1360, 1996)*.

- Definitions for in utero (early) vs intrapartum (late) transmission *(NEJM 327:1246, 1992)*
    - •• In utero: viral culture and/or PCR+ on blood within 48 hours of birth (peripheral blood samples)
    - •• Intrapartum: diagnostic studies negative during first week but + from days 7–90 and infant not breast-fed

- Untreated (no antiretroviral rx and no PCP prophylaxis): Symptomatic disease occurred at median age 8 months, 80% infants symptomatic by age 2. Median survival 22–38 months *(NEJM 321:1791, 1989; Ped IDJ 15:321, 1996)*. In children with minimal complications at diagnosis of AIDS median survival 66 months, whereas with serious complications at diagnosis median survival 9 months *(Ped IDJ 12:310, 1993)*. The rate of disease progression in infants is directly related to the severity of maternal disease at time of delivery *(NEJM 330:308, 1994)*, evidence of severe disease in 1st 2 weeks [hepatosplenomegaly, ↑ IgM, ↓ CD4, + HIV by culture, PCR *(JAMA 275:606, 1996)*, and high viral burden *(Abst 249, 3rd CRV, 1996)*.

- Treated: Perinatally infected children who receive ZDV at onset of symptoms, median survival 7–8 years *(Lancet 339:449, 1992; AIDS Clin Care 5:48, 1993)*. No data yet for combination therapy.

---

[1] *From Pediatric AIDS, D. Wara, Medical Management of AIDS, 5th Ed., Eds. M.A. Sande, P.A. Volberding, W.B. Saunders & Co., 1996.*

TABLE 6C
HIV INFECTION IN CHILDREN[2]

1. HIV-Infected
   - Child <18 months known to be HIV+ or born to HIV+ mother
     and
     has positive results on 2 separate determinations from one or more: HIV culture, HIV PCR, HIV p24 antigen.

   - Child ≥18 months born to HIV+ mother or infected by blood products, sexual contact who is HIV antibody + by ELISA and Western blot or + HIV culture, PCR or p24 antigen.

2. Perinatally Exposed (E): A child who does not meet criteria above but
   - is HIV seropositive and <18 months of age
   - unknown antibody status but born to HIV+ mother

3. Seroreverter:
   - (CDC definition): A child born to HIV+ mother: Documented HIV negative (2 or more neg. EIA at 6–18 months, or 1 neg. EIA at >18 months) and no other lab evidence of infection and not had an AIDS-defining condition

4. Viral reversion (very rare):
   - (Pediatric AIDS Foundation): + PCR assay or viral cultures on blood samples (not cord blood) on 2 occasions, no HIV infection evident, no HIV antibody on 2 tests at age >18 months, + genetic relatedness of viruses in mother and infant. Those not meeting these criteria classed as "ambiguous" *(NEJM 334:801, 1996)*.

1994 CDC PEDIATRIC HIV CLASSIFICATION[2]

Immunologic Categories	Clinical Categories			
	N: No signs/ symptoms	A: Mild signs/ symptoms	B: Moderate signs/ symptoms	C: Severe signs/ symptoms
1: No evidence of suppression	N1	A1	B1	C1
2: Evidence of moderate suppression	N2	A2	B2	C2
3: Severe suppression	N3	A3	B3	C3

Immunologic Categories

Immunologic Category	Age of Child					
	<12 months		1–5 years		6–12 years	
	CD4 μL	(%)	CD4 μL	(%)	CD4 μL	(%)
1: No evidence of suppression	≥1,500	(≥25)	≥1,000	(≥25)	≥500	(≥25)
2: Evidence of moderate suppression	750–1,499	(15–24)	500–999	(15–24)	200–499	(15–24)
3: Severe suppression	<750	(<15)	<500	(<15)	<200	(<15)

[2] 1994 revised classification system for HIV infection in children less than 13 years of age *[MMWR 43(RR-12):1–10, 1994]*

Clinical Categories for Children With Human Immunodeficiency Virus (HIV) Infection

CATEGORY N: NOT SYMPTOMATIC
Children who have no signs or symptoms considered to be the result of HIV infection or who have only one of the conditions listed in Category A.

CATEGORY A: MILDLY SYMPTOMATIC
Children with **two or more** of the conditions listed below but none of the conditions listed in Categories B and C.
- Lymphadenopathy (≥0.5 cm at more than two sites; bilateral = one site)
- Hepatomegaly
- Splenomegaly
- Dermatitis
- Parotitis
- Recurrent or persistent upper respiratory infection, sinusitis, or otitis media

TABLE 6C (2)
CATEGORY B: MODERATELY SYMPTOMATIC

Children who have symptomatic conditions other than those listed for Category A or C that are attributed to HIV infection. Examples include but are not limited to:

- Anemia (<8 gm/dL), neutropenia (<1,000/mm³), or thrombocytopenia (<100,000/mm³) persisting ≥30 days
- Bacterial meningitis, pneumonia, or sepsis (single episode)
- Candidiasis, oropharyngeal (thrush), persisting (>2 months) in children >6 months of age
- Cardiomyopathy
- Cytomegalovirus infection, with onset before 1 month of age
- Diarrhea, recurrent or chronic
- Hepatitis
- Herpes simplex virus (HSV) stomatitis, recurrent (more than 2 episodes within 1 year)
- HSV bronchitis, pneumonitis, or esophagitis with onset before 1 month of age
- Herpes zoster (shingles) involving at least 2 distinct episodes or more than 1 dermatome
- Leiomyosarcoma associated with EBV *(NEJM 332:12, 1995)*
- Lymphoid interstitial pneumonia (LIP) or pulmonary lymphoid hyperplasia complex
- Nephropathy
- Nocardiosis
- Persistent fever (lasting >1 month)
- Toxoplasmosis, onset before 1 month of age
- Varicella, disseminated (complicated chickenpox)

CATEGORY C: SEVERELY SYMPTOMATIC

- Serious bacterial infections, multiple or recurrent (i.e., any combination of at least 2 culture-confirmed infections within a 2-year period), of the following types: septicemia, pneumonia, meningitis, bone or joint infection, or abscess of an internal organ or body cavity (excluding otitis media, superficial skin or mucosal abscesses, and indwelling catheter-related infections)
- Candidiasis, esophageal or pulmonary (bronchi, trachea, lungs)
- Coccidioidomycosis, disseminated (at site other than or in addition to lungs or cervical or hilar lymph nodes)
- Cryptococcosis, extrapulmonary
- Cryptosporidiosis or isosporiasis with diarrhea persisting >1 month
- Cytomegalovirus disease with onset of symptoms at age >1 month (at a site other than liver, spleen, or lymph nodes)
- Encephalopathy (at least one of the following progressive findings present for at least 2 months in the absence of a concurrent illness: (a) failure to attain or loss of developmental milestones or loss of intellectual ability, (b) impaired brain growth or acquired microcephaly demonstrated by head circumference measurements or brain atrophy demonstrated by CT or MRI, (c) acquired symmetric motor deficit manifested by ≥2 of the following: paresis, pathologic reflexes, ataxia, or gait disturbance
- Herpes simplex virus infection causing a mucocutaneous ulcer that persists for >1 month; or bronchitis, pneumonitis, or esophagitis for any duration affecting a child >1 month of age
- Histoplasmosis, disseminated (at a site other than or in addition to lungs or cervical or hilar lymph nodes)
- Kaposi's sarcoma
- Lymphoma, primary, in brain
- Lymphoma, small, noncleaved cell (Burkitt's), or immunoblastic or large cell lymphoma of B-cell or unknown immunologic phenotype
- Mycobacterium tuberculosis, disseminated or extrapulmonary
- Mycobacterium, other species or unidentified species, disseminated (at a site other than or in addition to lungs, skin, or cervical or hilar lymph nodes)
- Mycobacterium avium complex or Mycobacterium kansasii, disseminated (at site other than or in addition to lungs, skin, or cervical or hilar lymph nodes)
- Pneumocystis carinii pneumonia
- Progressive multifocal leukoencephalopathy
- Salmonella (nontyphoid) septicemia, recurrent
- Toxoplasmosis of the brain with onset at >1 month of age
- Wasting syndrome: (a) persistent weight loss >10% of baseline OR (b) downward crossing of at least 2 of the following percentile lines on the weight-for-age chart (e.g., 95th, 75th, 50th, 25th, 5th) in a child ≥1 year of age OR (c) <5th percentile on weight-for-height chart on 2 consecutive measurements, ≥30 days apart PLUS (a) chronic diarrhea (i.e., at least 2 loose stools per day for ≥30 days) OR (b) documented fever (for ≥30 days, intermittent or constant)

TABLE 6D
INITIATION OF ANTIRETROVIRAL THERAPY, P. CARINII PROPHYLAXIS, AND SUPPORTIVE THERAPY
[MMWR 44(RR-4):1, 1995, or Ped IDJ 15:165, 1996, Working Committee 1997]

A. P. carinii Prophylaxis—**1995 Revised Guidelines**

1. In infants with perinatally acquired HIV, PCP occurs most frequently at 3–6 months, often acute in onset with poor prognosis. HIV+ infants <1 year of age at risk even with CD4 ≥1500.
    - Identify infants born to HIV+ mothers promptly (screen mothers during pregnancy), obtain PCR or viral culture at ≥1 month and at ≥4 months.

TABLE 6D (2)

- Recommendations *(Ped IDJ 15:165, 1996):*

Age	PCP Prophylaxis	CD4+ Monitoring
Birth to 4–6 wk	No	1, 3, 6, 9, 12 months of age
4–6 wk to 4 mos	Yes	3 months
4–12 mos		
HIV infected or indeterminate	Yes—continue thru 1st year or until HIV infection excluded	6, 9, and 12 months
HIV infection excluded*	No	None
1–5 yrs**	Yes if CD4 <500 or <15% or Category C	Every 3–4 months
6–12 yrs	Yes if CD4 <200 or <15% or Category C	Every 3–6 months

    * ≥2 negative HIV diagnostic tests (PCR or culture) at ≥1 month and ≥4 months or 2 negative HIV IgG antibody tests after 6 months, no clinical evidence of HIV disease
    ** If CD4 <750 in 1st year, continue prophylaxis until 2 years of age or otherwise indicated.
    Table adapted from Lancet 348:866, 1996

  2. Drug Regimens for PCP Prophylaxis in Children ≥4 Weeks of Age:
- TMP/SMX (150 mg TMP/M²/day) po divided twice daily 3x/week on consecutive days (i.e., Mon., Tues., Wed.). Alternatives: same daily dose 1x/day, divided bid 7 days/week or bid on alternate days.
- If TMP/SMX not tolerated:
  - •• Dapsone 2 mg/kg po 1x/day (not to exceed 100 mg)
  - •• Aerosolized pentamidine (children ≥5 yrs) 300 mg via Respirgard II inhaler monthly (or IV pentamidine 4 mg/kg q2 or 4 weeks)

B. Antiviral Therapy
  1. When should antiviral therapy be started?

Clinical trials in children have not kept pace with the rapid advances in antiviral therapy for HIV. Therefore, decisions about when to start antiviral therapy are based largely on knowledge about natural history, data from trials of combination therapy in children with advanced disease, extrapolation from adult trials, and intuition. Considerations which drive the decision to recommend aggressive therapy for children include: (1) the very high viral loads seen in the first year of life, (2) the lack of good immunologic control of viral replication in the first year of life, (3) the potential for immune reconstitution with control of viral replication, and (4) the early and often severe effects on growth and neurologic development. As in adults, viral RNA is an excellent prognostic marker, particularly when combined with CD4 percent *(JID 175:1029, 1997; NEJM 336:1337, 1997)*. CD4 count decreases normally with age during the first 4 years of life, and is harder to interpret in young children. Decreases in vRNA on therapy correlate with improved clinical outcome *(Palumbo 4th Conf on Retroviruses)*.

Early therapy with completely suppressive regimens is the goal in treating children with HIV infection. This must be balanced against the limited number of drugs available in pediatric formulation, limited knowledge about pharmacology and long-term safety, difficulty in complying with complicated regimens, especially with the other difficulties in HIV-affected families, and the real risk of "running out" of drugs. In the fall of 1997 a working group of experts in pediatric HIV disease and virology was convened which issued the first new guidelines for antiviral treatment in 4 years *(CDC Guidelines for the use of antiretroviral drugs in pediatric HIV infection. MMWR RR in press 1998)*. The recommendations below are adapted from those guidelines:

Therapy is recommended for:
a. All children with symptoms (Clinical Category A, B, or C) or evidence of immune suppression (Immune Category 2 or 3). Supported by clinical trials *(NEJM 336:1704, 1997, NIH PACTG 300 executive summary 1997)*.
b. Infants <12 months of age as soon as infection is confirmed, regardless of clinical status, immune status or viral load. Predictors of rapid progression (high viral load, positive PCR at birth, CD4 percent <30%) exist but are not adequate to identify a group who should not be treated.
c. For children >1 year without symptoms and normal CD4 counts, there are 2 approaches:
   (1) If adherence can be assured, treat all children to prevent immunologic deterioration.
   (2) Treat children at risk of progression: high viral load (vRNA >10,000–20,000), declining CD4 percentage, or rising viral load. Consider deferring treatment and closely following viral load and CD4 count for those with low viral load, normal CD4 percent, and no symptoms.

These decisions to start treatment and the choice of therapy must be made with an understanding of the critical importance of adherence in preventing the emergence of drug-resistant virus.

  2. Initial Therapy
Combination therapy is preferred over monotherapy for all children. ddI monotherapy provided benefits similar to ZDV + ddI and was superior to ZDV monotherapy in ACTG 152 *(NEJM 336:1704, 1997)*, combination therapy with ZDV + 3TC or ZDV + ddI led to better clinical outcome in ACTG 300 *(NIH PACTG 300 executive summary, 1997)*. Since dual nucleosides rarely result in long-lasting viral suppression and because of data from adult studies *(NEJM 337:725, 1997)*, most experts prefer triple combinations whenever possible. In adults with very high viral loads (>500,000 copies), which are relatively common in children, 4 drug regimens are increasingly used to achieve complete suppression. There are no data in children and the obstacles to adherence are high, but some would consider this approach if the family situation was appropriate.
a. Preferred regimen:
Protease inhibitor + 2 NRTIs. In preliminary study among experienced patients, up to 74% below 400 copies by week 12 *(ICAAC 1997, LB 7)*.
Protease inhibitor:
   Nelfinavir or ritonavir preferred for young children, FDA-approved for age >2 years
   Alternative:
     Indinavir for those who can swallow pills
     Saquinavir softgel for those who can swallow pills

Recommended NRTI combinations:
    ZDV + ddI
    ZDV + 3TC
    d4T + ddI
    d4T + 3TC
b. Alternative regimen: **Nevirapine + 2 NRTIs**. Less likely to produce sustained response (2/6 infants treated before 4 months, *NEJM 336:1343, 1997)* but preserves PI as a later option.
c. Secondary alternative: **2 NRTIs** from the list above. Good evidence for clinical benefit demonstrated in trials (ACTG 152, ACTG 300), but unlikely to sustain complete viral suppression and less effective than PI-containing regimen in adults (ACTG 320, Agouron 511). However, compliance is simpler, and PI may be used later.
d. NOT RECOMMENDED:
    Any monotherapy
    d4T + ZDV
    ddC + ddI
    ddC + d4T
    ddC + 3TC

3. Monitoring therapy: Viral load and CD4 count and percent should be monitored 4–6 weeks after beginning or changing antiviral therapy and at least every 3 months. Some experts, including the authors, prefer to monitor viral load 4 and 8 weeks after modifying therapy to detect suboptimal responses early *(Table 5A)*. Adherence and dosing issues can be addressed. Single measurements showing increasing viral load should be confirmed, since illness may cause transient increases, and viral load levels show slightly greater variability in children.

4. When to switch:
    The working group in 1997 completely changed the approach to changing therapy in children. A key change is the critical role of viral load monitoring in children. These recommendations have not been validated in pediatric trials, nor is it likely they will be. The general principles are those derived in adults, and most experts think these principles apply to all HIV-infected persons. Before assuming that progression is due to drug failure, it is critical to review adherence, tolerance, and dosing, and to educate the caregivers about these issues.

    There are 3 main reasons to change therapy:
    a. Failure of the regimen
        (1) Virologic failure
            • Lack of minimally acceptable response at 8–12 weeks. Generally a 1.0 log (10-fold) ↓ should be achievable
            • Lack of suppression to below 400–500 copies by 4–6 months. This goal may not be reasonable in children with over 1,000,000 copies, those treated with 2 drug regimens, and those with extensive prior treatment.
            • Rebound, e.g., persistently detectable levels in a child who was consistently undetectable, or >0.5–0.7 log increase in vRNA (3–5 fold).
        (2) Immunologic failure
            • Change in immunologic classification *(see Table 6C, page 22)*
            • For children in immunologic category 3 (<15% CD4), a consistent drop of >5 points in CD4 percent (e.g., 14% to 9%)
        (3) Clinical failure
            • Progressive neurodevelopmental deterioration
            • Growth failure (persistent decline in growth velocity despite adequate nutritional support, without other cause)
            • Clinical progression, defined as changing from one clinical category to another *(Table 6C, page 22)*
    b. Toxicity or intolerance: Given the limited number of available drugs, it is desirable to try to control some side-effects rather than change therapy. For instance, children with flank pain or nephrolithiasis on indinavir can often be managed with increasing hydration. Diarrhea should be managed with antidiarrheal agents if possible.
    c. New data showing that there is a better approach.

5. What to use as alternative therapy
    There are very limited data on sequencing of drug regimens in HIV-infected persons. Given the smaller number of available drugs for children and the difficulty in adhering to regimens, decisions on changing therapy are complex. Several general principles are useful:
    a. When changing due to treatment failure *(see above)*, assess the adherence to the treatment.
    b. If changing due to virologic failure and adherence was good, assume viral resistance. If possible, change all 3 drugs.
    c. Never add a single drug to a regimen that is clearly failing.
    d. Predicted cross-resistance should be taken into account.
    e. When changing due to clinical intolerance without evidence of virologic failure, it may be reasonable to stop all drugs, substitute a new agent for the suspected offending agent, and restart. In general, dose reduction below recommended ranges should be avoided unless levels can be measured.

TABLE 6D (4)

PREVIOUS REGIMEN	OPTIONS
1 NRTI	2 new NRTIs and PI 2 new NRTIs and NNRTI
2 NRTIs	2 new NRTIs* and PI 2 new NRTIs and dual PI**
2 NRTIs and NNRTI	2 new NRTIs and PI 2 new NRTIs and dual PI*
2 NRTIs and nelfinavir	2 new NRTIs and ritonavir + saquinavir** 2 new NRTIs and indinavir + NNRTI
2 NRTIs and ritonavir	2 new NRTIs and ritonavir + saquinavir**

*
Initial NRTIs	New NRTIs
ZDV + 3TC	d4T + ddI
ZDV + ddI	d4T + 3TC
d4T + 3TC	ZDV + ddI
d4T + ddI	ZDV + 3TC

** Pharmacokinetic data on dual protease combinations not available for children. Based on adult data, when used with ritonavir, saquinavir softgel capsule might be dosed at 20–30 mg/kg q12h up to 400 mg q12h. Additional dual protease combinations (nelfinavir + indinavir, nelfinavir + ritonavir, indinavir + ritonavir) are being evaluated in adults, but pharmacologic interactions should be determined in children before dosing can be determined.

Pediatric Dose of Nelfinavir to be Administered 3 Times Daily

Body Weight		Number of Level 1 Gm Scoops	Number of Level Teaspoons	Number of Tablets
Kg	Lbs			
7 to <8.5	15.5 to <18.5	4	1	—
8.5 to <10.5	18.5 to <23	5	1¼	—
10.5 to <12	23 to <26.5	6	1½	—
12 to <14	26.5 to <31	7	1¾	—
14 to <16	31 to <35	8	2	—
16 to <18	35 to <39.5	9	2¼	—
18 to <23	39.5 to <50.5	10	2½	2
≥23	≥50.5	15	3¾	3

C. Supportive Treatment and Prophylaxis
1. Intravenous immune globulin (IVIG)
   a. Not routinely used. Recommended for infants and children with evidence of humoral immune defects (hypogammaglobulinemia or significant recurrent infections despite antimicrobial therapy. IVIG 400 mg/kg q28 days is recommended. In 2 double-blind placebo-controlled trials, ↓ bacterial infections and hospitalization with early or late disease including children on ZDV *(NEJM 325:73, 1991; JAMA 268:483, 1992)*. In a more recent study, benefit shown only in a subgroup, not on TMP/SMX *(NEJM 331:1181, 1994)*. In this trial (ACTG 051), there was an ↑ in S. pneumoniae with IVIG + TMP/SMX. **Ages and "normal" Ig ranges** (mg/dl) *(Pediatrics 37:715, 1966)*:

Age:	Newborn	1–3 months	4–6 months	7–12 months	13–24 months	2–3 years	3–5 years	6–8 years
Ig:	1044±201	481±127	498±204	752±242	870±258	1024±205	1078±24	1112±293

   b. Thrombocytopenia (<20,000/mm³) on antiretroviral therapy: IVIG 0.5–1.0 gm/kg/dose x3–5 days *(See Table 10 for Winrho®)*
2. Immunization: *See Table 20, page 121*
3. Pneumocystis carinii: prophylaxis recommended for (1) infants aged 1–12 months with indeterminate infection regardless of CD4 count, (2) children aged 1–5 years with CD4 count <500 or CD4 % <15%, and (3) children 6–12 years with CD4 count <200 (as for adults). Regimens for PCP prophylaxis: TMP/SMX preferred (dose in Table 6F). Pentamidine and dapsone are second-line alternatives.
4. Mycobacterium avium complex: prophylaxis recommended *(MMWR 46:RR-12, 1997)*. Begin if CD4 <50 for children ≥6 years; for children 2–6 years, begin if CD4 <75; for 1–2 years if CD4 <500. Clarithromycin 7.5 mg/kg po bid or azithromycin 20 mg/kg po once weekly is preferred. Rifabutin now used as third-line, 5 mg/kg po once daily.
5. Psychosocial support *(see Am Acad Pediatrics, Red Book, 1994)*: School attendance, child/foster care, adolescent education

TABLE 6E
CLINICAL SYNDROMES, OPPORTUNISTIC INFECTIONS, IN INFANTS AND CHILDREN, WHICH DIFFER FROM ADULTS*

In HIV-infected infants and children, disease progression is manifest by decrements in growth and delayed neurodevelopment as well as opportunistic infections as occur in adults
(J Ped 128:58, 1996)

CLINICAL SYNDROME	INFANT/CHILD	ADULT	CLINICAL FEATURES (in children)/COMMENTS
Central Nervous System			
Encephalopathy			General: HIV encephalopathy is a syndrome that includes motor and cognitive dysfunction seen in pts with advanced HIV. Administration of zidovudine has been shown to be beneficial in treating children with HIV encephalopathy. ZDV can effectively reverse and improve neurologic symptoms. Its effect can be transient secondary to ↑ viral replication and emergence of drug-resistant HIV-1 variants within the CNS *(JID 174:1200, 1996)*.
Static course	Common	0	25% children show cognitive and motor deficits. Most have head circumference in 10–25th percentile. Problems with verbal expression, attention deficits, hyperactivity. Mild ↑ reflexes in legs to spastic diplegia. IQ stable.
Plateau course	Uncommon	0	Infant's or child's gain of cognitive or motor skills plateaus. Motor deficits are common. IQ usually only 50–79.
Subacute progressive course	Uncommon	AIDS dementia common	Gradual progressive decline in motor, language, adaptive function. Early, child is alert, wide-eyed, with a paucity of facial movements. Endstage: mute, dull-eyed, quadriparetic. CSF: mild pleocytosis, ↑ protein, may be + for HIV antibody and virus. CT: atrophy, progressive calcification in basal ganglia (most common in infants and young children).
Focal brain diseases: seizures, focal neurologic deficits			
Infections Toxoplasmosis	V. rare	Common	Toxo is uncommon in infants and children since it is most often due to reactivation.
Progressive multifocal leuko-encephalopathy (JC virus)	V. rare	Common	PML is uncommon in infants and children since it is most often due to reactivation.
Endocrine			
Failure to thrive and growth retardation	Common	Wasting syndrome common	33/36 HIV+ children showed failure to thrive, not purely related to diarrhea and malnutrition. Known causes of growth failure are growth hormone deficiency, hypothyroidism, and glucocorticoid excess. 1/3 of HIV+ children have abnormal thyroid function (↑ thyrotropin, ↑ TBG) which correlates with disease progression *(J Ped 128:70, 1996)*.
Eye			
Cytomegalovirus retinitis	Uncommon	Common	CMV chorioretinitis in 1.6% children vs 10–20% in adults *(Arch Ophthal 107:978, 1989)*. In children it usually occurs with generalized CMV infection, viremia and multiple organ involvement. When present, ocular lesions are same as in adults, *Table 9, page 45*.
Retinal depigmentation, on ZDV	~5%	0	Asymptomatic peripheral retinal depigmentation (dosages > 300 mg/M²/d)
HIV-associated "cotton wool" spots	Rare	Common	Seen only in children > 8–10 years, while seen in 60–70% of adults.
Gastrointestinal Tract			
Mouth Kaposi's sarcoma	V. rare	Common	21 cases have been reported. Clinical spectrum similar to adults.
Esophagus Dysphagia, odynophagia	Uncommon	Common	When pain/difficulty occur, children more likely to refuse to eat. CMV—odynophagia, Candida—dysphagia.
Diarrhea	Common	Common	Most common agents: rotavirus 24% (more common in inpatient setting), salmonella (19%), campylobacter (8%) (more common in outpatients). Presence of blood and/or WBC in stool has high positive predictive value for salmonella or campylobacter *(PIDJ 15:876, 1996)*.

* Much of the information in this table has been obtained from *Pediatric AIDS, 2nd Ed., Eds. P.A. Pizzo, C.M. Wilfert. Williams & Wilkins, 1994.*

TABLE 6E (2)

CLINICAL SYNDROME	INFANT/CHILD	ADULT	CLINICAL FEATURES (in children)/COMMENTS
Heart	Common	Common	Abnormal ECG changes (ventricular hypertrophy and non-specific ST-T changes) in 55–93% HIV+ children.
Cardiomyopathy	Common	Uncommon	Left ventricular dysfunction 29–74% (most important cardiac change). 20% transient or chronic congestive failure. Unexpected cardiorespiratory arrests in 8/81 *(JAMA 269:2869, 1993)*. Pericardial effusions and tamponade have been noted frequently in children *(PIDJ 15:819, 1996)*.
Hematologic Hypergammaglobulinemia	Common	Uncommon	By age 6 months, almost all HIV+ children have ↑ gamma-globulins.
Protein S (coagulation inhibitor)	Common	Common	19/26 children had ↓ levels, but risk of thrombosis low *(Ped IDJ 15:106, 1996)*. Adults, ↓ protein S in 27–73%, thrombotic complications in 12%.
Hepatobiliary	Rare	Common	Very few reports relating to children. Etiologies such as AIDS cholangiopathy, peliosis hepatis (bacillary angiomatosis) not reported. 2 cases of fatal hepatic necrosis associated with adenovirus reported *(Rev Inf Dis 12:303, 1990)*.
Lung Tuberculosis	Uncommon	Common	Virtually all are primary infections. Clinical: fever, cough. X-ray: often focal infiltrates with hilar adenopathy, cavitation uncommon.
Lymphocytic interstitial pneumonitis (LIP)	Common	V. rare	LIP occurs in 40% of children with perinatally acquired HIV. HIV and EBV antigens have been demonstrated in lung tissue. Usually diagnosed in children >1 year as compared with PCP which is most common in first year. LIP has better prognosis than PCP. Median survival is ~5x shorter in children diagnosed with PCP than in children with LIP *(Lancet 348:866, 1996)*. Clinical: slowly progressive tachypnea, cough, wheezing, hypoxemia. Rales are infrequent. Clubbing of digits is characteristic. Generalized lymphadenopathy, hepatosplenomegaly and parotid swelling. X-ray: diffuse reticulonodular infiltrates associated with hilar lymphadenopathy. Bacterial suprainfection is common. Diagnosis by lung biopsy. Rx: steroids may be of some benefit.
Cryptococcosis	Uncommon		Disseminated infection or localized process of the lungs. Intermittent fever is most common presenting manifestation. All pts have low CD4, history of previous OIs, and onset of cryptococcosis most commonly in 2nd decade of life *(PIDJ 15: 796, 1996)*.
Congestive heart failure	Common	Uncommon	*See Heart, above*
Leiomyosarcoma	Rare (but ↑)	V. rare	EBV demonstrated by PCR in tumors *(NEJM 332:12, 1995)*
Renal Nephropathy	Common	Rare	Nephropathy observed in 29% children with perinatal AIDS *(Kidney 31:1167, 1987)*. In children may present with nephrotic syndrome with a course of 12–18 months *(NEJM 321:625, 1989)*. Steroid rx may be of value.
"Sepsis"	Common	Uncommon	25% of symptomatic HIV+ children will have bacteremic episodes, most due to bacteremic pneumonia or bacteremia without a focus *(Pediatric AIDS, Eds. P.A. Pizzo, C.M. Wilfert, Ch. 13, page 199, 1991)*.
Fungemia (a nosocomially-acquired infection)			Risk factors: central venous catheter (>90 days), prior antibiotic therapy (>3 different antibiotics, parenteral ↑ risk), parenteral hyperalimentation, hemodialysis, prolonged neutropenia, colonization by Candida species *(CID 23:515, 1996)*
Skin Impetigo	Common	Uncommon	Due to Staph. aureus or Group A strep. Clinical: areas of erythema with "honey crusting." May be widespread and evolve into "cellulitis."

TABLE 6F
SELECTED DRUGS COMMONLY USED IN CHILDREN WITH HIV INFECTION

INDICATION/DRUG	DOSAGE	FORMULATIONS	COMMENTS
Antifungal Drugs			
Amphotericin B	0.25–1.0 mg/kg/d IV *(same as adult, see Table 11)*	No pediatric formulation	
Ampho B lipid complex	5 mg/kg/d IV as for adults		
Fluconazole		Oral suspension (orange-flavored), 50 mg/5 ml (teaspoon)	<u>Adult Dose</u> <u>Pediatric Equivalent</u>
Oral/esophageal candidiasis	6 mg/kg po 1st day, then 3 mg/kg/d po		100 mg 3 mg/kg
Systemic candidiasis	6–12 mg/kg/d po		200 mg 6 mg/kg
Cryptococcal meningitis			400 mg 12 mg/kg (not to exceed 600 mg/d)
Treatment	12 mg/kg po 1st day, then 6 (to 12) mg/kg/d po		
Suppression	6 mg/kg/d po		
Itraconazole	3 mg/kg po qd		Efficacy and safety not established
Anti-HIV Drugs[1]			
Nucleoside reverse transcriptase inhibitors (NRTIs)			
Didanosine (ddl)	Usual dose: 90 mg/M^2 q12h Neonatal dose: 50 mg/M^2 q12h	Pediatric powder for oral solution 10 mg/ml with antacid 25, 50, 100, 150 mg chewable/dispersible tablets	Taken on empty stomach. Oral solution should be refrigerated. If using tablets, should take 2 tablets at once. Full daily dose given once daily in adults but no data for children. FDA-approved.
Lamivudine (3TC)	Usual dose: 4 mg/kg q12h Neonatal dose (<30 days): 2 mg/kg q12h	Solution 10 mg/ml 150 mg tablet Combined tablet 150 mg 3TC with 300 mg ZDV (Combivir)	Can be administered with or without food. Should never be used alone. Demonstrated activity with ZDV or d4T. FDA-approved
Stavudine (d4T)	Usual dose: 1 mg/kg q12h up to 30 kg 30–60 kg: 30 mg q12h >60 kg: 40 mg q12h Neonatal dose: under investigation	Solution 1 mg/ml 15, 20, 30, 40 mg capsules	Can be administered with or without food. Solution should be refrigerated. FDA-approved.
Zalcitabine (ddC)	Usual dose: 0.01 mg/kg q8h Neonatal dose: unknown	Syrup 0.1 mg/ml (investigational) 0.375 and 0.75 mg tablet	Rarely used in children. Not FDA-approved for children
Zidovudine (ZDV)	Usual dose: 160 mg/M^2 q8h IV 120 mg/M^2 q6h Neonatal dose: 2 mg/kg q6h	Syrup 10 mg/ml 100 mg capsule 300 mg tablet	Doses used in trials range from 90 mg/M^2 q6h to 180 mg/M^2 q6h. FDA-approved
Non-nucleoside reverse transcriptase inhibitors (NNRTIs)			
Delavirdine	Usual dose: unknown Neonatal dose: unknown	100 mg tablet	Inhibitor of CYP 3A. No pediatric data. Not FDA-approved for children
Nevirapine	Usual dose: 120–200 mg/M^2 q12h Neonatal dose: 5 mg/kg once daily for 14 d. followed by 120 mg/M^2 q12h for 14 d. followed by 200 mg/M^2 q12h	Suspension 10 mg/ml (investigational, available from manufacturer) 200 mg tablets	Begin at half dose for 14 days (induces its own metabolism). CYP 3A inducer. Not FDA-approved for children

[1] Adolescents ≥ Tanner 4 should be dosed according to adult dosing *(see Table 5B)*

TABLE 6F (2)

INDICATION/DRUG	DOSAGE	FORMULATIONS	COMMENTS
Anti-HIV Drugs[1] *(continued)*			
Protease Inhibitors			
Indinavir	Usual dose: 500 mg/M^2 q8h Neonatal dose: unknown, not currently recommended in neonates	200 and 400 mg capsules	Must be taken on empty stomach and must not be taken with ddI. Inhibitor of CYP 3A. Not FDA-approved for children
Nelfinavir	Usual dose: 20–30 mg/kg tid Neonatal dose: 10 mg/kg tid (under investigation in PACTG 353)	Powder for oral suspension 50 mg/gm (1 gm scoop) *(see Table 5B)* 250 mg tablet	Powder may be mixed with water, milk, formula, pudding or ice cream. Acidic juices such as orange or apple result in bitter taste. Take with food. FDA-approved
Ritonavir	Usual dose: 350–400 mg/M^2 q12h Neonatal dose: under investigation	Solution 80 mg/ml Capsules 100 mg	Oral solution is unpleasant tasting. May be mixed with chocolate milk, pudding. Peanut butter or popsicle before dose helps. Very potent inhibitor of CYP 3A. FDA-approved
Saquinavir	Usual dose: Softgel capsule 33 mg/kg q8h Neonatal dose: unknown	200 mg softgel capsule	Inhibitor of CYP 3A. Not FDA approved for children
Antimycobacterial Drugs			
M. tuberculosis			
Ethambutol	15–25 mg/kg/d po	No pediatric formulation	Not recommended in children <13 yrs
Isoniazid	Neonates: 10 mg/kg po qd. Infants/Children: 10–14 mg/kg po qd (maximum 300 mg/day)	50 mg/5 ml syrup	Can give IM
Pyrazinamide	15–30 mg/kg po qd as 1 or more doses (maximum 2.0 gm/day)	No pediatric formulation	
Rifampin	10–20 mg/kg po qd (maximum 600 mg/day)	No pediatric formulation	Can give po or IV
Streptomycin	20–30 mg/kg IM qd, divided q12h (maximum 1.0 gm/day)		
MAC—Mycobacterium avium-intracellulare complex			
Azithromycin	5 mg/kg/d for treatment 20 mg/kg once weekly, not to exceed 1200 mg	Oral suspension 100 or 200 mg/5 ml	
Clarithromycin	15 mg/kg/d divided q12h po (not to exceed 300 mg bid)	Granules for oral suspension (125 or 250 mg/5 ml) (DO NOT refrigerate suspension)	
Clofazimine	1–2 mg/kg/d po to max. of 100 mg/day	No pediatric formulation	
Rifabutin	5 mg/kg/d po	No pediatric formulation	

[1] Adolescents ≥ Tanner 4 should be dosed according to adult dosing *(see Table 5B)*

TABLE 6F (3)

INDICATION/DRUG	DOSAGE	FORMULATIONS	COMMENTS
Antiparasitic Drugs			
P. carinii			
Prophylaxis *(See Table 6D—after 4 weeks of age)*			
TMP/SMX or	150 mg/M^2 TMP component po divided bid on 3 consecutive days (M, T, W) each week. Abbreviated schedules: *Table 6D*	Oral suspension (cherry or grape flavored), 40 mg TMP/ 200 mg SMX/5 ml (teaspoon)	Breakthrough episodes of PCP: TMP/ SMX 3%, dapsone 15% or higher, aerosol pentamidine 15%, IV pentamidine 25% *(J Ped 122:163, 1993)*
Dapsone or	2 mg/kg/day po (not to exceed 100 mg)	No pediatric formulation	
Aerosolized pentamidine—only if ≥5 yrs old	300 mg with Respirgard II inhaler 1x monthly		Used as young as 8 months *(Ped IDJ 12:958, 1991)*
Treatment			
Atovaquone suspension	30–40 mg/kg po qd. Dosing interval not established	Not FDA-approved for pediatric use	Efficacy in children not established. CNS levels <1%.
Pentamidine isethionate	4 mg/kg/d IV or IM x12–14 d		
TMP/SMX	Children >2 months 20 mg TMP/100 mg SMX/kg/d divided q6h po or IV in same dose q6–8h		Start with IV in all but mildest cases
Antiviral Drugs—other than anti-HIV			
Cytomegalovirus			
Cidofovir	No studies in children	IV solution only	See guidelines for hydration and probenecid
Foscarnet Induction Maintenance	180 mg/kg/d divided q8h 90 mg/kg/d q24h	No pediatric formulation	No studies reported in children. Deposited in teeth & bone of growing animals.
Ganciclovir Induction Maintenance	2.5 mg/kg IV q8h 6.0 mg/kg IV qd	Adult capsule or IV solution	Has potential carcinogenicity
Herpes simplex virus			
Acyclovir	250 mg/M^2 IV q8h. Infuse over 1 hour	200 mg/5 ml oral suspension (banana flavored) available if appropriate	Daily urine output should be 1 ml/1.3 mg of acyclovir
Varicella zoster (<2 yrs old)			
Acyclovir	500 mg/M^2 IV q8h		

TABLE 6G
PROPHYLAXIS FOR FIRST EPISODE OF OPPORTUNISTIC DISEASE IN HIV-INFECTED INFANTS AND CHILDREN

PATHOGEN	INDICATION	PREVENTIVE REGIMENS*	
		FIRST CHOICE	ALTERNATIVES
Pneumocystis carinii	HIV-infected or HIV-indeterminate infants aged 1–12 months	TMP/SMX 150/750 mg/M²/d in 2 div. doses po 3x/wk on consecutive days (A2)	Aerosolized pentamidine (children aged ≥5 yrs) 300 mg 1x monthly via Respirgard II nebulizer (C3); dapsone (children aged ≥1 mo.) 2 mg/kg (max 100 mg) po qd (C3); IV pentamidine 4 mg/kg every 2–4 weeks (C3)
	HIV-infected children aged 1–5 yrs with CD4 count <500 or CD4 percent <15%	Acceptable alternative dosage schedules: (A2) Single dose po 3x/wk on consecutive days	
	HIV-infected children aged 6–12 yrs with CD4 <200 or CD4 percent <15%	2 div. doses po qd; 2 div. doses po 3x/wk on alternate days	
Mycobacterium tuberculosis			
Isoniazid-sensitive	TST reaction ≥5 mm OR prior positive TST result without treatment OR contact with case of active tuberculosis	Isoniazid 10–15 mg/kg (max. 300 mg) po OR IM qd x12 mos. (A1) OR 20–30 mg/kg (max. 900 mg) po 2x/wk x12 mos. (B3)	Rifampin 10–20 mg/kg (max. 600 mg) po or IV qd x12 mos. (B2)
Isoniazid-resistant	Same as above; high probability of exposure to isoniazid-resistant tuberculosis	Rifampin 10–20 mg/kg (max. 600 mg) po or IV qd x12 mos. (B2)	Uncertain
Multidrug (isoniazid and rifampin)-resistant	Same as above; high probability of exposure to multidrug-resistant tuberculosis	Choice of drug requires consultation with public health authorities	None
Mycobacterium avium complex	For children aged ≥6 yrs, CD4 <50; 2–6 yrs, CD4 <75; 1–2 yrs, CD4 <500; <1 yr, CD4 <750	Clarithromycin 7.5 mg/kg (max. 500 mg) po bid (A2) OR azithromycin 20 mg/kg (max. 1200 mg) po 1x/wk (A2)	Children aged ≥6 yrs, rifabutin 300 mg po qd (B1); <6 yrs, 5 mg/kg po qd when suspension becomes available (B1); azithromycin 5 mg/kg (max. 250 mg) po qd (A2)
Varicella zoster virus	Significant exposure to varicella with no history of chickenpox or shingles	Varicella zoster immune globulin (VZIG), 1 vial (1.25 ml)/10 kg (max. 5 vials) IM, administered ≤96 hrs after exposure, ideally within 48 hrs (A2)	None

* See page 9 for HIV classification

TABLE 7
MANAGEMENT OF OCCUPATIONAL EXPOSURES TO HIV-1
(Excellent references: NEJM 332:444, 1995; MMWR 44:929, 1995; AnIM 125:497, 1996)

I. Immediate Measures (optimally should be done by exposed individual before seeking medical consultation):
   Decontaminate:
   Skin: Wash thoroughly with soap and water
   Eye: Rinse thoroughly with sterile saline, eye irrigant, clean water flush (analogous to chemical splash to the eye)
   Mouth, nose: Clean water rinse/flush

II. Evaluation of Exposure Severity [should be done by an individual trained/experienced in such evaluations; evaluation should be thorough and standardized, information including the immediate measures taken should be documented. ALL RECORDS MUST BE CONFIDENTIAL!] *(MMWR 44:929, 1995)*:

   A. Nature of exposure
      Needlestick: Site of injury (draw location)
            Gauge of needle if known (if not, estimate) (risk ↑ with large-bore hollow needles)
            Needle device in use (no documented transmission by sticks with suture needles, to date)
            Mechanism of occurrence (i.e., recapping a needle)
            Depth of needlestick (deep, OR 16.1)
            Visible bleeding at needlestick site
            Volume injected, if any
      Laceration/cut: Site of injury
            Instrument involved (i.e., scalpel blade, test tube)
            Mechanism of occurrence
            Depth of laceration or cut
      Mucosal Splash: Site of splash, volume and duration of contact
            Volume (estimate)
      Non-intact skin (i.e., eczema, previous burn, blister, scratch):
            Site of exposure and mechanism of occurrence
            Nature of underlying skin injury/disease
      Intact skin: Transmission not documented (0/2712)

FACTORS PREDICTING TRANSMISSION OF HIV TO HCWs AFTER PERCUTANEOUS EXPOSURE *(NEJM 337:1485, 1997)*	Adjusted Odds Ratio (95% CL)
Deep (IM) injury	16.1 (6.1–44.6)
Visible blood on device (needle)	5.2 (1.8–17.7)
Needle used to enter blood vessel	5.1 (1.9–14.8)
Source pt with terminal AIDS	6.4 (2.2–18.9)
ZDV prophylaxis used	0.2 (0.1–0.6)

      [NOTE: Average hollow-bore needlestick transmission risk is 0.2–0.5%, but individual risk may be higher (if large volume exposure or source with high level viremia, i.e., seroconversion or late stage disease) or lower (if needlestick is superficial and source is asymptomatic)]. Best estimate of mucosal transmission is 0.1% *(NEJM 332:444, 1995)*.

   B. Source fluid/secretion
      Fluids with known risk of HIV transmission: blood, bloody body fluids, semen, vaginal fluids, concentrated HIV materials in research labs
      Fluids with suspected risk of HIV transmission: pleural fluid, cerebrospinal fluid, peritoneal fluid, synovial fluid, pericardial fluid, amniotic fluid
      Materials with doubtful risk of HIV transmission: feces, vomitus, urine, saliva, sweat, tears (unless bloody)

   C. Source individual (record name; if patient, record number)
      Known HIV positive: record stage of illness (terminal, OR 6.4), CD4 count (if known), antiretroviral rx history
      HIV risk behaviors [male homosexual/bisexual, injection or crack cocaine drug use, multiple sex partners (male or female), multiple transfusions before 1985, hemophiliac]: request consent to test (HIV and hepatitis B)
      HIV risk factors not present: testing is low yield, especially in low prevalence areas

III. Post-Exposure Care:

   A. Counseling: Address anxiety (recognize stress syndromes), where appropriate discuss safer sex/third party risks, HIV pre- and post-test counseling

   B. HIV testing:
      Baseline serum is essential to document occurrence of infection. If HIV testing is refused, bank serum for later testing if indicated. Obtain specimen before HBIG is given if HBIG is required since HBsAg testing is usually performed.
      Follow-up: repeat HIV tests at 6 weeks, 3 months, and 6 months. If negative at 6 months, assume HIV infection did not occur (because seroconversion window is rarely more than 6 months; assurance cannot be absolute, but nearly so). All reported HCW seroconversions have occurred before 6 months, even with ZDV rx. The sensitivity of PCR, bDNA, p24 antigen or viral culture to detect infection in exposed HCW is too low to be of use in the initial management.

   C. Chemoprophylaxis: Although ZDV has been used for post-exposure prophylaxis since the drug became available, only recently have data supporting its efficacy become available *(see table above)*. In a case control study, the risk for HIV infection was ↓ 79% among HCW who used ZDV *(MMWR 44:929, 1995)*. Adverse effects were GI and fatigue. At least 8 treatment failures have been documented. Current recommendations at San Francisco General Hospital are based on exposure level and stage of source patient:

TABLE 7 (2)

ADVICE ABOUT PROPHYLAXIS AFTER EXPOSURE TO HIV AT SAN FRANCISCO GENERAL HOSPITAL

Attributes of the Exposure	Attributes of the Source Patient		
	Asymptomatic, Known Low Titer	AIDS, Symptomatic Infection	Preterminal AIDS, Acute Infection, Known High Titer
Percutaneous injuries			
Superficial injury	Offer	Recommend	Strongly encourage
Visibly bloody device used in artery or vein	Recommend	Recommend	Strongly encourage
Deep intramuscular injury or actual injection	Recommend	Strongly encourage	Strongly encourage
Mucosal contacts			
Small volume and brief contact	Offer	Offer	Offer
Large volume or prolonged contact	Offer	Recommend	Recommend
Large volume and prolonged contact	Recommend	Recommend	Strongly encourage
Cutaneous contacts			
Small volume and brief contact	Offer if obvious portal of entry	Offer if obvious portal of entry	Offer if obvious portal of entry
Large volume or prolonged contact	Offer (recommend if obvious portal of entry)	Offer (recommend if obvious portal of entry)	Offer (recommend if obvious portal of entry)
Large volume and prolonged contact	Offer (recommend if obvious portal of entry)	Recommend (especially with portal of entry)	Recommend (especially with portal of entry)

Adapted from Gerberding: AnIM 125:497, 1996

THE RECOMMENDED PROPHYLAXIS REGIMEN

> The Revised Collaborative Zidovudine Chemoprophylaxis Study Group Protocol is: ZDV 200 mg po tid + 3TC 150 mg po bid + indinavir 800 mg po q8h (Ind. only for massive exposure) for 28 days (start as soon as possible, ideally within 1 hour of exposure).

Treatment is deferred for women who are pregnant or breast feeding and for women who decline contraception during the follow-up period (6 months). To date, objective toxicity has not been observed. Treatment usually not provided if >72 hours post-exposure.

D. Early HIV Infection: The acute retroviral syndrome [fever, rash (usually morbilliform), pharyngitis, lymphadeno-pathy (an infectious mononucleosis syndrome)] occurs in 50–70%, normally 3–6 weeks, in the subset of health care workers who become infected. If such occurs, obtain serum for ELISA and Western blot, but patient will probably be antibody (ELISA)-negative, need plasma HIV PCR (*see Table 5A, page 15*).

Abbreviations: HCW = health care workers, **OR** = odds ratio

TABLE 8
PROPHYLACTIC ANTIMICROBIAL AGENTS AGAINST OPPORTUNISTIC PATHOGENS IN ADOLESCENTS AND ADULTS [WJM 165:67, 1996; CID 25(Suppl.3):S299, 1997]
Prevention of First Episode of Disease

LOWEST CD4 COUNT[1]	PATHOGEN	PREVENTIVE REGIMENS		COMMENTS
		PRIMARY	ALTERNATIVE	
All patients regardless of CD4 level	Mycobacterium tuberculosis: TST[2] ≥5 mm or prior untreated pos. TST or contact with case of active TB	[INH 5 mg/kg/d po, maximum 300 mg po + pyridoxine 50 mg po qd x12 mos.] or [INH 900 mg po + pyridoxine 50 mg po x12 mos.. 2x/wk]	Rifampin 600 mg po qd x12 mos.[3]	See Table 9, page 59
	As above but high probability of exposure to INH-resistant TB	Efficacy of various regimens not established. Regimens include rifampin 600 mg po qd x12 mos.[3] OR rifabutin 300 mg po qd x 12 mos.[3]	(PZA + ETB + ciprofloxacin 750 mg bid po) or ofloxacin 400 mg bid po x6–12 mos. OR ETB [(15–25 mg/kg/d po) (at 25 mg/kg ETB monitoring for retrobulbar neuritis required)] + PZA (25–30 mg/kg/d po) for 12 months.	
	Exposure to multi-drug resistant TB	Consultation recommended		
CD4 <200/mm[4]	Pneumocystis carinii (see Table 9, page 62)	Trimethoprim/sulfamethoxazole-DS (160 TMP) (TMP/SMX-DS) one tab po 3x/week or qd OR Dapsone 100 mg po qd	Aerosolized pentamidine 300 mg q month via Respirgard II nebulizer (if toxo pos., see below) OR [Dapsone 200 mg po + pyrimethamine 75 mg po + leucovorin 25 mg po], all 1x/week.	Clindamycin/primaquine is less effective (CID 23:718, 1996). ACTG 081—failure rates for 2° prophylaxis with dapsone 50 mg po bid 18%, TMP/ SMX 18%, aerosolized pentamidine 21%; dapsone 100 mg po qd, 100 mg po biw or tiw or 200 mg qw also effective.
CD4 <100/mm[4] [Note: in high prevalence areas, institution at <150/mm[4] being considered (Ann Int Med 122:730, 1995)]	Toxoplasma gondii (in patients with + IgG toxo, antibody titer)	TMP/SMX-DS one po qd	(TMP/SMX-SS one tab po qd) or [dapsone 50 mg po qd + pyrimethamine 50 mg po q week + leucovorin (folinic acid) 25 mg po q week]	Clindamycin is less effective than sulfadiazine or TMP/SMX for prophylaxis (Ann Int Med 122:730, 1995)
CD4 <50/mm[4]	Mycobacterium avium-intracellulare[3] (see Table 9, page 64)	Clarithromycin 500 mg po twice daily or azithromycin 1200 mg po weekly	Rifabutin 300 mg po qd[3] OR azithromycin 1200 mg po weekly + rifabutin 300 mg po qd	See Table 12, page 80
	Cytomegalovirus—Authors feel it is reasonable to observe patients closely, treat active CMV retinitis, and then institute chronic suppression (see Table 12, page 93)	Oral ganciclovir 1 gm po tid. Consider only if pt is seropositive for CMV & has positive plasma PCR for CMV (see Comment).	None	See Table 12, page 93, chronic suppression. Prophylaxis decision should include risk group: gay males 35% vs IVDA 4.7% risk of CMV during life. If plasma PCR for CMV pos., 43% risk of disease (↓ to 26% on oral ganciclovir); if PCR neg., 14% risk ↓ to 1% on oral ganciclovir (NEJM 334:1491, 1996). Therefore, use prophylaxis in gay males when PCR pos.
	Candida species[4], cryptococcus Not routinely recommended prior to 1st fungal infection.	100–200 mg fluconazole po qd (see Comment)	100–200 mg fluconazole po once weekly; 200 mg tiw	Recent study of fluconazole 200 mg tiw: 18% candida, 0.4% cryptococcal meningitis (CID 23: 1282, 1996).

[1] Until data assessing risk for OIs available, following the ↑ in CD4 counts associated with initiation of antiretroviral rx (esp. protease inhibitors), most experts recommend prophylaxis be initiated and continued based on the lowest CD4 count recorded (pre-antiretroviral rx CD4 count); [2] TST = tuberculin skin test (Mantoux); [3] Interaction with protease inhibitors to be considered; see Table 12, page 79; [4] Authors feel it is reasonable to observe patients closely, treat strongly suspected or active MAC, then institute chronic suppression (see Table 12, page 80); [5] Fluconazole 200 mg po qd decreased cryptococcal infection from 8% to 1% (NEJM 332:700, 1995). Whether 100 mg qd will be effective has not been determined.

TABLE 9A[1]

DIAGNOSIS AND DIFFERENTIAL DIAGNOSIS OF CLINICAL SYNDROMES, OPPORTUNISTIC INFECTIONS AND NEOPLASMS *(For Treatment, see Table 12)*

CLINICAL SYNDROME/MAJOR DIAGNOSTIC CONSIDERATIONS	DIAGNOSTIC CLUES/COMMENTS
Acute retroviral (HIV) syndrome (symptomatic primary HIV infection): Differential diagnosis includes: EBV mononucleosis, CMV mononucleosis, toxoplasmosis, rubella, viral hepatitis, syphilis, primary HSV, drug reactions NOTE: During acute retroviral syndrome, individuals have very high plasma and genital secretion viral titers and are highly infectious both from sexual activity and needlesticks. Mathematical models predict that 56–92% of all HIV infections may be transmitted during this period of acute infection *(NEJM 333:1783, 1995; J AIDS 7:1169, 1994) (See Fig. 1, page 4, & Table 5A, page 15)*	**Clinical:** Occurs in 50–90%, others have asymptomatic seroconversion. Time from exposure to sx usually 2–6 weeks. Symptoms: Fever >95%, lymphadenopathy 74%, pharyngitis 70%, maculopapular rash (5–10 mm lesions on face, trunk, sometimes palms/soles) 70%, myalgia/arthralgia 54%, diarrhea 32%, headache 32%, nausea/vomiting 29%, hepatosplenomegaly 14%, neuropathy 6%, encephalopathy 6% *(AnIM 125:257, 1996)*. **Laboratory:** thrombocytopenia 45%, lymphopenia followed by lymphocytosis (↓ CD4, ↑ CD8, often atypical lymphs), ↑ hepatic enzymes 21% *(Brit MJ 297:1363, 1988; JID 168:1490, 1993)* **Viral burden:** high-level HIV viremia (10^5–10^8 copies/ml plasma), high p24 antigen (+75%), high titers in PBMC, standard HIV antibody tests usually neg., **false-positive viral RNA in low titers reported**. **Course/Prognosis:** symptoms usually resolve in 1–2 weeks. The occurrence of the acute retroviral syndrome and duration of illness >14 days correlate with more rapid progression to AIDS. May benefit from antiretroviral rx *(NEJM 333:450, 1995 & 333:408, 1995). See Table 5 for recommendations.*

Central Nervous System (includes myelopathy, neuropathy, meningitis) *(Excellent references: AnIM 121:769, 1994; NEJM 332:934, 1995)*

Cognitive Disorders, Diffuse Brain Dysfunction

Declining mental acuity (difficulty in memory, concentration, mathematical calculations) with **preservation of alertness**

HIV-1 associated cognitive-motor complex *[J AIDS 7(Suppl 2):538, 1994]*, also known as AIDS dementia complex. Frequency: 1/3 of adults, 1/2 children with AIDS.	Process is slowly progressive, weeks to months (usually occurs after AIDS defining diagnosis) and CD4 count usually <200/mm³ [mean 61/mm³, median 18/mm³ *(AnIM 124:633, 1996)*]. Degree of intellectual impairment and stage of ADC appears to correlate with CSF HIV RNA *(5th Conf. Retrovir & Ols 1998, Abst. 460)*.

AIDS dementia complex (Price & Worley, 1998)[2] (HIV-1 associated cognitive/motor complex, *Ln 348:445, 1996*)
 Stage 0: normal
 Stage 1: mild, can work
 Stage 2: moderate but cannot work
 Stage 3: severe, cannot work, major intellectual disability
 Stage 4: vegetative (In AIDS dementia complex, a "vegetative" patient can be aroused to a level of alertness. This is an important distinction between AIDS dementia complex and many other potential etiologies.)

[CSF abnormalities: pleocytosis, ↑ protein or ↑ immunoglobulin levels reported in 30% asymptomatic HIV+ individuals *(JID 158:193, 1988)*]

Progressive clinical signs occur without direct infection of neurons by HIV-1 or autoimmunity. HIV-1 binds to brain macrophages, which overrespond to 2° stimuli with release of neurotoxic substances (glutamate-like neurotoxins, free radicals, arachidonic acid). The toxins overstimulate N-methyl-D-aspartate (NMDA) receptors, resulting in ↑ levels of neuronal calcium ion (similar to injury in stroke, trauma). Memantine & nitroglycerins are NMDA antagonists which are being studied *(NEJM 332:934, 1995)*.

Neuro exam: non-focal

	Early	Late
Cognition	Inattention ↓ concentration Forgetfulness, slowing of thought processing	Global dementia
Motor	Slowed movements Clumsiness Ataxia	Paraplegia
Behavior	Apathy Blunting of personality Agitation	Mutism

CSF: Normal 30–50%, ↑ WBC (monos) 5–10%

MRI scan: Early are typically normal. Cerebral atrophy, occasionally with diffuse fluff ("spilled milk"), edema of antral white matter and basal ganglii, best seen on T-2 weighted imaging. No mass effect. Normal gadolinium rules out most cases of primary brain lymphoma and toxo but does not rule out other infections (neurosyphilis, cryptococcal meningitis, MAC encephalitis)

FIGURE 3

COURSE OF NEUROLOGIC DISEASE AND HIV INFECTION IN ADULTS

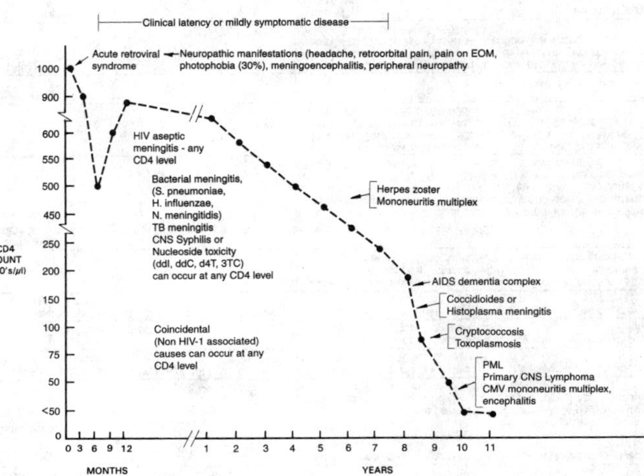

CLINICAL SYNDROME/MAJOR DIAGNOSTIC CONSIDERATIONS	DIAGNOSTIC CLUES/COMMENTS
Central Nervous System/Cognitive Disorders/Declining mental acuity with preservation of alertness *(continued)*	
Progressive multifocal leucoencephalopathy (PML) in early-stage disease *(see page 40)*	Dementia is rare, occurs only late
Depression or anxiety	Sleep inversion, neuropsychiatric testing (Beck Depression Inventory)—most helpful in equivocal cases. *See Table 9C, pages 72–73*
Concomitant **depression of alertness**	
AIDS dementia complex *(as above, Stage 3 or 4)*	Course: ZDV can reduce prevalence of dementia in pts with HIV brain lesions but benefits disappear after about 12 months rx *(J AIDS 6:42, 1993)*. The role of combination retroviral rx not defined and could be ineffective if ZDV not included *(Ln 346:1244, 1995)*.
Cryptococcal disease *(see Meningitis, page 41; Eye, page 46)* Frequency 8–10%, CD4 usually <100/mm³	Clinical: Only ¼ of pts have nuchal rigidity. Extraneural disease in 20–60%. Skin lesions resembling Molluscum contagiosum in 3–10%.
Toxoplasmic encephalitis Frequency 3–10% (in U.S.), CD4 <100/mm³ in 80%	Clinical: Usually subacute. Serum antibody titer positive (>85%) MRI: *See below: focal brain disease*
Progressive multifocal leucoencephalopathy (PML). *See Focal brain disease, page 40.* Frequency 2–4%, CD4 usually <50/mm³	Pts usually alert in early stages of disease; can become depressed later *(see page 40)*.
Primary CNS lymphoma Frequency 3%, CD4 usually <50/mm³	Clinical: Rare without focal findings, which occur when deep structures in brain involved MRI: Single (most often) or multiple, hypodense, contrast-enhancing lesions. Both clinical presentation, CT, and MRI frequently indistinguishable from toxoplasmic encephalitis.
Cytomegalovirus (CMV) encephalitis Frequency not well defined. Overall CMV ~20%, clinical encephalitis occurs in 1% of CMV cases, probably much higher	
Diffuse micronodular encephalitis	Clinical: Onset of symptoms subacute (mean 3.5 weeks): delirium/confusion 90%, apathy and withdrawal 60%, focal neurologic signs 50%. Metabolic abnormalities: hyponatremia 54%, hyperkalemia 23%, hypo-osmolality 38%, hypernatremia secondary to dehydration 30%. CSF: usually 0 cells. MRI with contrast: meningeal enhancement *(CID 20:747, 1995)*, also focal ring-enhancing, space-occupying lesions *(CID 22:626, 1996)*; PCR for CMV DNA shows promise for dx & prognosis *(JID 172:527 & 1087, 1995)*.
Ventriculoencephalitis	Clinical: Onset of symptoms acute (mean 2 weeks): lethargy, disorientation, cranial nerve palsies, nystagmus. Antecedent CMV retinitis in 11/22 pts and 7/11 on anti-CMV rx. CSF: uniformly abnormal (↑ cells, ↑ protein, ↓ glucose). MRI: ventriculomegaly *(CID 20:747, 1995; AJM 96:415, 1994)* with periventricular enhancement with gadolinium *(AnIM 125:577, 1996)*..
Tuberculosis. *See Meningitis, page 41* Frequency 0.5–1.0%	
Bartonella henselae encephalitis Frequency undetermined	Clinical: 16/50 CSF samples from 50 HIV+ pts with neurologic disease + for B. henselae antibodies. Clinical data available on 14/16 pts: confusion 8, subacute progressive dementia 6, hallucinations 5. No data on rx *(Neurol 44:1312, 1994)*. Presence of antibodies strongly associated with ADC: odds ratio 3.59 *(5th Conf. Retrovir & Ols 1998, Abst. 461)*
Neurosyphilis (general paresis, meningovascular) Frequency undefined, any CD4	Serum VDRL and FTA/ABS + in >90%. CSF VDRL sensitivity ranges from 10–89% *(CID 18:288, 1994)*. MRI: cortical atrophy, infarcts.
Herpes simplex virus (HSV) encephalitis Frequency and role still undefined	CSF: Virus seldom cultured from CSF. Definitive dx requires brain biopsy or CSF PCR test for HSV DNA (now available at commercial labs) [98% sensitive during 1st week of disease, antibody neg. early but ↑ after 10–14 days *(CID 20:414, 1995)*].
Neuropneumocystosis	7 cases reported *(CID 25:82, 1997)*. Most receiving aerosolized pentamidine, most had headache and confusion without focal findings. Dx at postmortem in all.

See page 70 for abbreviations and footnotes

CLINICAL SYNDROME/MAJOR DIAGNOSTIC CONSIDERATIONS	DIAGNOSTIC CLUES/COMMENTS
Central Nervous System/Cognitive Disorders/Concomitant depression of alertness *(continued)*	

Causes not directly related to HIV:
    Drugs: sedative/hypnotic, alcohol, "street drugs"
    Hypoxemia
    Sepsis
    Metabolic: hypothyroidism, vitamin B_{12} deficiency, electrolyte imbalance
	Exclude systemic factors

Focal brain dysfunction: seizures and/or focal neurologic findings (hemiparesis, cerebrovascular abnormalities, blindness)	

Abrupt onset
    Cerebrovascular event
        Transient ischemic attack (TIA)
        Cerebrovascular accident (stroke, CVA)
	Clinical: Most TIAs are "benign"; cause is unknown but may be associated with hypercoagulable state *(AJM 101:257, 1996)*. Exclude meningovascular syphilis. Inquire as to cocaine use with resulting risk of vasospasm ischemic events.

Subacute course (days)	

Toxoplasmosis [In U.S., occurs in 3–10% of patients with AIDS; in Europe and Africa occurs in 25–50% *(NEJM 329:995, 1993)*. Frequency ↓ with use of TMP/SMX prophylaxis vs P. carinii (Remington in *MEDICAL MANAGEMENT OF AIDS*, 1998).]	Clinical: Altered mental status (70%), hemiparesis and/or other focal signs (60%), headache (50%), seizures (30%). Fever, confusion, coma also seen. CD4 <100/mm³ in 80%.
	Toxoplasma serum IgG antibody titer predictive of toxoplasmic encephalitis:
	        IgG Incidence/yr.
	        <150 7.4%
	        >150 21.5%
	
	Scan: MRI more sensitive than CT. MRI not always necessary if multiple lesions seen on CT. Multiple spherical ring-enhancing lesions in basal ganglia and cortex, mass effect common. Lesions often identified without concomitant neurologic findings.
	Course: >85% will respond to specific anti-toxo treatment. In one series, 86% responded by day 7 *(NEJM 329:95, 1993)*. If no improvement after 7–10 days of rx—biopsy. In 22 "non-responsive" cases, primary lymphoma in 10; treatable diagnosis in 16 *(West J Med 158:249, 1993)*. Brain biopsy indicated earlier (in <7 days) in patients with early AIDS or if negative toxo antibody titer, single lesion and progression of symptoms on antitoxo rx. If improvement, biopsy not required *(Ln 340:1135, 1992)*.

Primary CNS lymphoma
    Frequency 3% but becoming more frequent cause of focal brain disease
    as toxoplasmic encephalitis ↓ 2° to TMP/SMX prophylaxis
	Clinical: Usually afebrile. Often alert, but with mass effect may have more global mental dysfunction (60%), seizures (15%).
	CSF: Normal 30–50%, protein 10–150 mg%, cells (monos) 0–40/ml, cytology + in <5%.
	Scan: White matter more often involved than gray matter. One or a few weakly enhancing irregular lesions, typically in periventricular region with mass effect. Thick-walled lesions are more common in lymphoma than in toxo *(Radiol 179:823, 1991)*.
	Biopsy necessary for diagnosis.

Tuberculous brain abscess *(Meningitis, page 41)*	Clinical: Evidence of extracranial infection may be absent.
Cryptococcoma *(Meningitis, page 41)*	Clinical: Usually concomitant with cryptococcal meningitis, CRAG of CSF and serum often positive. But when an isolated occurrence, CRAG (serum and CSF) may be negative.
Varicella zoster virus (VZV) encephalitis	Clinical: Often associated with dermatomal zoster (71%) *(Abst 168, 3rd Clinical Retroviral Conference, 1996)*. CSF: Mean WBC 127/mm³, predom. lymphs, protein 157. PCR sensitive and specific. Virus may be isolated. Scan: Multifocal infection of white matter similar to PML or vasculitis resulting in other findings.
Cytomegalovirus (CMV) infection	MRI: May show focal ring-enhancing space-occupying lesions *(CID 22:626, 1996)*.

See page 70 for abbreviations and footnotes

CLINICAL SYNDROME/MAJOR DIAGNOSTIC CONSIDERATIONS	DIAGNOSTIC CLUES/COMMENTS
Central Nervous System/Focal brain dysfunction/Subacute course *(continued)*	
Herpes simplex virus (HSV) encephalitis	*See page 70 for CSF PCR test.* Asymmetric encephalitis, positive MRI, virus rarely isolated from CSF.
Bacillary angiomatosis, intracerebral *(see B. henselae encephalitis, page 38)*	Clinical: Very rare but treatable. Associated with other lesions (skin, liver). Scan: Contrast-enhancing mass lesion. Course: Responds to erythromycin *(AnIM 116:740, 1992)*
Chagas' Disease (Trypanosoma cruzi)	Clinical: One case report with hemiparesis. Born in El Salvador, in U.S. 6 years before onset of illness *(AJM 92:429, 1992)*. Rare causes such as this emphasize the importance of brain biopsy.
Chronic course (weeks) *(see CID 20:1305, 1995)*	
Progressive multifocal leucoencephalopathy (PML) Frequency 4–7% of AIDS patients. Caused by JC virus (a papovavirus) (CD4 usually ≤100/mm³, mean 85/mm³)	Clinical: **Develops insidiously with a single focus** (limb weakness 1/3, ataxia 13%, visual defects 1/3, altered mental status 1/3) *(J Infect 32:97, 1996)*. With progression, multiple foci occur. **Preservation of alertness** until late into disease course and without fever *(AIDS Clin Care 5:17, 1992)*. Seizures found in 20% in one series *(AJM 99:64, 1995)*. CSF: Normal (pleocytosis in 20%, ↑ protein 30%) MRI Scan: Multiple fluffy or diffuse hypodense non-contrast enhancing lesions in **subcortical white matter**, no mass effect. High signal intensity on T-2 images in hemispheric white matter, ill-defined margins (CT/MRI—clinical dissociation, images worse than pt. symptoms). Lab: JC IgM antibody and PCR of CSF for JCV 82% sensitive, 100% specific *(JID 169:1138, 1994)*. Brain biopsy is definitive diagnostic procedure (demyelination, JCV on electron microscopy), sensitivity 40–96%, but not required if MRI is characteristic. Course: Mild response to cytarabine seen in only 3 of 8 patients with no effect on survival *(CID 23:1066, 1996)*. Camptothecin, a topoisomerase inhibitor which blocks DNA in human cancer cells, was used in 1 non-AIDS patient with clinical response *(Ln 349:1366, 1997)*. Reports of improvement with triple drug (2 RTIs and PI) antiretroviral regimens. Death usual within 6 months but spontaneous sustained remissions occur in 5–10% *(Neurol 38:1060, 1988)*. Prolonged survival and remission reported with effective antiretroviral rx *(Ln 349:850, 1997 & 5th Conf Retrovir & Ols 1998, Abst. 463, 464, 465)*.
Seizures *(See causes of focal brain dysfunction)*	
Cerebral mass lesions (32%) Encephalopathy (24%) Meningitis (16%) Other or undetermined cause (28%)	Cerebral mass lesions: majority were toxoplasma *(AJM 87:173, 1989)*, now ↑ lymphoma.
Headaches	
Chronic *(see Focal brain dysfunction)*	
HIV-associated, early disease	May be a presenting symptom. Not AIDS dementia complex or HIV-associated aseptic meningitis, CSF: 0 pleocytosis *(Neurol 43:1098, 1993)*.
Nucleoside therapy (ZDV 50–60% in controlled trial, 3% in open study; ddI 1–7%, ddC 2–12%, stavudine 95% in controlled trial, 3% in parallel track program)	

See page 70 for abbreviations and footnotes

CLINICAL SYNDROME/MAJOR DIAGNOSTIC CONSIDERATIONS	DIAGNOSTIC CLUES/COMMENTS
Central Nervous System (continued)	
Meningitis (headache, fever, lethargy with or without nuchal rigidity)	
Cryptococcal meningitis (CD4 usually $\leq$ 100/mm^3)	Clinical: Stiff neck in only 1/4 of patients, focal findings in 1/5. The presence of headache, nausea & vomiting & cranial nerve abn. correlates with meningitis (ArlM 155:2231, 1995). Extraneural disease in 20–60%. Skin lesions resembling Molluscum contagiosum in 3–10%. Lab: CRAG* (serum) >99% positive—excellent screening test. CSF: LP opening pressure >200 in 60% pts. Often non-inflammatory. Median of 4 lymphs/mm^3, glucose normal to low, protein normal to ↑. India ink prep 75% sensitive. CSF CRAG >90% sensitive (NEJM 321:794, 1989). Increased intracranial pressure may be associated with blindness and ↑ mortality. If opening pressure >300 mmH$_2$O, urgently rx with CSF drainage (10–20 ml CSF). Lumbar drainage and selective placement of lumbar-peritoneal shunts have also been effectively used to control persistent ↑ CSF pressure (J AIDS & Human Retro 17:137, 1998). Dexamethasone or mannitol of questionable value [Saag, MEDICAL MANAGEMENT AIDS, 6th Ed; CID 22(Suppl 2):S119, 1996)].

Bacterial meningitis (occurs at any CD4 level)
   Streptococcus pneumoniae
   Haemophilus influenzae
   Neisseria meningitidis
	Clinical: Presentation similar to non-HIV+ population. Blood cultures usually positive.

Listeria monocytogenes	Incidence of listeriosis (meningitis and bacteremia) 65–145X more common than in general population (CID 17:224, 1993). Yield from blood cultures ↑ by "cold shock" of cultures, i.e., refrigerate overnight before incubation. HIV+ persons should avoid soft cheeses, undercooked chicken (J AIDS 8:466, 1995).
Tuberculous (Mycobacterium tuberculosis) Occurs at any CD4 level	Clinical: HIV+ at ↑ risk but clinical manifestations are similar to HIV– patients (NEJM 326:668, 1992) except intracerebral mass lesions more common (AJM 93:520, 1992). CSF: Lymphocytic pleocytosis, glucose normal or ↓. May resemble cryptococcal meningitis but CRAG* neg.
Coccidioidal or histoplasmal meningitis CD4 usually <100/mm^3	Clinical: Common in endemic areas (see page 63)
HIV aseptic meningitis Occurs at any CD4 level	Clinical: May occur early in HIV infection or relapsing throughout course. CSF: Mild lymphocytic pleocytosis, modest ↑ protein. These findings may be present in asymptomatic patient.
Meningovascular syphilis	Clinical: May present with focal neurologic findings due to active endarteritis. Lab: CSF VDRL positive (serum VDRL negative in 5–10%). >20 cells, CSF glucose may be ↓.
Most Common Peripheral Nerve Syndromes in HIV Disease by Stage: **Clinical Syndrome/Diagnostic Considerations/Major Clinical Features**	**Diagnostic Procedures/Comments**

The following are organized according to stage of HIV infection and relative prevalence

Acute retroviral syndrome:	See Acute retroviral syndrome, page 36
Clinical: headache/retro-orbital pain, often ↑ with eye movement (30%), photophobia. Myelopathy, peripheral neuropathy, brachial neuritis, facial palsy, cauda equina and Guillain-Barre syndrome reported. Course: Usually self-limited, but persistence reported.	
Neuropathy (6–8%) Course: Usually self-limited, but persistence reported.	

CLINICAL SYNDROME/MAJOR DIAGNOSTIC CONSIDERATIONS	DIAGNOSTIC CLUES/COMMENTS
Central Nervous System/Most Common Peripheral Nerve Syndromes in HIV Disease by Stage *(continued) (See Intl J STD & AIDS 8:16, 1997)*	
Clinical Syndrome/Diagnostic Considerations/Major Clinical Features	**Diagnostic Procedures/Comments**
Early (asymptomatic HIV):	
Mononeuritis, multiplex (also occurs late) (rare) 　Facial weakness, foot or wrist drop	EMG, multifocal axonal neuropathy
Multiple sclerosis-like syndrome (rare) 　Waxing and waning course, multifocal defect	
Demyelinating polyneuropathy (occurs <5%)	
Subacute (Guillain-Barre syndrome) or acute inflammatory demyelinating polyradiculoneuropathy (AIDP) 　Ascending paralysis with preservation of sensory function	Demyelination, CSF ↑ lymphocyte count (<50 cells/ml), EMG: ↓ nerve conduction and signs of acute denervation of muscles
Chronic (chronic inflammatory demyelinating polyneuropathy) (CIDP) (may also occur late) 　Weakness in arms and legs, paresthesias with minor sensory loss, may be asymmetrical, absent DTRs	Demyelinating polyneuropathy, CSF ↑↑ protein, mild to moderate lymphocytic pleocytosis, EMG shows demyelination.
Late (symptomatic HIV):	
Weakness/spasticity:	
Vacuolar myelopathy (occurs in as many as 40% of patients at autopsy) 　Progressive painless gait disturbance with ataxia and spasticity. Also rarely occurring in upper extremities, + Babinski, may involve bowel and bladder	CSF normal or ↑ protein, 5–10 cells/mm³. Imaging usually normal.
CMV lumbosacral polyradiculopathy/myelitis (occurs <5%) (cauda equina syndrome) 　Subacute onset. Back and radicular pain, ascending weakness, areflexia, bladder and sphincter dysfunction, variable sensory loss	CSF pleocytosis, (avg. 500/mm³ with 71% PMNs), ↑ protein (270 mg/dl), ↓ glucose (29 mg/dl); EMG-multilevel nerve involvement. Cultures + for CMV in 50–60%
Mononeuritis multiplex due to CMV 　Multifocal sensory and motor deficits in major peripheral or cranial nerves (esp. laryngeal nerves and upper > lower extremities—acute onset over 1 month). CD4 <50	CMV blood culture usually positive.
Numbness/burning:	
Distal predominantly sensory symmetrical polyneuropathy (DSP) (occurs >5%) 　Burning feet, painful, may affect walking, distal numbness with ↓ ankle DTR, stocking/glove sensory loss	EMG: axonal neuropathy
Toxic axonal neuropathy from nucleosides (ddI, ddC, d4T, 3TC) (occurs >5%) 　Often aching feeling of feet, occasional burning sensation	EMG: axonal neuropathy; symptoms may worsen for up to 4 weeks after discontinuation of rx.
Weakness/myalgias:	
Myopathy: HIV, zidovudine 　Weakness without sensory finding, DTRs intact with myalgias	EMG: irritative myopathy, ↑ CPK, muscle biopsy, myofibril degeneration + inflammation

See page 70 for abbreviations and footnotes

TABLE 9A (8)

CLINICAL SYNDROME/MAJOR DIAGNOSTIC CONSIDERATIONS	DIAGNOSTIC CLUES/COMMENTS
Electrolyte and Metabolic Abnormalities	

Hyponatremia
  Volume depletion 2° to diarrhea
  Syndrome of inappropriate secretion of antidiuretic hormone (SIADH) (2° to pulmonary or CNS infections)
  Adrenal insufficiency, primary
  Hyporeninemic hypoaldosteronism
  Nephrotoxic drugs: pentamidine, amphotericin B
  Nephrogenic diabetes insipidus: ganciclovir
	Clinical: About 20% of ambulatory and 50% of hospitalized patients have serum Na of <135 mmol/L. On admission ½ due to GI loss and hypovolemia. During hospitalization ½ due to SIADH (PCP, bacterial pneumonias, CNS infection). Patients are edema-free, with hypertonic urine with low serum osmolality and high urinary sodium (*AJM 94:169, 1993*).

Hyperkalemia
  Trimethoprim
  Adrenal insufficiency
  Hypoaldosteronism
  Ketoconazole
	Clinical: 20–53% pts on TMP/SMX or TMP + dapsone for treatment of PCP develop hyperkalemia. TMP is a sodium channel inhibitor and functions as a K-sparing diuretic agent (*NEJM 328:703, 1993*).

Hypercalcemia Lymphoma	Lab: ↑ serum 1,25-dihydroxy vitamin D concentrations.
Hypocalcemia Drug-related: Foscarnet, ketoconazole, amphotericin B, aminoglycosides	Clinical: Neuromuscular irritability, carpal or pedal spasm. Foscarnet forms complex with ionized calcium. Ketoconazole can block formation of 1,25-dihydroxy vitamin D (*NEJM 327:1360, 1992*). Ampho B and aminoglycosides may lead to Mg^{++} wasting with inhibition of parathyroid hormone release and action (*ArIM 151:1441, 1991*).

Lactic acidosis
  Dideoxynucleoside (zidovudine, ddl, ddC) associated lactic acidosis (? idiopathic)
  Tissue hypoxia
	Clinical: Nausea, vomiting, fever, tachypnea with dyspnea. Arterial O_2 saturation normal. Blood lactate >5 mmol/L. Hepatomegaly with steatosis reported. Occurs disproportionately in obese women, *see Table 5B, page 16.* Resembles adult Reye's syndrome. Mortality ~50% (*AnIM 118:37, 1993; AIDS 7:379, 1993*).

Protein catabolism	Clinical: In patients with AIDS and secondary infections, caloric intake ↓ but there is no compensatory ↓ in energy expenditure (*NEJM 327:329, 1992*). *See Systemic, wasting syndromes, page 76.*
Endocrine System (*see M. Schambelan, in* MEDICAL MANAGEMENT OF AIDS, *Eds. M.A. Sande, P.A. Volberding, W.B. Saunders & Co., 1998; The Endocrinologist 7:32, 1997*)	
Pituitary gland Infectious involvement of anterior pituitary: CMV, P. carinii, Toxoplasma gondii	Clinical: 25% of advanced but non-AIDS HIV+ patients have ↓ pituitary reserve (*AJM Sci 305:321, 1993*). Functional pituitary insufficiency is very uncommon but reported (*AJM 77:760, 1984*). Useful diagnostic tests: Corticotropin-releasing hormone (CRH) test; testing for several hormones simultaneously: insulin + thyrotropin-releasing hormone (TRH) + gonadorelin (GnRH); measure glucose, cortisol, GH, TSH, prolactin, LH, FSH and ACTH.
Thyroid gland (clinical hyper- or hypothyroidism not reported) Chronic illness	Lab: ↓ T_3 with reciprocal ↑ rT_3, T_4 usually normal. Useful diagnostic tests: T_3, T_4, thyroid-binding globulin, rT_3 (reverse T_3).
HIV infection	Lab: Normal thyroid function reported. Serum T_3 concentrations less low than seen in patients equally ill with other diseases. Thyroxine-binding globulin ↑ (*NEJM 327:1360, 1992*).

TABLE 9A (9)

CLINICAL SYNDROME/MAJOR DIAGNOSTIC CONSIDERATIONS	DIAGNOSTIC CLUES/COMMENTS
Endocrine System (continued)	
Adrenal gland (the most commonly affected endocrine gland) Primary adrenal failure differential diagnosis: • CMV adrenalitis (found in 33–88% of AIDS pts at autopsy) • HIV infection of adrenal • Infiltration by Kaposi's sarcoma, lymphoma or infection (MAC, crypto, histo, pneumocystis) • Drug-induced: ketoconazole (impairs steroid synthesis), rifampin (induces hepatic enzymes which ↑ metabolism of steroids), megestrol (prolonged use) (AnIM 122:843, 1995) • Pituitary insufficiency (see page 43)	Overt Addison's disease is uncommon, although blunted responses to ACTH are common (AJM Sci 305:321, 1993). Another study reports adrenal insufficiency in 16% of 49 pts tested (J Infection 31:1, 1995). Clinical: Addison's disease: fever, hypotension, abdominal pain, hyponatremia, hyperkalemia. Addisonian crisis may be precipitated by excessive stress or ketoconazole. Patients with suboptimal response to ACTH stimulation should receive stress doses of corticosteroids where there is infection, trauma, etc. Useful diagnostic tests: AM, PM plasma cortisol levels [AM level <275 μmol/L suggests adrenal insufficiency (Clin Endo 45:97, 1996)]; single dose cosyntropin stimulation test; plasma ACTH levels. Pos. blood culture for CMV may indicate CMV adrenalitis.
Pancreas	
Pancreatitis Drug-associated: pentamidine, didanosine (ddI) 2–6%, zalcitabine (ddC) <1%, stavudine (d4T) 1%, lamivudine (3TC) 1% but 15% in children	Clinical: Type I diabetes mellitus may develop.
Hyperglycemia Drug-induced [especially protease inhibitor 6%, megestrol acetate, and corticosteroids (J AIDS & Human Retro 17:46, 1998)]	Other diabetogenic drugs frequently taken by HIV+ patients: dapsone, rifampin, sulfamethoxazole in patients with renal failure, octreotide, ganciclovir (AnIM 118:529, 1993). Protease inhibitors produced symptomatic diabetes mellitus in 6/105 pts (ICAAC 1997, LB-8).
Hypoglycemia Drug-induced [Pentamidine (IV), 2%]	During destruction of islets, insulin release may cause hypoglycemic coma.
Gonads	
Testes Primary testicular failure Drug-associated: ketoconazole	Clinical: ↓ libido and impotence common. Gynecomastia. May be a factor in generalized wasting. Lab: ↓ testosterone levels, ↑ LH and FSH, normal GnRH response.
Ovaries	Clinical: Amenorrhea very common with advanced AIDS, especially with severe wasting. Information on gonadal function is not available.
Eye (see JAMA 275:142, 1996): **Acute loss of vision**—diff. dx: CMV papillitis, VZV, syphilis, cryptococcal meningitis, endophthalmitis (bacterial or fungal)	
Eyelids (Ln 348:525, 1996)	
Herpes zoster ophthalmitis, Kaposi's sarcoma, Molluscum contagiosum	
Anterior Segment Infections	
Fungal keratitis, candida sp.	Clinical: Often no history of trauma, spontaneous & bilateral ulcers. Dx based on corneal scrapings & culture.
Herpes simplex virus keratitis	Clinical: Predilection for peripheral rather than central involvement. Lesions take longer to heal and recurrences common. Dx: Fluorescein + epithelial "dendrites".
Varicella zoster virus keratitis	Clinical: Most patients have H. zoster lesions in trigeminal nerve (1st division) distribution. 2/3 have keratitis, usually punctate.
Corneal microsporidiosis (Encephalitozoon hellum) (J Infect 27:229, 1993)	Clinical: Photophobia, dry eyes, foreign body sensation, blurred vision. Punctate keratopathy. Pets, especially birds, suspected source. Nasal sinus epithelium occasionally involved. Dx: epithelial scrapings (Am J Ophth 115:285, 1993).
Chronic follicular conjunctivitis due to Molluscum contagiosum	Clinical: Lesions larger, more numerous, more rapid in onset than in immunocompetent individuals.

See page 70 for abbreviations and footnotes

CLINICAL SYNDROME/MAJOR DIAGNOSTIC CONSIDERATIONS	DIAGNOSTIC CLUES/COMMENTS
Eye *(continued)*	
Posterior Segment Infections [At least 12 infectious agents identified as causes of retinal or choroidal disease in HIV+ patients *(ID Clin NA 6:909, 1992)*. Considerations include more common or major entities. Prompt ophthalmologic consultation indicated, etiologic diagnosis usually dependent on clinical characteristics rather than laboratory findings.	
HIV-associated "cotton wool" spots (CWS)	CWS occurs in about 50% of patients with non-infectious microvascular retinopathy. Clinical: Usually asymptomatic but occur more in late-stage disease. Ophthal. exam: Small fluffy white lesions with indistinct margins without exudates or hemorrhages. Lesions do not progress and usually regress spontaneously, do not require treatment. CWS may indicate ↑ risk for onset of CMV retinitis.
Cytomegalovirus (CMV) retinopathy Peripheral retinitis	Clinical: Occurs in 20–30% of AIDS patients. CD4 count is <50/mm³ (has occurred with >200/mm³ on HAART). Course: Usually begins with unilateral "floaters" to ↓ visual acuity to blindness. Ophthal. exam: Findings are usually initially in the periphery, moving centrally until macula and/or optic disc involved. Lesions are large creamy to white areas with granular borders and perivascular exudates and hemorrhages ("cottage cheese and ketchup" appearance) with little overlying vitreous reaction. If redness or pain of the eye, photophobia or irregular-shaped pupil develops, suspect infection other than CMV retinopathy. Dx: Based on clinical features, not on cultures or antibody test. Rx: *See Table 12, page 93.* Mortality from CMV correlates with CMV DNA in plasma *(JCI 101:Y97, 1998).*
Primary CMV papillitis	Clinical: **Rapid ↓ in visual acuity**. Swelling of optic nerve head, atrophy within 4 weeks. Consider pulsed systemic steroids + ganciclovir or foscarnet *(Am J Ophth 108:691, 1989).* Dx and rx: *See CMV peripheral retinitis, above, and Table 12, page 93.*
Herpes zoster/simplex virus (VZV) retinitis (mean CD4 24)	Clinical: May not be associated with cutaneous zoster. (1) **Acute retinal necrosis (ARN) syndrome:** rapidly progressive necrosis of peripheral retina (often 360°) with occlusive vasculopathy, marked vitreous and anterior chamber inflammation, optic neuritis and scleritis. Complete visual loss in involved eye. In 1/2 pts both eyes involved *(Am J Ophth 112:119, 1991; Am J Ophth 110:341, 1990; Ln 348:525, 1996; CID 26:34, 1998).* (2) Ill-defined areas of peripheral retinal whitening without granular borders, minimal vitreous reaction, no pain or foveal lesions (confused with CMV).
Toxoplasmic chorioretinitis	Clinical: Ocular involvement uncommon in AIDS. Lesions may be single or multifocal, usually discrete, perivascular in location. Pre-existing chorioretinal scars usually absent. Hemorrhages are absent or minimal. Vitreitis and iridocyclitis (red, painful eye) are common. May occur without intracranial lesions. Lab: Antibody titers unreliable. Course: Response to rx usually good, prolonged suppression required. Oral steroids not used.
Syphilis: iridocyclitis, vitreitis, optic neuritis, chorioretinitis, or combinations of these **Uveitis in HIV: Think syphilis**	Clinical: In HIV+, syphilitic ocular disease is more common, more severe and often bilateral. Necrotizing retinitis with hemorrhage may be confused with CMV. Cream-colored posterior plaques may be seen with mucocutaneous lesions in 2° syphilis. Rule out neurosyphilis. Lab: Positive VDRL and FTA/ABS on serum. Course: Rx failures reported.

See page 70 for abbreviations and footnotes

TABLE 9A (11)

CLINICAL SYNDROME/MAJOR DIAGNOSTIC CONSIDERATIONS	DIAGNOSTIC CLUES/COMMENTS
Eye, Posterior Segment Infections *(continued)*	
Choroidal pneumocystosis	Clinical: Almost all patients have had P. carinii pneumonia and prophylaxis with aerosolized pentamidine. Creamy to orange choroidal lesions, usually bilateral without vitreous inflammation. Visual acuity usually not affected. Course: Response to systemic rx usually good.
Iritis secondary to cidofovir *(CID 25:337, 1997)*	Common with intravitreal injection but recurrent episodes with IV also reported.
Cryptococcosis: choroiditis, endophthalmitis	Clinical: In one series 9/27 (33%) pts with crypto meningitis had neuro-ophthal. signs *(Ophth 96:1092, 1989)*. Rapid visual loss with optic nerve involvement. May be due to ↑ intracranial pressure, a medical emergency—rx with CSF drainage. Multifocal white lesions with optic nerve edema usually without vitreous inflammation seen. Dx usually based on systemic and/or meningeal crypto. With rx, progressive optic atrophy may occur.
Candidal endophthalmitis	Clinical: Prevalence in HIV+ pts unclear. It is rare with only mucocutaneous candidiasis, but may be associated with candidemia with IV lines and neutropenia. Well-demarcated yellow to white lesions which protrude into vitreous, not associated with hemorrhage and usually unilateral.
Bacterial retinitis: Mycobacterium avium-intracellulare, Rhodococcus equi reported	
Rifabutin-associated uveitis	Reported in 1–2% pts on 600 mg/d *(NEJM 330:438, 1994)*. Also rarely on 300 mg/d *(AnIM 121:510, 1994)*. Becoming ↑ common with use of protease inhibitors *(see Table 17, Drug/Drug Interactions)*.
Retinal depigmentation	Clinical: 5% of children on didanosine (ddI) at >300 mg/M^2/day developed retinal depigmentation. Asymptomatic.
Retinal deposits of clofazimine	Clinical: Clofazimine deposits in pigmented tissues. May result in brownish refractile crystals in retina.
Fever of Unknown Origin (FUO) Etiology of fever in AIDS: Pneumocystis carinii pneumonia (14%), MAC (11%), bacterial pneumonia (9%), sinusitis (6%), lymphoma (5%), catheter infection (1–10%), drug allergy (2–5%), Bartonella (8.5% of 250 bc pos. for B. henselae or B. quintana), & occ. CMV (5%) *(excellent reviews: ID Clin NA 10:149, 1996; ID in Clin Pract 5:412, 1996))*, unexplained in 15–30% (but fever in 80–90% of these patients resolved in 2 weeks). In Spain, TBC identified in 42%, leishmaniasis in 14% and MAC in 14% *(CID 20:872, 1996)*.	In 704 HIV+ pts with fever at SFGH *(F.M. Hecht, in press)*, 18% blood cultures + in hospitalized pts. Predictors of + culture: pneumonia, UTI, abscess, central line or neutropenia. Without 1 predictor, only 1.5% were +. Sensitivity of AFB bc related to CD4 count: <100 19% +, 101–200 7% +, >200 0% +. **Fungal bc of no value:** only 1.7% + and in all 5 fungus (3 crypto, 2 histo) either isolated 1st from routine bc or from other site. Serum CRAG + in 3%; all <200 CD4. Chest x-ray of value when respiratory sx present 85–95% sensitive but specificity only 16–30%. Urine culture of value with dysuria. In pts with abn LFTs, liver bx revealed cause of fever in 13/24 pts *(CID 20:606, 1995)*. Bone marrow bx pos. in 52/123 FUO pts in Spain but could have probably been dx through other means *(ArIM 157:1577, 1997)*. When fever remains unexplained, think MAC, lymphoma, Bartonella, PCP or fungus. In endemic areas—babesiosis *(CID 22:809, 1996)*.
Gastrointestinal Tract	
Mouth[3] *(AnIM 125:485, 1996)*	
Oral lesions with or without soreness	
Acute retroviral syndrome	Clinical: Oral ulcerations (aphthous) in 12/30 pts (40%), enanthemas (40%), 5 pts had both *(CID 17:59, 1993)*. Oral candidiasis (12%) *(JID 168:1490, 1993)*. Lab: Thrombocytopenia 74%. HIV antibody test initially + in 7/30 (23%).
Candidiasis CD4 200–500 *(J AIDS 4:770, 1991)*	
Pseudomembranous form (thrush) (most common form)	Clinical: Small 1–2 mm to large white plaques on any mucosal surface. Can be wiped off, leaving erythematous to bleeding base. Lab: Dx established by KOH prep of scraping and culture.

See page 70 for abbreviations and footnotes

TABLE 9A (12)

CLINICAL SYNDROME/MAJOR DIAGNOSTIC CONSIDERATIONS	DIAGNOSTIC CLUES/COMMENTS
Gastrointestinal Tract/Mouth, Oral lesions with or without soreness, Candidiasis, CD4 200–500 *(continued)*	
Erythematous form	Clinical: Smooth red patches on soft or hard palate, dorsal tongue and/or buccal mucosa. Lab: Dx established as above.
Angular cheilitis	Clinical: Erythematous cracks and fissures at corner of mouth. Lab: Dx established as above.
Hyperkeratotic form (candidal leukoplakia)	Clinical: White lesions on tongue, palate and/or buccal mucosa that cannot be wiped off. Clinically resembles hairy leukoplakia *(see below)*. Lab: Biopsy of lesion will show fungi.
Kaposi's sarcoma	Clinical: Red to purple macules, papules or nodules, occasionally the same color as adjoining tissue, on tongue, palate or buccal mucosa. Usually asymptomatic but may become painful with ulceration and inflammation. Lab: Biopsy
Hairy leukoplakia	Clinical: A sign of advancing HIV infection. Lesions usually asymptomatic. White thickening of oral mucosa and/or lateral tongue margins with vertical folds or corrugations. Lesions range from few mm to covering entire dorsal surface of the tongue. Has been associated with Epstein-Barr virus (EBV) and human papillomavirus (HPV). Occasionally mixed with candida. ↑ frequency in smokers. Lab: Biopsy; epithelial hyperplasia with thickened parakeratin layer with hair-like projections and vacuolated prickle cells. Cannot be cultured on routine viral cultures. Rx: Usually not treated, but can be rx with high-dose acyclovir *(see Table 13, page 104)*. Lesions respond but recur. 10/10 pts responded to one application of topical podophyllin resin within 4–5 days; remissions of 2–28 weeks *(J AIDS 4:543, 1991)*.
Warts [human papillomavirus (HPV)]	Clinical: Usually asymptomatic. Present as single or multiple papilliform warts with multiple white spike-like projections, or as pink cauliflower masses, or as flat lesions resembling focal epithelial hyperplasia. Lab: Biopsy. Types 7, 13 & 32, but usually not 6, 11, 16 & 18 which are associated with anogenital warts.
Lymphoma	Clinical: Poorly demarcated swelling on alveolar ridges and/or discrete oral masses. Lab: Biopsy
Carcinoma, squamous cell	Clinical: Squamous cell carcinoma of tongue reported in HIV disease. Lab: Biopsy
Cytomegalovirus (CMV) oral ulcers	Clinical: A rare manifestation of CMV *(AnIM 119:924, 1993)*. Usually with disseminated infection. Lab: Biopsy and immunohistochemistry
Histoplasmosis, Geotrichosis, Cryptococcosis	Clinical: Rare in occurrence. Lesions are not clinically typical. Lab: Biopsy; organism identified on culture and stains.
Sore mouth without discrete lesions HIV-associated gingivitis and periodontitis	Clinical: Common with advanced HIV. Marked halitosis, spontaneous bleeding and deep-seated gingival pain are usual. Gingiva show fiery red margins with necrosis and ulceration of interdental papillae. May rapidly progress to loss to gingival soft tissue and destruction of supporting bone leading to loss of teeth and necrotizing stomatitis. Is similar to noma (gangrenous stomatitis). Dx: Based on clinical features. Cultures not helpful. Rx: Start with curettage/debridement, followed by topical povidone-iodine (Betadine) irrigation, then chlorhexidine gluconate (Peridex) mouthwash + oral antibiotics effective against anaerobes (metronidazole, clindamycin, AM/CL).

See page 70 for abbreviations and footnotes

TABLE 9A (13)

CLINICAL SYNDROME/MAJOR DIAGNOSTIC CONSIDERATIONS	DIAGNOSTIC CLUES/COMMENTS
Gastrointestinal Tract/Mouth (continued)	
Oral lesions, painful	
Recurrent aphthous ulcers (RAU)	Clinical: RAU may be more common in HIV disease. Recurrent crops of superficial painful ulcers (1 mm to 1 cm) on non-keratinized oral or oropharyngeal mucosa. Lab: Biopsy; shows only non-specific inflammation. Rx: Topical steroids in 50% Orabase may ↓ pain and swelling. Thalidomide (200 mg po qd x14d), 13/14 pts responded (CID 20:250, 1995). In ACTG 251, 14/23 healed with thalidomide rx vs 1/22 on placebo but ¼ had significant side-effects.
Herpes simplex virus (HSV)	Clinical: Recurrent crops of small painful vesicles that ulcerate, usually on palate or gingiva. Usually heal but tend to recur. Herpetic geometric glossitis [extremely tender longitudinal fissures occur, heal with acyclovir IV (NEJM 329:1859, 1993)]. Lab: Smears from lesions reveal multinucleate giant cells, + for HSV on immunofluorescent staining.
Drug-associated lesions	Clinical: Painful mouth lesions occur in 10–15% of patients on zalcitabine (ddC), dapsone.
Xerostomia (dry mouth)	
Sjogren's-like syndrome	Clinical: Dry mouth occurs in 2% of patients on didanosine (ddI). See Salivary gland enlargement, below.
Drug-associated	Rx: Saliva substitutes (Orex®, Xero-Lube®, Moi-Stir®, Salivart®) (electrolytes in carboxymethylcellulose base) and nasal spray may help.
Salivary gland enlargement	
Benign parotid lymphoepithelial lesions (diffuse infiltrative CD8 lymphocytosis syndrome or DILS)	Clinical: Presents as painless (80%) bilateral parotid swelling due to infiltration with CD8 + T lymphocytes. Submandibular glands not involved. CD4 counts 200–500/mm³. 80% have generalized lymphadenopathy, bilateral cervical. Resembles Sjogren's syndrome with sicca symptoms (dry mouth and eyes). Associated findings may include lymphocytic interstitial pneumonia (60%), aseptic meningitis. Most black pts were HLA-DR5. In contrast to Sjogren's, none had anti Ro/SS-A or anti La/55-B antibodies, rheumatoid factor usually negative. Dx based on fine needle aspiration. Rx with zidovudine (AnIM 112:3, 1990; Am J Surg 162:324, 1991). More common in children. All initially responded to radiation but 11/12 relapsed after 5 months.
Other possibilities: CMV (17%), PCP, adenovirus, lymphoma, Kaposi's sarcoma, tuberculosis, MAC, sarcoid	Uni- or bilateral painful parotid swelling (CID 19:1045, 1994; CID 22:369, 1996).
Esophagus⁴ (also see AnIM 122:143, 1995)	
Dysphagia (difficulty swallowing with a sensation of food sticking)	
Candidiasis Frequency 50–70% In HIV+ pt with new onset dysphagia/odynophagia, especially if oral thrush present, fluconazole 100 mg po qd x2 weeks, followed by 200 mg po qd x2 weeks in non-responders. If no response, then endoscope (AJM 92:412, 1992; ArIM 154:2705, 1994).	Clinical: The most common cause of dysphagia in HIV+ patients (42–79% of pts). X-ray: Barium swallow; typically evidence of plaques and ulceration ("moth-eaten" appearance). Findings supportive but not diagnostic. Endoscopy: Large yellow-white plaques usually seen throughout the esophagus. Biopsy/brushing: Will show tissue-invasive pseudomycelia. Secondary prophylaxis: Recurrence rates (20–80%) in 45–90 days. Fluconazole: dosage not defined; 100 mg po biweekly, 10% recurrence over median of 9 months (32nd ICAAC Abst 1116:297, 1992). 150 mg po weekly, 42% recurrence over 6 months (Med J Aust 158:312, 1993).
Drug-associated	Clinical: Dysphagia occurs in 2–3% of patients on zalcitabine (ddC).

See page 70 for abbreviations and footnotes

CLINICAL SYNDROME/MAJOR DIAGNOSTIC CONSIDERATIONS	DIAGNOSTIC CLUES/COMMENTS
Esophagus *(continued)*	
Odynophagia (pain on swallowing) or esophagospasm (retrosternal episodic pain without swallowing)	
Cytomegalovirus (CMV) esophagitis Frequency 5–15%	Clinical: Common 8–13% HIV+ pts. Symptoms are odynophagia, usually without dysphagia, weight loss. Endoscopy: Large solitary (>10 cm^2 in surface area), shallow, superficial ulcers especially in the distal esophagus *(AnIM 113:589, 1990)*. Histology necessary to establish diagnosis. If no inclusions, rx as aphthous ulcer. Present in 24/74 pts who had failed antifungal rx for odynophagia *(AJM 101:599, 1996)*. Rx: Therapeutic trial with ganciclovir in symptomatic patient may be warranted. 27/35 pts responded, relapse rate was high. 5/8 non-GCV responders responded to foscarnet *(AJM 98:169, 1995)*. Stricture may occur after healing.
Idiopathic (aphthous) esophageal ulceration (IEU) Frequency 10–30%	Clinical: In one series, ½ pts with esophageal ulcers due to IEU. Pts present with odynophagia. Differential diagnosis: CMV, HSV, drug-induced ulcers. Found in 25/74 pts who failed antifungal rx for odynophagia *(AJM 101:599, 1996)*. Endoscopy: Large discrete ulcers. Rx: Prednisone 40 mg po qd, taper by 10 mg/week, total course 4 weeks. 11/12 pts responded clinically *(AJM 93:131, 1992)*. Thalidomide (200 mg po qd x14 d), 5 of 5 pts healed or improved, 1 relapsed *(CID 20:250, 1995)*. To obtain thalidomide, call Andrulis Corp., 301-419-2400.
Herpes simplex virus (HSV) esophagitis Frequency 5–10%	Clinical: Acute onset, intense pain, widespread involvement. May be associated with oral herpes *(AIDS Clin Care 7:2, 1995)*. Median CD4 15/mm^3 *(CID 22:926, 1996)*. Endoscopy: Shallow erosive ulcers (like reflux esophagitis) Rx: Acyclovir
Esophageal ulcers associated with acute HIV infection	Clinical: Acute retroviral syndrome (fever, myalgia, maculopapular rash) *(page 36)* + odynophagia or dysphagia *(JAMA 263:2318, 1990)*. Lesions heal spontaneously. These pts are not predisposed to recurrent esophageal ulceration. Endoscopy: One or more discrete ulcers. On biopsy: retroviral virions. Rx: Viscous lidocaine may ↓ symptoms.
Lymphoma, Kaposi's sarcoma, squamous cell carcinoma, histoplasmosis	Clinical: Occur occasionally in esophagus in HIV.
Stomach: nausea, vomiting, early satiety, hematemesis, melena	
Kaposi's sarcoma (KS)	Clinical: Occurs in 40% of patients with cutaneous or nodal KS. Usually asymptomatic, occasional hematemesis. Endoscopy: Submucosal reddish nodules with intact overlying mucosa. Biopsy necessary to confirm dx but many lesions (3/4) cannot be biopsied because of submucosal location and limited depth of endoscopic biopsies.
Lymphoma	Clinical: May produce obstructed gastric outlet syndrome or hemorrhage (hematemesis, melena). In HIV lymphomas often multifocal with disease throughout abdomen. X-ray: Larger masses often show "target lesions" with central umbilicated ulcerations. Endoscopy: Mass lesions, biopsy
Cytomegalovirus (CMV) gastritis	Endoscopy: See CMV esophagitis above, lesions are similar
Drug-induced abdominal pain	Consider antiretroviral drugs as the cause: zidovudine (500 mg/d, dyspepsia 6%), didanosine (250 mg bid, abdominal pain 7%), zalcitabine (0.75 mg q8h, abdominal pain 3%), foscarnet (60 mg/kg IV q8h, abdominal pain ~5%); drugs for opportunistic infection: TMP/SMX, ketoconazole, fluconazole, neomacrolides (abdominal pain 2–3%); other drugs, especially NSAIDs.

See page 70 for abbreviations and footnotes

CLINICAL SYNDROME/MAJOR DIAGNOSTIC CONSIDERATIONS	DIAGNOSTIC CLUES/COMMENTS
Gastrointestinal Tract/Stomach (continued)	
Leishmaniasis (stomach, duodenum)	Dysphagia, odynophagia, epigastric and abdominal pain, diarrhea, GI bleeding reported in AIDS pts with CD4 <100/mm³ in endemic areas (CID 19:48, 1994).
Abdominal pain, acute onset	
Pancreatitis	Drug-associated; e.g., didanosine, pentamidine, lamivudine (3TC) in children
Bowel perforation/peritonitis Most common cause is CMV in advanced HIV infection	AIDS pts with perforation usually febrile, with rigid abdomen, rebound tenderness. Perforations most common in large bowel. Also lymphoma, typhlitis, KS, tuberculosis, salmonellosis (Emerg Med Clin NA 7:575, 1989).

Small bowel disease: cramping paraumbilical abdominal pain, weight loss, large volume diarrhea

Diarrhea

Diarrhea occurs in 30–60% of U.S. and European HIV+ pts and approx. 90% in developing countries. If diarrhea persists for >5 days, evaluation should include microscopic exam of stool (wet mount for Isospora and E. histolytica, modified acid-fast stain for cryptosporidia and cyclospora, modified trichrome for microsporidia), cultures for routine pathogens and C. difficile toxin. If above negative, consider endoscopy of colon and small bowel for treatable causes such as CMV, MAC, KS, lymphoma (COID 8:398, 1995; Ln 346:352, 1995; J AIDS & HR 13:33, 1996).

Acute infectious diarrhea in patients with AIDS[5] (for specific treatment, see Table 12) (Major site of infection may be small bowel or colon) (Gastro Clin N.A. 26:259, 1997; The AIDS Reader, Nov/Dec, 1997)

Agent	Prevalence/CD4 Stage	Clinical Features	Diagnostic Clues/Comments
Campylobacter jejuni, C. coli, C. upsaliensis	4–15% (isolated from 7/43 pts with diarrhea, CID 24:1107, 1997) Any CD4	Watery or bloody diarrhea, fever, fecal WBC ±	Stool culture, most labs cannot detect C. cinaedi, C. fennelli, ↑ sensitivity using membrane filter technique on non-selective blood agar.
Clostridium difficile	3–15% Any CD4	Watery diarrhea, fecal WBC ±, fever, leucocytosis, cramps, hypoalbuminemia; disease spectrum: nuisance diarrhea, colitis, megacolon. Endoscopy usually shows pseudomembranous colitis but may be normal. C. difficile toxin usually pos. CT scan shows colitis with thickened mucosa.	Antibiotic exposure: most common—cephalosporins, clindamycin, ampicillin; rare—TMP/SMX, ZDV, albendazole, rifampin
Enteric viruses: rota, adeno, corona, astro, picobirna, & calicivirus	4–15% Any CD4	Acute watery diarrhea but ⅓ become chronic	Stool electronmicroscopy (detection of viral particles has limited value because viruses produce a self-limiting infection and are untreatable (NEJM 329:14, 1993; J AIDS & HR 13:33, 1996)
Enteroadherent E. coli	10–20% Any CD4, mean 26	Watery diarrhea, weight loss, ↓ D-xylose absorption, acute but may be chronic, usually in right colon, most pts on TMP/SMX prophylaxis	Adherence to Hep-2 cells (research labs only)
Idiopathic	25–40% Variable CD4. Non-infectious causes, rule out medicines, diet, inflammatory bowel disease, anxiety, food poisoning		Negative studies include culture, ova & parasites, C. difficile toxin assay

Salmonella
    S. enteritidis
    S. typhimurium
	5–15%
	100x ↑ when compared to general population, any CD4 count, more common with lower CD4
		Watery diarrhea, fever, fecal WBC ±	Blood culture, stool culture (sensitivity approx. 90%)

Shigella	2% Any CD4	Watery or bloody diarrhea, fever, fecal WBC +	Stool culture

See page 70 for abbreviations and footnotes

CLINICAL SYNDROME/MAJOR DIAGNOSTIC CONSIDERATIONS		DIAGNOSTIC CLUES/COMMENTS	
Chronic infectious diarrhea in patients with AIDS			
Agent	**Prevalence/CD4 Stage**	**Clinical Features**	**Diagnostic Clues/Comments**
Cryptosporidia	20% CD4 <150	Enteritis; watery diarrhea, noninflammatory diarrhea (fecal WBC neg.), afebrile, malabsorption, wasting, large stool volume with abdominal pain, remitting symptoms for months, years	Water-borne, low infectious dose, in healthy adults only 132 oocysts *(NEJM 332:855, 1995)*. AFB smear of stool to show **oocyst 4–6 µm**. In pts with CD4 >180/mm³, C. parvum cleared spontaneously in 7–28 days; with CD4 <180, 87% persisted *(AnIM 116:840, 1992)*. Rx with HAART was associated with clearance of organism from stools except when cholangitis *(5th Conf Retrovir & Ols 1998, Abst 480)*. Pet exposure not a risk for acquisition of cryptosporidia *(J AIDS & Human Retro 17:79, 1998)*.
Cyclospora cayetanensis	US <1%, Haiti 11% CD4 <100	Enteritis, watery diarrhea	Stool AFB smear, **oocyte 8–10 µm**, resembles cryptosporidia *(CID 23:429, 1996; NEJM 328:1308, 1993; AnIM 121: 654, 1994)*
Cytomegalovirus (CMV)	20% CD4 <100	Fever +, fecal WBC +, blood ±, enteritis, colitis, perforation with toxic megacolon, solitary rectal ulcer, small bowel mass	Sigmoidoscopy with rectal biopsy (best initial invasive test), 10–30% of CMV colitis will affect only right side, further steps include colonoscopy with small bowel biopsy, CT—segmental lesions or pancolitis.
Entamoeba histolytica	1–3% Any CD4 count	Colitis, bloody stool, cramps, pos. fecal WBC, most are asymptomatic carriers	Travel history (Latin America). Stool ova and parasites.
Giardia	1–5% Any CD4 count	Enteritis, watery diarrhea, flatulence, bloating, malabsorption	History of drinking mountain stream water. Stool ova and parasites.
Idiopathic	More common with lower CD4 (<200)	Watery diarrhea, malabsorption, no fecal WBC	Biopsy shows villous atrophy, crypt hyperplasia, no identifiable cause despite endoscopy with biopsy and electronmicroscopy for microsporidia.
Isospora belli	U.S. 1.5%, developing countries 10–12% CD4 <100	Enteritis, watery diarrhea, wasting, noninflammatory diarrhea (no fecal WBC), no fever	AFB stool smear, **oocytes 20–30 µm**

Microsporidia
  Septata intestinalis
  Enterocytozoon
    bieneusi
    hellum
	20%
	CD4 <50
		Enteritis; watery diarrhea, noninflammatory diarrhea (fecal WBC neg.), fever is uncommon, remitting disease over years, malabsorption, wasting common *(5th Conf Retrovir & Ols 1998, Abst. 482)*.	Food/water-borne infection **spores 1–2 µm**, fluoresce with calcofluor (excellent screening test), confirmation with Giemsa stain. Special trichrome stain also diagnostic. Complications: disseminated disease, biliary disease.

Mycobacterium avium
  (cause and effect for
  diarrhea not always clear)
	10%
	CD4 <50
		Enteritis, watery diarrhea, no fecal WBC, common fever and wasting, diffuse abdominal pain in late stage	Stool culture unreliable, colonization may occur without diarrhea. Diagnosis: positive blood cultures, biopsy may show changes like Whipple's disease, hepatosplenomegaly, adenopathy, thickened small bowel

Small bowel overgrowth		Watery diarrhea, malabsorption, wasting, often associated with hypochloridia.	Hydrogen breath test, culture of small bowel aspirate

See page 70 for abbreviations and footnotes

CLINICAL SYNDROME/MAJOR DIAGNOSTIC CONSIDERATIONS	DIAGNOSTIC CLUES/COMMENTS
Gastrointestinal Tract/Small Bowel Disease (continued)	
Diarrhea due to alternative mechanisms	Considerations: HIV disease per se, autonomic denervation, Crohn's disease, overgrowth of normal microbial bowel flora.
Typhlitis (acute cecitis, inflammation of cecum)	Clinical: Clinically resembles acute appendicitis, but involves the cecum, which is ulcerated, edematous, necrotic. Associated with Clostridium septicum and Pseudomonas aeruginosa (AnIM 116:998, 1992). Can be a manifestation of C. difficile.
Colorectal disease: left lower quadrant and/or suprapubic cramping, rectal urgency (tenesmus), frequent small volume stools, occasional proctalgia and dyschezia (painful defecation)	
Drug-associated diarrhea	See adverse effects, Tables 5 and 13. Diarrhea is a common complication of rx with antimicrobial agents (including antiretroviral agents). May be a direct effect of drug on GI motility (macrolides), overgrowth of GI flora (clinda), C. difficile
Infectious agents (as above)	
Idiopathic (aphthous) proctitis	Clinical: Endoscopy—large, discrete ulcers. Biopsy to exclude other causes. Thalidomide (200 mg po qd x21 d), improvement in 2/2 pts (CID 20:250, 1995). See Table 12, page 89.
Cytomegalovirus (CMV)	Endoscopy: Focal ischemic colitis with submucosal hemorrhages and discrete shallow ulcers in distal colonic mucosa. Ganciclovir is effective in most patients (JID 167:278, 1993).
Herpes simplex virus (HSV) Types 1 & 2	Clinical: Painful recurrent small to persistent progressive large necrotizing ulcers in perirectal area. Emergence of acyclovir-resistant strains on rx is common. Lab: Smears from lesions reveal multinucleate giant cells, + for HSV on immunofluorescent staining.
Mycobacterium tuberculosis	Clinical: Tuberculosis in ileocecal area and colon may be seen in HIV patients without evidence of pulmonary TBc on chest x-ray. 14% of diarrhea caused by TBc in India (CID 23:482, 1996).
Other considerations: Idiopathic inflammatory bowel disease (ulcerative colitis), Kaposi's sarcoma, lymphoma, epidermoid carcinoma and other neoplasms	

Proctitis
   Neisseria gonorrhoeae
   Herpes simplex virus
   Syphilis, primary or secondary
   Lymphogranuloma venereum (LGV)
   Chlamydia trachomatis (non-LGV immunotypes)
   Human papillomaviruses
   Cytomegalovirus
   Enteric pathogens, e.g., Shigella, Entamoeba histolytica, Campylobacter
	Lab: Numerous PMNs on smear of exudate. Specific diagnosis depends on laboratory studies.

Genital Tract (See new USPHS STD Treatment Guidelines, MMWR, Jan. 1998)	
Anogenital warts (Condylomata acuminata)	
Genital warts [human papillomavirus (HPV) types 6, 11, 16 and 18]: The most common STD in the U.S. in 1998 (NEJM, in press, 1998) Secondary syphilis, condyloma lata Carcinoma	Clinical: Soft, moist, pink or red swellings that grow rapidly. Usually several in same area and look like cauliflower. Identified clinically. Exclude condyloma lata of secondary syphilis. If atypical or persistent, biopsy to exclude carcinoma. Women with cervical warts should not be treated until result of Pap smear available. Rx: Podophyllin or podofilox (See Table 12, page 89)

TABLE 9A (18)

CLINICAL SYNDROME/MAJOR DIAGNOSTIC CONSIDERATIONS	DIAGNOSTIC CLUES/COMMENTS
Genital Tract (continued)	
Cervical dysplasia Cervical intraepithelial neoplasia (CIN) associated with human papillomavirus (type 16, 18, or 31 in 80–90%)	Clinical: In one study 14/35 HIV+ had intraepithelial lesions vs 3/32 HIV– women (*J AIDS 3:896, 1990*). May be missed on Pap smear, colposcopy better (*Ob Gyn 78:84, 1991*). Cervical cancer ↑ (*see Table 6, page 19*) and is the most common cause of sexually transmitted disease-related deaths among females.

Chancroid (Haemophilus ducreyi)
    Culture from edge of lesion or bubo on medium supplemented with patient's own serum
    See primary syphilis
	Clinical: Genital ulcers are exquisitely tender. Usually associated with suppuration of inguinal nodes. Upon exposure to HIV+ contact, HIV seroconversion occurred in 2.9% of men with genital ulcers vs 1.0% in those without ulcers (*AnIM 119:1181, 1993*).
	Rx: *See Table 12, page 78*

Genital herpes simplex (HSV) [usually type 2, but may be type 1 (~5%)] *See primary syphilis*	Clinical: Small painful vesicles, usually in clusters. Ulcerate and may coalesce into large lesions. Inguinal nodes usually slightly enlarged and tender. Usually heal in 10–20 days without scarring. In AIDS pt, recurrent genital herpes may be of ↑ severity with severe local pain, prolonged viral shedding and symptoms lasting weeks. Frequently result in large chronic ulcers in advanced HIV infection. Acyclovir resistance is common. Rx: *See Table 12, page 84*
Gonorrhea (urethritis, cervicitis) Gonorrhea (↑ in gay men in western U.S. cities, 1996)	Clinical: Spontaneous purulent discharge Lab: Urethral smear usually shows >95% PMNs. 50% of patients with gonorrhea have concomitant C. trachomatis. Rx: *See Table 12, page 82* (↑ resistance to ciprofloxacin in SE Asia, 1996)
Granuloma inguinale (Calymmatobacterium granulomatis) *See primary syphilis*	Clinical: Rare in the U.S. Initially a painless red nodule which slowly increases in size and ulcerates. No associated lymphadenopathy. Lab: Giemsa stain of scraping: Donovan bodies, intracytoplasmic bacilli in macrophages. Rx: *See Table 12, page 77*
Idiopathic genital ulcers: "Aphthous-like" (*J AIDS & Human Retro 13:343, 1996*)	Clinical: Painful, shallow ulcers with negative workup including bx for syphilis and herpes simplex. 37% had coexistent oral ulcers and 19% of genital ulcers progressed to fistula formation. Rx: Most responded to topical, intralesional or systemic steroids.

Lymphogranuloma venereum (LGV)
    "Viral syndromes"; influenza (predominance of constitutional symptoms)
    Ulcerative proctitis
	Clinical: Small, transient non-indurated vesicular lesion which heals quickly and may be unrecognized. 1st symptom usually unilateral tender enlargement of inguinal nodes (avoid biopsy—may fistulate) which progresses to inflammation of overlying skin, multiple sinuses. Constitutional symptoms: fever, malaise, headache, joint pains are common. If rectum involved, bloody purulent rectal discharge. Rx: *Table 12, page.* 78.

Non-gonococcal urethritis, cervicitis Non-gonococcal urethritis: C. trachomatis (50%), other known causes (10–15%); Ureaplasma urealyticum. In women: Herpes simplex virus, trichomoniasis, candidiasis	Clinical: Urethral discharge usually not spontaneous (no "drip"), thin, watery in character. Lab: Urethral smear usually shows <80% PMNs + epithelial cells. Positive fluorescent antibody (FA) test vs C. trachomatis. Rapid EIA tests have sensitivity of only 52–74% (do not warrant widescale use) (*JAMA 273:9, 1995*). 6–10% of ureaplasma are resistant to tetracycline (doxycycline).
Pediculosis pubis (Phthirus pubis) (crabs)	Clinical: Itching in anogenital region. Scrotal dermatitis (excoriation) usually present. Ova (nits) attach to the skin at the base of the hairs. Minute brown spots on undergarments (louse excreta) may be seen.
Reiter's syndrome *See Musculoskeletal System, page 66*	

CLINICAL SYNDROME/MAJOR DIAGNOSTIC CONSIDERATIONS	DIAGNOSTIC CLUES/COMMENTS
Genital Tract (*continued*)	
Salpingitis-pelvic inflammatory disease (PID), salpingitis, tuboovarian abscess • Pelvic inflammatory disease: gonococcus, chlamydia, anaerobes (Bacteroides fragilis and other species), enterobacteriaceae, streptococci (especially Group B), mycoplasma • Appendicitis • Ectopic pregnancy	Clinical: PID is more serious in HIV+ women (7–17% require hospitalization). Indications for hospitalization: compliance as an outpatient unlikely, pregnant, peritonitis, suspected pelvic (tuboovarian) abscess, diagnosis uncertain, need for laparoscopy to clarify diagnosis, failure to respond on outpatient rx in 72 hours.
Scabies (Sarcoptes scabiei) (Norwegian scabies) See *Skin, pages 69, 70*	
Syphilis (*see G. Bolan, MEDICAL MANAGEMENT OF AIDS, 6th Edition, 1998).* Syphilis cases are at an all-time low in U.S. in 1997.	
(Syphilis in the HIV+ pt has been described with fulminant presentations, rapid progression, irregular serologic findings, and failure of standard penicillin therapy. Yet others have reported that HIV has not altered clinical syphilis *(AnIM 118:350, 1993).* Uveitis, retinitis more likely in HIV+.)	
Primary syphilis (chancre): other etiologies that cause ulcerative lesions—herpes, chancroid, scabies, granuloma inguinale, trauma. Uncommon: tuberculous ulceration, Behçet's, CMV. Drug reaction: foscarnet. Idiopathic (aphthous) genital ulcers reported in women; ½ had similar lesions in mouth *(J AIDS & HR 13:343, 1996).*	Clinical: Syphilitic chancre not exquisitely tender. Dual infections, syphilis and herpes, not uncommon. All genital ulcers should be considered syphilitic until proven otherwise. Lab: RPR does not become + until 3–6 weeks after initial infection. An early negative test does not exclude syphilis. If negative, repeat at 6 weeks. The FTA/ABS becomes + at 3–4 weeks. Rx: *Table 12, page 84*
Secondary syphilis: Can mimic most skin diseases. Common misdiagnoses include: drug-induced eruption, rubella, infectious mononucleosis, fungal infection, acute HIV. Condyloma lata confused with warts. Alopecia areata, scalp lesions resembling ringworm.	Clinical: Usually associated with generalized lymphadenopathy. Patient often febrile. May show findings of hepatitis and/or nephritis. Ulceronodular syphilis with vesicular lesions (Lues Maligna) reported *(CID 20:387, 1995).* Lab: Positive darkfield. The RPR and FTA/ABS are virtually always positive. In pts with suggestive clinical findings and non-reactive RPR or VDRL dilute serum to exclude possible prozone phenomenon *(ArIM 153:2496, 1993).* Biological false-positive VDRL 4–6% in HIV+ vs 0.2–0.8% in HIV–, but in some (5%), BFP proved to be true pos. active syphilis *(JID 176:1397, 1997).*
Latent [early, <1 year's duration; late, >1 year's duration], indeterminate, neurosyphilis	The diagnosis of neurosyphilis in HIV+ individuals is problematic. All HIV+ patients with or without neurologic symptoms, or individuals with serum FTA/ABS antibody titer ≥ 1:32, or individuals who will not be rx with penicillin should have an LP. *See Table 12, page 84. (MMWR 42:(RR-14) 39, 1993).* Pts with reactive CSF VDRL tests are considered to have proven neurosyphilis (but sensitivity is 9–89%), so neg. VDRL on CSF does not rule out neurosyphilis. Pts with reactive serum RPR and FTA/ABS (or VDRL and MHA-TP) and CSF pleocytosis or ↑ levels of protein are considered to have presumptive neurosyphilis. But in HIV+ individuals with no evidence of syphilis, 30% have CSF pleocytosis or ↑ protein *(CID 18:288, 1994).* Therefore, if rx based on pleocytosis or ↑ protein alone, many pts without syphilis will be treated *(for rx issues, see Table 12, page 84).*
Vaginitis	
Candidiasis	Candida vaginitis, recurrent and/or refractory, initial symptom of HIV infection in about ¼ of women *(AJM 89:142, 1990).* Pruritus; thick cheesy discharge; pH 4.5; hyphae on KOH prep
Trichomoniasis	Copious foamy discharge, pH 5–7, T. vaginalis on isotonic saline prep
Bacterial vaginosis	Malodorous discharge; pH 5–6; wet prep shows cells covered with organisms "clue" cells. Fishy odor when secretions rx with KOH

See page 70 for abbreviations and footnotes

TABLE 9A (20)

CLINICAL SYNDROME/MAJOR DIAGNOSTIC CONSIDERATIONS	DIAGNOSTIC CLUES/COMMENTS
Heart	
Incidence of cardiovascular disease specifically related to HIV is low; pericarditis and pulmonary hypertension most common)	
Pericarditis/Pericardial effusion	Clinical: Usually asymptomatic (↑ cardiac silhouette on CXR), may have chest pain, rub, tamponade in ~30%. Pericardial effusion is sign of poor prognosis (6 mos. mortality 64%) *(Circ 92:3229, 1995)*. Echocardiogram: Pericardial effusion in 30–38%. Etiology: Infection—viral, HIV, M. tbc (37%); tumor; Kaposi's sarcoma, lymphoma
Primary pulmonary hypertension	Estimated incidence 0.5% *(Circulation 89:2722, 1994)*. Clinical: Dyspnea, right-sided heart failure *(S Med J 87:357, 1994)*. Lung biopsy: Lesions similar to lupus erythematosus (possibly due to cytokines). Etiology: Likely multiple; seems to be related to chronic HIV infection in most cases (83%) but not to CD4 count or hx of pulmonary infections *(Mayo Clin Proc 73:37, 1998)*. HIV not found in vascular endothelium by PCR *(Am Rev Resp Dis 145:1196, 1992)*.
Myocarditis/Cardiopathy Infectious: Toxoplasmosis, CMV, EBV reported	Prevalence depends on definition. Autopsy: focal myocarditis 15–50% *(Curr Prob Cardiol 15:575, 1990)*. Echo: 0–40% develop evidence of LV dysfunction. Clinical cardiomyopathy in 1–3% AIDS pts. Rule out alcohol, cocaine.
Idiopathic	Biventricular dilatation with pathologic features of myocarditis. Average ejection fraction 33% *(J Am Coll Cardiol 13:1030, 1989)*. Etiology is unknown. Causal relationship to Coxsackie B, CMV and HIV not proven. No causal relationship to malnutrition, immunologic mechanisms. Rx is after load reduction and diuretics.
Drug-associated	Clinical: ZDV and ddl—6 cases reported; and chemotherapeutic agents, esp. adriamycin. CHF after 16 mos. rx, 2 associated with skeletal myositis *(AnIM 116:311, 1992)*. Patients improved after antiretroviral drugs discontinued. Recommend: Pts developing CHF, withdraw dideoxynucleoside rx for 1 month, then perform invasive cardiac function evaluation. Reversible cardiac dysfunction reported with interferon alfa *(NEJM 321:1246, 1989)*, also with IL-2, foscarnet *(Am Heart J 125:1439, 1993)*.
Endocarditis; non-bacterial, thrombotic (marantic) *(see SANFORD GUIDE TO ANTIMICROBIAL THERAPY, 1998)*	Sterile thrombi common, may be on any valve and embolize systemically. Opportunistic pathogens not a common cause of endocarditis in HIV+ patients (although there are case reports). Response of HIV+ patient to rx is similar to non-HIV+ patient.
Infective	Consider in injection drug users, reported in 4–10%. B. henselae reported.

Malignancy
   Kaposi's sarcoma
   Lymphoma
	Lesions are clinically silent but may produce irritability with arrhythmias. Cardiac involvement with Kaposi's sarcoma or lymphoma usually occurs only with widespread disease.

Hematologic Abnormalities[6]	
Anemia (occurs in up to 85% of AIDS patients)	
Anemia of chronic disease (impaired erythropoiesis) due to HIV, OI, malignancy	• Normochromic, normocytic • ↓ reticulocyte counts • ↓ erythropoietin levels (inappropriately low for degree of anemia) • ↓ serum iron, ↓ total iron-binding capacity (TIBC), normal to ↑ serum ferritin • ↑ bone marrow iron stores
Iron deficiency anemia secondary to GI bleeding (Kaposi's sarcoma, lymphoma, carcinoma)	• Microcytic, hypochromic • ↓ serum iron, ↑ TIBC, ↓ serum ferritin • ↓ bone marrow iron stores

See page 70 for abbreviations and footnotes

TABLE 9A (21)

CLINICAL SYNDROME/MAJOR DIAGNOSTIC CONSIDERATIONS	DIAGNOSTIC CLUES/COMMENTS
Hematologic Abnormalities, Anemia *(continued)*	
Infiltration of the bone marrow (especially Mycobacterium avium-intracellulare)	Anemia often profound (hematocrit 15–20%), WBC and platelets might be ↓.
Decreased B_{12} levels	Occur in 20%. Most likely due to altered serum transport. Anemia usually not due to or compounded by B_{12} deficiency.
Antibody-mediated hemolysis	Direct Coombs test commonly positive. Hemolysis is rare.
Pure red cell aplasia due to parvovirus B-19. Found in 16% of autopsies in 1 series. Can also cause neutropenia *(Abst 172, 3rd CRV, 1996)*.	Bone marrow shows maturation arrest at pronormoblast stage. Rx with IV immune globulin has resulted in cure or remission in most patients, enabling administration of full ZDV dosage *(MEDICAL MANAGEMENT OF AIDS, 5th Edition, page 241)*.
Drug-induced anemia • G6PD deficient hemolysis; common: dapsone, primaquine; uncommon: INH, sulfonamides, TMP/SMX • Zidovudine produces megaloblastic anemia • Myelosuppression: ganciclovir, foscarnet, flucytosine, sulfonamides, trimethoprim, trimetrexate, pyrimethamine, pentamidine, interferon alfa, anti-neoplastic drugs	Zidovudine: May respond to epoetin alfa if endogenous serum erythropoietin levels ≤ 500 mU/ml and ZDV dose is ≥ 4200 mg/week. Patients with erythropoietin levels >500 mU/ml do not respond. With ZDV 500–600 mg/day, erythropoietin alfa is seldom required *(Table 10, page 75)*. Foscarnet: anemia in 1/3 pts but <1% required discontinuation.
Granulocytopenia (occurs in up to 50% of AIDS patients) Ineffective granulopoiesis Antineutrophilic antibodies Drugs: • Zidovudine ≫ddC and ddl, • Ganciclovir, • Flucytosine, • Foscarnet, • Sulfonamides, • Dihydrofolate reductase inhibitors: trimetrexate, pyrimethamine, trimethoprim, • Pentamidine, • Antineoplastic therapy, • interferon alfa	May respond to granulocyte-colony stimulating factor (G-CSF) or granulocyte-monocyte stimulating factor (GM-CSF). Suggest determining cause of granulocytopenia and using alternative agents rather than G-CSF or GM-CSF. These growth factors may be of particular value in antineoplastic chemotherapy regimens during nadir of neutropenia. Use may be associated with Sweet's syndrome and activation of HIV *(see Table 10, page 75)*. Infection most likely when profound neutropenia (<100 neutrophiles/mm³) associated with chemotherapy or lymphoma *(Abst 194, 3rd CRV, 1996)*.
Thrombocytopenia (occurs in 11%) Early stage HIV-associated thrombocytopenia (ITP) *(CID 21:415, 1995)* Drugs: • Antineoplastic therapy • Interferon alfa • Beta-lactam antibiotics • Most other drugs above that cause neutropenia	Clinical: Usually occurs in early HIV infection and platelet counts increase as HIV infection progresses. Studies show ↓ platelet production and ↓ platelet survival *(Ln 343:479, 1994)*. A common epitope demonstrated on HIV p24 and human platelets *(Ln 342:1274, 1993)*. Pseudothrombocytopenia due to EDTA-induced platelet clumping reported *(West J Med 157:668, 1992)*. Rx: • Treatment may not be necessary; incidence of significant bleeding is low, spontaneous remissions in 10–20%. • In a Swiss study, ZDV therapy increased platelet counts by 50,000 to 100,000/mm³ • IV immune globulin (400 mg/kg qd x 5 days) will usually lead to transient ↑ in platelet counts, but is expensive. IV anti-D (anti-Rh) antibody: response in 75% (may take 3 weeks) but sustained in <10%. Not effective in Rh-negative or pts with splenectomies *(Transfusion 34:759, 1994)*. See Table 10, page 75. • Splenectomy: Rarely indicated; 2/3 of patients will respond if other therapies fail.
Thrombotic thrombocytopenia (TTP), hemolytic uremic syndrome (HUS) TTP and HUS described in HIV+ individuals, cause unknown	Clinical: Fever, neurologic abnormalities, renal abnormalities, microangiopathic hemolysis (schistocytes on peripheral smear), and thrombocytopenia [was found in 7% of 350 consecutive AIDS pts admitted to Johns Hopkins Hospital 1996-97 *(5th Conf. Retrovir & OIs 1998, Abst. 503)*] *(Blood 80:1890, 1992)*. Rx: Primary—plasma exchange. Splenectomy, steroids, dextran for salvage rx.

See page 70 for abbreviations and footnotes

CLINICAL SYNDROME/MAJOR DIAGNOSTIC CONSIDERATIONS	DIAGNOSTIC CLUES/COMMENTS

Hematologic Abnormalities *(continued)*
Eosinophilia [HIV infection itself may induce proliferation of eosinophils *(JID 174:615, 1996; Immunology and Allergy Clin N.A. 17:207, 1997)*]
  Allergic diseases, drug reactions: Zalcitabine (3–5% pt), ganciclovir (≤1% pts), IL-2, other drugs such as TMP/SMX, dapsone. Zidovudine: 2 pts reported with fever, eosinophilia (8%, 19%) and cutaneous leukocytoclastic vasculitis after 2–4 weeks of ZDV *(ArIM 152:850, 1992)*. Eosinophilic vasculitis reported before ZDV *(ArIM 146:2059, 1986)*. Extensive workup of pts with eosinophilia and cutaneous disease not warranted since diagnostic yield vanishing low *(AJM 102:449, 1997)*.
  Parasitic infections: Strongyloides, Isospora belli (in contrast to cryptosporidia and giardia which are not associated with ↑ eos).
  Ecto-parasitic infections: Norwegian scabies
  Neoplasms: Hodgkin's disease
  Pulmonary lymphoid hyperplasia, seen in children
  Fungal infections: coccidioidomycosis	

Coagulation abnormalities: prolonged partial thromboplastin time (PTT), lupus anticoagulant/antiphospholipid antibodies (present in 20–66% HIV+, *Blood Rev 7:121, 1993)*	Clinical: An incidental finding in HIV+ patients, not associated with either excessive bleeding or thrombosis in this population. Invasive procedures have been performed without bleeding complications.
Hepatobiliary Disease (↑ transaminase levels in 2–3.8% asymptomatic HIV+ pts)	

Acalculous cholecystitis
  Pseudocholelithiasis
  Infectious
  Idiopathic (55%)
	Clinical: Prevalence ↑ in AIDS patients. Right upper quadrant pain, fever in 2/3 but jaundice uncommon (18%). R/O "pseudocholelithiasis" 2° to ceftriaxone, symptomatic in 9% pts with "sludge" in gallbladder by ultrasound. More likely in pts on ≥2.0 gm/d, on total parenteral nutrition, or younger patients on ≥28 days rx.
	Lab: Increase in alkaline phosphatase >other LFT abnormalities.
	Biopsy: In some cases, histologic sections have shown CMV, cryptosporidium, Isospora belli *(AnIM 121:663, 1994)* and Cyclospora cayetanensis *(CID 21:1092, 1995)*.
	Rx: Appropriate surgical intervention when indicated.

AIDS cholangiopathy (sclerosing cholangitis, intra- and extrahepatic) (obstructive biliary tract disease). Cause is uncertain; the following have been associated:
  Cryptosporidium
  Cytomegalovirus
  Microsporidia
  Kaposi's sarcoma
  Mycobacterium avium-intracellulare (MAC)
  Lymphoma
	Clinical: Fever, pain, right upper quadrant tenderness. Median survival of 20 pts was 7 months *(Gut 34:116, 1993)*.
	Lab: Alkaline phosphatase ↑ 2–20x normal.
	Ultrasound or ERCP: Prominent or dilated intrahepatic and/or extrahepatic bile ducts down to periampullary area with marked thickening of ductal walls. Papillary stenosis in ½ patients, sphincterotomy may relieve symptoms in these patients *(AJM 99:600, 1995)*.
	Cryptosporidia or CMV in 9/15 patients (60%) *(NEJM 328:95, 1993)*. Another series (20 pts): cryptosporidia 13, CMV 6.
	Enterocytozoon bieneusi found in 8/8 patients in whom cryptosporidia or CMV not found *(NEJM 328:95, 1993)*.

Hepatic parenchymal disease, *see Viral hepatitis, page 58*
  Causes identified in about 40% of patients.
    Infections: Cytomegalovirus 1–14%, MAC 11–17%, chronic active hepatitis 12%, C. neoformans 2%, H. capsulatum 1%, M. tuberculosis 1–3%, C. albicans 0.6%, Penicillium marneffei *(see Comments)*
    Neoplasms: Kaposi's sarcoma 0.4–9%, non-Hodgkin's lymphoma 1–2.5%
	Clinical: Hepatocellular abnormalities usually reflect systemic infection or malignancy. Histologic findings rarely of diagnostic value *(CID 23:1302, 1996)*. Hepatic histology abnormal in 90% of pts with AIDS: steatosis 42%, portal inflammation 35%, congestion 22%, poorly formed granulomata 14% *(Hepatology 7:927, 1987; AJM 52:404, 1992; J AIDS 11:170, 1996)*. Fever, weight loss, hepatosplenomegaly in pt with travel to Southeast Asia: consider Penicillium marneffei *(CID 23:125, 1996)*.

Hepatomegaly with severe steatosis, lactic acidosis in patients on antiretroviral therapy	Clinical: Occurs predominantly in women, majority overweight, at least 4 months of antiretroviral rx (zidovudine, ddI, or ddC). Abdominal pain, hepatomegaly. Lab: Hepatic transaminases 3–10X normal, ↑ triglycerides, ↓ serum HCO_3, ↑ arterial ammonia, lactic acidosis, ↑ PTT. Biopsy: severe macrovesicular steatosis. Prevalence: at least 40 cases, mortality >50%. Incidence <0.4% *(AIDS Clin Care 6:17, 1994)*.

CLINICAL SYNDROME/MAJOR DIAGNOSTIC CONSIDERATIONS	DIAGNOSTIC CLUES/COMMENTS
Hepatobiliary Disease *(continued)*	
Peliosis hepatis (bacillary angiomatosis) *(see J. Koehler in MEDICAL MANAGEMENT OF AIDS, 6th Edition, 1998)*	Clinical: Fever, abdominal pain, weight loss, hepato- and splenomegaly. About ½ pts will have skin lesions: painful, erythematous plaques or nodules. ½ have lymphadenopathy. 2/3 pts give history of cat bite or scratch *(JAMA 269:770, 1993).* Lab: Alkaline phosphatase ↑ >hepatocellular tests. Etiologic agent: Bartonella henselae (usual), B. quintana (uncommon). Can be isolated from blood, 5–15 days incubation of lysis-centrifugation cultures on blood agar under CO_2 *(J Clin Micro 30:275, 1992).* Rx: Can be rx with erythromycin, clarithromycin, azithromycin. Doxycycline may also be effective *(NEJM 323:1581, 1990).* Patients respond clinically (↓ fever, ↓ symptoms) in 3–4 days, but require up to 2 months for LFTs to become normal. Lifelong suppression with macrolide or doxy may be necessary *(see Table 12).* X-ray: May be associated with bone lesions (punched-out appearance). CT/MRI findings: characteristic intrahepatic vascular lakes. Rx: *Table 12, page 77.*
Drug-associated hepatic dysfunction (avoid acetaminophen)	Clinical: Multiple drugs used in HIV patients are associated with abnormalities in LFTs; among these are: TMP/SMX (½ pts), acyclovir, didanosine (ddI), ZDV, ddC, ganciclovir, foscarnet, ketoconazole, fluconazole, INH, rifampin *(see Table 13).* Most require dose reduction or discontinuation if abnormalities exceed about 5x normal values.
Viral hepatitis	
Hepatitis A (HAV) Hep A in HIV-infected persons is clinically indistinguishable from Hep A in HIV-uninfected persons *(5th Conf Retrovir & Ols 1998, Abst. 498)*	Risk factors include homosexual activity, injection drug use *(JID 171(S1):519, 1995).* HAV has ↑ in frequency in homosexual men in U.S., Canada, Australia *(MMWR 45:155, 1992).* Outbreaks also reported in IDUs *(Am J Pub Health 79:463, 1989).* Hepatitis A vaccine, inactivated, licensed in U.S. in 1995. FDA-approved indications include: persons engaged in high-risk sexual activity (homosexually active men), IDUs. Coinfection with Hep A may ↑ HIV RNA in plasma and ↓ CD4 counts.
Hepatitis B (HBV)	Clinical: Risk factors for HIV and hepatitis B are the same (80–90% HIV+ pts are + for HBV markers *(AnIM 117:837, 1992).* ↑ risk of becoming Hep B chronic carrier (23%). HIV+ pts respond less well to Hep B vaccine and about ½ lose antibody after 4 years *(NEJM 316:630, 1987; CID 18:339, 1994).* Rx: *Table 12, page 93.*
Hepatitis C (HCV)	Clinical: HCV infection may be more frequent: Italy 60% HIV+ IDUs, Denmark 4% in HIV+ homosexual men *(AJM 92:404, 1992; CID 23:1117, 1996).* Higher degree of HCV viremia and ↑ rate of HCV antibody loss. Co-infection with HCV and HIV ↑ risk of perinatal transmission of HIV to infant. Hepatitis C does not accelerate course of HIV but HIV appears to accelerate course of Hep C *(5th Conf Retrovir & Ols 1998, Abst 493).* Hep C + HIV associated with porphyria cutanea tarda *(Arch Dermatol 132:1503, 1996).* Rx: *Table 12, page 93.*
Hepatitis D (delta agent)	Clinical: Antibodies to delta agent in 25% of HIV+, HBV– individuals. Prolonged antigenemia. ↑ liver injury *(CID 18:339, 1994).*
Hepatitis E (HEV)	HEV antibodies by EIA found in 33/162 (20%) homosexual men (Italy), 60/198 (30%) (Spain) *(Ln 344:1433, 1994; ibid. 345:127, 1995).* Despite some technical non-specificity, an ↑ prevalence of HEV in endemic areas is suggested. In the U.S., where HEV prevalence is <1%, this may not be true.
Hepatitis, viral, other	There are isolated reports of hepatitis associated with other viruses: EBV *(Ped IDJ 7:383, 1988),* HSV *(JID 157:597, 1988);* VZV *(J Inf 25:107, 1992),* adenovirus *(RID 12:303, 1990).*

See page 70 for abbreviations and footnotes

TABLE 9A (24)

CLINICAL SYNDROME/MAJOR DIAGNOSTIC CONSIDERATIONS	DIAGNOSTIC CLUES/COMMENTS

Lung

Most common causes are Pneumocystis carinii pneumonia, bacterial pneumonia, tuberculosis *(Ln 348:307, 1996) (See Sanford Guide to Antimicrobial Therapy, 1998 for non-HIV pulmonary infections)*

CLINICAL SYNDROME/MAJOR DIAGNOSTIC CONSIDERATIONS	DIAGNOSTIC CLUES/COMMENTS
Bronchitis, bronchiectasis	In addition to mycoplasma and respiratory viruses, consider H. influenzae, S. pneumo, and P. aeruginosa, cultured from sputum *(ArIM 154:2087, 1994)*. Mean CD4 600/μl. Response to rx rapid, but recurrences in 4/10 pts. In pts with chronic productive cough or recurrent pneumonia in same site, consider bronchiectasis. Dx based on CT scan, not evident on CXR in 84% *(Quart J Med 85:875, 1992; J Comp Asst Tomo 17:260, 1993)*. Whether prevalence is ↑ has not been defined but suspected *(ArIM 154:2086, 1994)*.
Emphysema-like bullous disease	On high-resolution CT scan, 42% pts had bullous lesions *(Radiol 173:23, 1989)*. Pulmonary function tests: ↑ residual volume, ↑ functional residual capacity, ↓ diffusing capacity but no airflow obstruction *(AnIM 116:124, 1992)*. Cause is unknown, could be P. carinii.

Pneumonia (infiltrate on CXR) *(Good review of lab evaluation of OIs of lung: AnIM 124:585, 1996; Clinics in Chest Dis 4:713, 1996)*

Any CD4 level

Community-acquired bacterial

CLINICAL SYNDROME/MAJOR DIAGNOSTIC CONSIDERATIONS	DIAGNOSTIC CLUES/COMMENTS
Mycobacterium tuberculosis[7] (common)	Tuberculosis often occurs before pt has AIDS defining illness. Most cases due to reactivation but primary tuberculosis being recognized with increasing frequency. 10% of HIV+ individuals are tuberculin +. In U.S., ~4% AIDS pts have had TB, in Italy 11% *(J Infect 28:261, 1994)*. Rate of development of TB is 8%/year in PPD+ patients. Average CD4 count is 375/mm³. TBc has been shown to accelerate the course of HIV *(Am J Resp Crit Care Med 151:129, 1995)*. Clinical presentation varies with stage of HIV infection:

Multidrug Resistant (MDR) Tuberculosis. **ANY PT SUSPECTED OF TB SHOULD BE ISOLATED** [private room, negative pressure, health care workers (HCW) and visitors entering should wear high efficiency disposable masks] [*See Table 25, pages 16–17*]. By September 1992 clusters of MDR TB reported in 14 U.S. hospitals and 1 prison system *(Ann Int Med 118:77, 1993)*. Some organisms resistant to 7 drugs (INH, RIF, KM, ETB, ethionamide, SM, rifabutin). Nosocomial transmission in 7 hospitals and prison. MDR TB diagnosed in 241 pts, 17 HCW. Most transmission among AIDS pts. Acquisition of MDR reported in HIV+ pts being treated for sensitive M. tbc *(NEJM 328:1137, 1993)*. Interval between exposure and diagnosis 1–3½ months, diagnosis to death 4–16 weeks, mortality 72–89%. TBn skin test conversions in 18–50% HCW. 1 HIV-neg. HCW has died *[MMWR 41(RR-11):52, 1992]*. The number of new cases of MDR-TBc has declined in recent years (1994-95), likely due to the implementation of rigorous infection control measures and Directly Observed Therapy (DOT) *(CID 21:1265, 1995; MMWR 45:N053, 1997)*.

Early HIV infection (CD4 >400/mm³): Reactivation. Typical presentation with upper lobe cavitary disease most common. Extrapulmonary disease uncommon. PPD (5 TU) is + (≥ 5 mm induration) in 80%.

Later HIV infection (CD4 <400/mm³): Either reactivation or progressive primary disease (30–50%). Clinical: Fever, cough (may be absent), shortness of breath, weight loss, night sweats. ½ to ⅔ involve extrapulmonary sites, especially lymph nodes and bone marrow (granulomas in 50% of bone marrow biopsies). Mycobacterial blood cultures + in ¼ to ½ of patients. (BACTEC system is sensitive and rapid.) Caution: patients reported with blood + for both M. tbc and MAC. Cultures of urine, joint fluid, CSF, liver, GI mucosa and ascites may also be +. Mass lesions of brain (tuberculoma) may mimic CNS toxoplasmosis. PPD (5 TU) positive (≥ 5 mm induration in <25% with clinical AIDS).

X-ray: Mediastinal-hilar adenopathy most common with progression to diffuse, somewhat coarse interstitial densities or localized infiltrates, especially in mid or lower lung fields. Pleural effusion in 10–20%. Disseminated (reticulonodular infiltrates, not classic "miliary" since "millets" are granulomata, usually not seen in HIV with low CD4) the most common with CD4 <200/mm3. Hilar/peritracheal adenopathy uncommon with PCP or bacterial pneumonia, common in TB.

Sputum: Smears positive for AFB in 40–50% pts with pulmonary TB, BAL + in 50–60%, culture + in 80–90%.

Rx: *Table 12, page 78*

FIGURE 4

COURSE OF PULMONARY DISEASE AND HIV INFECTION IN ADULTS

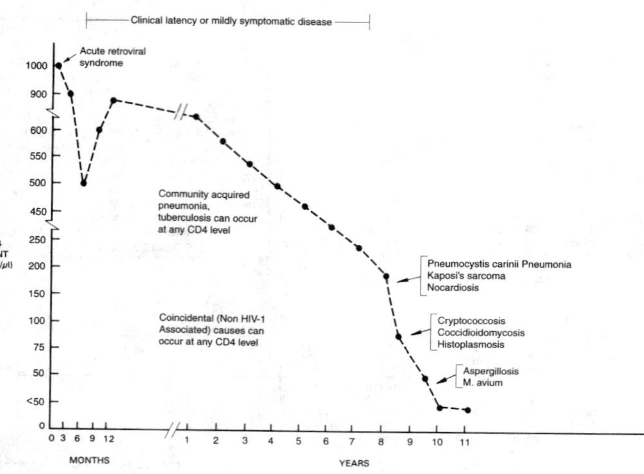

CLINICAL SYNDROME/MAJOR DIAGNOSTIC CONSIDERATIONS	DIAGNOSTIC CLUES/COMMENTS
Lung, Pneumonia/Any CD4 level/Community-acquired bacterial *(continued)*	

• Etiologies:
  Streptococcus pneumoniae (common, 35–70%)
  Haemophilus influenzae (common, 3–40%)
  Staphylococcus aureus (7%) (uncommon except with IDU, right-sided endocarditis)
  Pseudomonas aeruginosa (3–10%)
  E. coli (6–7%)
  Other Gram-negative (7–9%)
  Prevalence not defined:
    Mycoplasma pneumoniae, Chlamydia pneumoniae, Legionella sp. (rare)
• Multiple etiologies not uncommon; early bronchoscopy encouraged *(The AIDS Reader, July/Aug 1997, p. 112)*
 	
• Bacterial pneumonia ↑ in HIV (5.5 cases/100 person years vs 0.9/100 person years), mortality 4x ↑; TMP/SMX prophylaxis ↓ pneumonia by 67% *(NEJM 333:845, 1995)*.
 	
• Cigarette smoking ↑ risk of bacterial pneumonia *(RR:1.57)*, oral candidiasis *(RR:1.37)* and AIDS dementia complex *(RR:1.80)* *(J AIDS & Human Retro 13:374, 1996)*
 	
• HIV RNA copies: ↑ from a median of 60,000 copies/ml plasma to 245,000 copies/ml in 13 pts with bacterial pneumonia. Titers dropped to baseline after recovery *(J AIDS & HR 13:23, 1996)*.
	(Am J Epidem 138:909, 1993; ArIM 154:2589, 1994; NEJM 333:845, 1995; Clinics in Chest Med 17:713, 1996)
	Pneumococcal pneumonia is common in HIV+ patients (86% S. pneumo serotypes isolated included in pneumococcal vaccine, *Table 22*). Annual incidence of invasive disease due to S. pneumoniae is 1100 per 100,000 men with AIDS, age 25–44 years *(JAMA 265:3275, 1991)*. ↑ in African-Americans and CD4 <200 *(JID 173:857, 1996)*. Prevalence of penicillin-resistant Strep. pneumoniae among HIV+ individuals is same as in general population *(CID 23:577, 1996)*.
	Clinical: Typical presentation with fever, chills, productive cough, pleuritic chest pain and dyspnea can be seen at all stages of HIV infection. Most (up to 85%) of HIV+ patients with pneumococcal pneumonia will have positive blood cultures. Leucocytosis may not occur *(JID 173:870, 1996)*, but look for left shift bands.
	X-ray: Usually consolidation (homogeneous densities) with either segmental or lobar distribution.
	Course: Response to appropriate antibiotics is usually prompt (48–96 hours to become afebrile, radiographic resolution is much slower, as it is in non-HIV+ patients). If patient fails to respond as above, consider concomitant PCP or TBc.
	Rx: *Table 12, page 84.*
	Haemophilus influenzae pneumonia/bacteremia: occurs with ↑ frequency. Incidence of invasive disease is 80/100,000. In one series, most pts had pneumonia, in another only 30% had pneumonia. ⅓–½ isolates are type b, 15/15 reported were ß-lactamase negative. Response to appropriate antibiotics is prompt. Role of immunization against Hib can be questioned, incidence of disease ↑ but not striking, HIV+ pts do respond to vaccine *(NEJM 325:1837, 1991)* *(See Table 22)*.
	Pseudomonas aeruginosa: Pneumonia 8.7%/year. Clinical: median CD4 9/μl. ½–¾ community-acquired but ½ pts had been hospitalized in prior 30 days. CXR: 60–80% segmental, 40% bilateral infiltrates, 10–50% cavities. Respond to rx but relapse recurs in 1/3. Mortality 33%. *(CID 18:886, 1994; ibid. 19:417, 1994; J AIDS 7: 823, 1994; JID 171:930, 1995)*. Risk ↑ with advanced HIV, central venous and urinary caths, prior antibiotics & steroids.
	Legionella sp.: 77% community-acquired. Risk in AIDS 42x ↑ *(ArIM 154:2417, 1994)*. Nosocomial Legionella pneumophila pneumonia uncommon but reported in several small series *(CID 18:227, 1994)*.

Selected other HIV-associated pneumonias Aerobic Gram-negative bacilli	HIV infection/disease not reported to alter the prevalence or course of nosocomial, usually ventilator-acquired, Gram-negative bacillary pneumonia. M. avium may be acquired from hot water systems *(Ln 343:1137, 1994)*.
Influenza virus, A or B (common in outbreaks)	No evidence that influenza is more severe in HIV-infected patients.
Mycoplasma pneumonia (uncommon)	No evidence that mycoplasma infection is more severe in HIV-infected patients.
Ehrlichiosis (Ehrlichia chaffeensis)	In a case report, pt presented with fever, tachypnea, neutropenia with 17% bands, thrombocytopenia, ↑ hepatic enzymes. Chest x-ray: diffuse bilateral infiltrates. Arterial blood gases: ↓ PaO_2. Patient deteriorated. Diagnosis suspected on last day, optimal antibiotic rx not given *(NEJM 329:1164, 1993)*.
Measles	In U.S., 9 of 11 patients had pneumonitis; 3 had no rash and 8 had atypical exanthems; mortality 3/11 *(JAMA 267:1237, 1992)*. Immunization of HIV+ children recommended, although immune responses may be ↓. Ribavirin aerosol has been used but efficacy not proven *(ibid.)*.
Adenovirus	Based on lack of reports, no apparent ↑ in susceptibility. Adenovirus diarrhea important *(see page 70)*.
Human herpesvirus 6 (HHV-6)	HHV-6 infected cells detected in tissues obtained at necropsy in 9/9 pts. In one pt, probably primary cause of fatal pneumonitis. Relevance is that HHV-6 infections may be treatable with ganciclovir and foscarnet *(Ln 343: 577, 1994)*.

See page 70 for abbreviations and footnotes

CLINICAL SYNDROME/MAJOR DIAGNOSTIC CONSIDERATIONS	DIAGNOSTIC CLUES/COMMENTS

Lung/Pneumonia (continued)

CD4 <200/mm³

Pneumocystis carinii[8] (common)

Abst 190, 3rd CRV, 1996, Pomerantz et al: Predicting etiology of community-acquired pneumonia:

Dx (OR=Odds Ratio)	Bact Pn (94)		PCP (101)		TBC (37)	
	%	OR	%	OR	%	OR
Fever >7 d	11%	1.0	34%	4.3[†]	54%	9.9[†]
Cough >7 d	20%	1.0	50%	3.9[†]	51%	4.2[†]
Yellow-green sputum	54%	2.8[†]	30%	1.0	30%	1.0
DOE	43%	1.5	81%	9.0[†]	32%	1.0
Weight loss	23%	1.0	44%	2.2[†]	68%	6.8[†]
Night sweats	23%	1.0	46%	2.7[†]	54%	3.9[†]
Tachycardia	57%	2.8[†]	39%	1.3	32%	1.0
Tachypnea	18%	1.1	43%	3.8[†]	16%	1.0
Abn auscultation	77%	3.5[†]	62%	1.8	49%	1.0
LDH >400	29%	1.0	62%	4.0[†]	43%	1.9
pO₂ <75	36%	1.8	66%	6.0[†]	24%	1.0
Interstitial infiltrate	17%	1.3	69%	14.5[†]	14%	1.0
Lobar infiltrate	54%	59[†]	22%	1.0	32%	24.8[†]

OR: 95% CI does not include 1.0 when indicated by †

CD4: 1st episode mean CD4 79/mm³, med. 36/mm³; 2nd episode mean 34/mm³, med. 10/mm³

Clinical: dry cough, fever, progressive dyspnea

Laboratory: Arterial blood gas—$\downarrow$ pO₂ (<70 mmHg in 80% patients); pulmonary function tests— restrictive type defect with $\downarrow$ vital capacity and $\downarrow$ total lung capacity. Diffusion abnormalities common; single breath diffusing capacity for CO <80% of predicted (90% sensitivity but only 25% specificity).

Chest x-ray:[9] 5–10% have normal chest x-ray (in these pts, CO diffusing capacity, $\downarrow$ PaO₂ with exercise may be of particular value.

Most common: diffuse bilateral symmetrical fine heterogeneous reticular infiltrates

Less common: Unilateral/focal distribution of same quality infiltrates or focal alveolar consolidation (especially upper lobe in patients on aerosolized pentamidine prophylaxis) or an interstitial pattern with fine nodular infiltrates or miliary lesions or focal nodules without cavitation, thick-walled cysts or pneumatoceles or pneumothorax

Rare: pleural effusion and/or intrathoracic adenopathy

After 4 days of treatment with trimethoprim/sulfamethoxazole, there is commonly an $\uparrow$ infiltrate resembling pulmonary edema. This complication is significantly reduced when corticosteroid rx used with TMP/SMX in patients with low pO₂ *(see Table 12, page 90).*

Response: with effective rx, improvement is expected in 7–10 days.

Sputum, induced *(see Table 30, page 133)*: detection of P. carinii—sensitivity 77%, negative predictive value 64%; use of fluorescent antibody technique markedly improves detection over that with Giemsa stain.

Bronchoalveolar lavage (BAL): do not delay initiation of rx if BAL not immediately available. Treatment for several days does not $\downarrow$ diagnostic sensitivity. Detection of P. carinii—sensitivity 85–89%.

Transbronchial biopsy: detection of P. carinii—sensitivity 88–97%. P. carinii rarely found on transbronchial biopsy if not found on BAL. Pneumothorax is a common complication of PCP pneumonia and is associated with a high mortality *(CID 23:624, 1996).*

Kaposi's sarcoma (KS)[10] (common)

DNA sequences of a herpesvirus, HHV-8, have been identified in >90% of AIDS-associated Kaposi's sarcoma and in classic endemic African, Mediterranean KS, suggesting a role in pathogenesis of KS *(Science 266:1865, 1994; Ln 345:722, 759, 761, 1043, 1995; NEJM 332:1181, 1995)*

Clinical: Usually but not always associated with cutaneous and/or mucosal KS. May present with cough, bronchospasm and shortness of breath *(Thorax 50:407, 1995).*

X-ray: Findings are somewhat distinctive: coarse, poorly defined nodular densities throughout the lungs with concomitant coarse linear densities in the perihilar regions. Nodules increase slowly in size, rapid $\uparrow$ suggests hemorrhage. Pleural effusions common (up to 50%). Hilar adenopathy rare (<10%).

Dx: Bronchoscopy will usually show typical violaceous endobronchial lesions.

Rx: *Table 19, page 118.*

Lymphoma: HHV-8 also identified in body cavity lymphomas *(NEJM 332:1186, 1995)—see above*

Lymphomas associated with advanced HIV infection are becoming increasingly common, are usually non-Hodgkin's B cell type, with extranodal involvement the rule. Thoracic involvement is uncommon (10%) but when it occurs produces pleural effusion in 50%, hilar and/or mediastinal adenopathy in ¼ and either reticulo-nodular interstitial infiltrates or alveolar consolidation in 25%.

See page 70 for abbreviations and footnotes

TABLE 9A (28)

CLINICAL SYNDROME/MAJOR DIAGNOSTIC CONSIDERATIONS	DIAGNOSTIC CLUES/COMMENTS
Lung, Pneumonia/CD4 <200/mm³ *(continued)*	
Lymphoid interstitial pneumonia (LIP) (children)	A disease of unknown etiology which may present with shortness of breath in children with HIV infection *(see Table 6E, page 28)*. X-ray: Resembles PCP with diffuse or focal, fine to medium reticular interstitial infiltrate. Findings gradually worsen over months. Dx: Lung biopsy is necessary for dx; shows an accumulation of lymphocytes and plasma cells in interstitial areas. Rx: Corticosteroids may be beneficial.
Nocardiosis (Nocardia asteroides)	Uncommon, 43 cases reported *(Med 71:128, 1992)*. CD4 <200/mm³. Clinical: Fever, malaise, cough, weight loss. Chest x-ray: 83% abnormal, cavitation 62%, lobar consolidation 52%, pleural effusion 33%, reticulonodular infiltrates 33%. Lab: Blood cultures rarely +.
CD4 <100/mm³ *(For ATS statement on fungal infection in HIV+ persons, see Am J Resp Crit Care Med 152:816, 1995)*	
Cryptococcosis (Cryptococcus neoformans) (common)	C. neoformans is a ubiquitous soil fungus which usually affects the CNS *(see Meningitis)* in patients with CD4 <100/mm³. Site of entry is usually the lungs and pneumonia has been reported. X-ray: Variable pattern; single *(CID 23:810, 1996)* or multiple well-defined nodules with or without cavitation or diffuse reticular infiltrates and/or hilar/mediastinal adenopathy. Occasionally a reticulonodular pattern may occur. Dx: Isolation of C. neoformans from respiratory secretions. Serum CRAG may be positive. Rx: *Table 12, p. 86*.
Coccidioidomycosis (Coccidioides immitis) (common—endemic areas) (see *CID 23:563, 1996*)	A common reactivation or primary infection in patients from "cocci belt" (southwest U.S.) with CD4 <150/mm³. In HIV-negative individuals, annual incidence of symptomatic infection is 0.43%, in HIV+ individuals 25% developed symptomatic cocci over 41 months *(AJM 94:235, 1993)*. Cases of cocci have ↑ 10x in central California valleys in 1992, 1993 vs 1990 *[CID 19(S1):S14, 1994]*. 15% pts had simultaneous PCP *(Med 69:384, 1990)*. Clinical: Presentation is similar to histoplasmosis—fever, chills, night sweats and weight loss; severe shortness of breath is common. X-ray: Diffuse bilateral reticulonodular infiltrate (65%) similar to histoplasmosis or focal pulmonary infiltrate (14%) or normal (16%) *(CID 23:563, 1996)*. Dx: While complement fixation antibody tests are frequently positive (68%), dx is established by identification of large spherules of C. immitis in sputum, BAL, biopsy or on culture. Rx: *Table 12, page 86*.
Histoplasmosis (Histoplasma capsulatum) (common—endemic areas) (see *CID 24:1195, 1997*)	A common reactivation infection when CD4 <200/mm³ in pts with geographical history of having been in the "histo belts" (Ohio-Mississippi River Valley, southeastern U.S., St. Lawrence River Valley, Central America and northern South America) *(IDCP 4:300, 1995)*. Annual incidence in Missouri 4.7% in HIV-infected. Clinical: Usually presents with nonspecific systemic complaints: fever, weight loss, night sweats, but lungs commonly involved with shortness of breath. Hepatosplenomegaly and rarely focal cutaneous pustules or ulcers may be presenting findings. Pts may also present with "septic shock" including DIC. CD4 count <150. X-ray: Commonly shows diffuse, bilateral poorly defined small (1–2 mm) nodular infiltrates with or without hilar/mediastinal adenopathy. Dx: Identification of H. capsulatum in WBC on peripheral blood smear or bone marrow (PAS or silver stain) and culture (about 90% are positive). If suspected and blood/bone marrow not positive, biopsy lymph node, liver, lung or lesions. About 80% will have positive immunodiffusion or complement fixation test for antibodies. Measurement of H. capsulatum antigen in urine + in 95% AIDS pts with disseminated histo, test also useful in following rx and relapse *(CID 19(S1):S19, 1994)*. (Available at Histoplasmosis Reference Lab (1-800-HISTO-DG). However, cross-reactivity with paracocci, blastomyces, cocci, and penicillium has been detected *(CID 24:1169, 1997)*. Rx: *Table 12, page 87*.

See page 70 for abbreviations and footnotes

CLINICAL SYNDROME/MAJOR DIAGNOSTIC CONSIDERATIONS	DIAGNOSTIC CLUES/COMMENTS
Lung, Pneumonia/CD4 <100/mm³ *(continued)*	
Blastomycosis (uncommon)	Uncommon, largest series is 15 cases *(AnIM 116:847, 1992)*. CD4 <200/mm³. Pulmonary (7 cases): 4 dyspnea, 2 chest pain, CXR 3 focal, 3 diffuse reticulonodular. BAL cultures +. Disseminated (8 cases): CNS involvement (5 cases), multiple organs (6 cases). Rx: *Table 12, page 85.*
Mycobacterium kansasii (uncommon)	X-ray: Infiltrates "atypical"; alveolar, interstitial or diffuse parenchymal or pleural effusion. Upper lobe cavities. ½ have extrapulmonary dissemination *(Rev Inf Dis 13:789, 1991)*.
Penicillium marneffei	Primarily presents as fever, anemia, weight loss & skin lesions (70%) with lymphadenopathy but ½ have cough & organism cultured from lung in 15%. Pulmonary infiltrates (densities, abscesses and cavities) have been seen. Essentially all cases from SE Asia. Dx by isolation from skin, blood or bone marrow *(CID 23:125, 1996)*. Rx: *Table 12, page 88.*
Rhodococcus equi (uncommon)	One-half of pts with Rhodococcus equi present with slowly progressive mass lesion which cavitates *(Rev Inf Dis 13:91, 1991)*. Has tendency to relapse, may require surgery and long-term suppressive rx. Rx: *Page 83.*
Toxoplasma gondii (uncommon)	Clinical: Rare in U.S., in France represents up to 5% of cases of suspected PCP. Febrile illness, minimal cough, ↑ dyspnea. Reported to be associated with ARDS *(CID 19:169, 1994)*. Chest x-ray: Diffuse interstitial or diffuse coarse nodular (resembles PCP). Pleural effusion in 2/6 patients. Lab: ↑ transaminase, ↑ LDH. Sputum: BAL + for T. gondii *(CID 23:1249, 1996)*. Rx: *Table 12, page 90.*
CD4 <50/mm³	
Aspergillosis (uncommon)	Aspergillus sp. are commonly isolated from respiratory sites (4%), but invasive aspergillosis developed in only 15% of colonized patients, more common in pts with AIDS and associated neutropenia *(CID 14:141, 1992; ibid., 19(S1):S41, 1994)*. Clinical: 33 patients reported in one series. 64% had an episode of infectious pneumonia ≤ 1 year before. CD4 <50/mm³. All were febrile, cough 97%, dyspnea 80%, chest pain 20%, hemoptysis 17%. 21% CNS signs. Chest x-ray: cavities 42% (most upper lobe), bilateral interstitial infiltrates 54%, pleural effusion 15%. Despite rx, mean time to death was 8 weeks *(AJM 95:177, 1993)*. Rx: *Table 12, page 85.*
M. avium (pulmonary findings uncommon) • Infection due to Mycobacterium avium-intracellulare complex [M. avium 52%, M. intracellulare 21%, M. xenopi 7%, M. fortuitum 2% *(CID 20:73, 1995)*] [M. genavense, an unrelated organism which clinically behaves like MAC, antibiotic susceptibilities not known *(CID 18:455, 1994)*] • Following initiation of highly active antiretroviral rx, pts with MAC infection have developed unusual systemic and pulmonary syndromes: painful generalized lymphadenopathy-like scrofula, massive abdominal and thoracic adenopathy with pulmonary infiltrates, fever, leucocytosis, and cutaneous nodules *(Ln 351:252, 1998) (Table 9B)*	Clinical: CD4 usually ≤ 50/mm³ *(see Table 12, page 80)*. Usually presents as disseminated infection with symptoms of fever, weight loss, night sweats, diarrhea, anemia and neutropenia, but may be asymptomatic even with positive blood cultures. Highest concentration of organisms (6.7 $\log_{10}$/gm) in mesenteric nodes *(JID 173:942, 1996)*. Lab: Colonization of respiratory secretions and GI tract is common and may precede disseminated disease. When symptomatic, blood cultures are usually positive for MAC (BACTEC system is very sensitive). Dual infection with M. tbc recognized. X-ray: When lungs involved, heterogenous interstitial infiltrates with or without hilar lymphadenopathy. Rx: *Table 12, page 80.*
Cytomegalovirus (CMV) (uncommon)	CMV pneumonitis in HIV+ pts is rare but 90% of AIDS pts have evidence of CMV at autopsy. Viral cultures of BAL fluid are frequently positive. CMV has been isolated from 30% of pts with PCP, and associated with ↑ mortality *(AJM 78:429, 1985)*, but rx with ganciclovir does not appear to affect outcome *(NEJM 314:801, 1986)*. Consider lung bx when CMV infection elsewhere, fever, cough and dyspnea, persistent interstitial/ alveolar infiltrates *(Abst 158, 3rd CRV, 1996)*. Syndrome of ↑ dyspnea (over 1–3 months), interstitial infiltrates, hypoxemia, hemolytic anemia, siderophages on BAL reported *(CID 22:616, 1996)*. Would rx if biopsy revealed interstitial inflammation with CMV inclusions and no other pathogens.
Mass lesion ± necrosis (abscess) Histoplasmosis, coccidioidomycosis, cryptococcosis, anaerobes, S. aureus, M. kansasii, Rhodococcus equi, Mycobacterium tuberculosis, Pneumocystis carinii, lymphoma, Kaposi's sarcoma, aspergillus, MAC, Nocardia asteroides, P. aeruginosa	Cavitary lesions: PCP uncommon manifestation of common disease. Frequent: aspergillosis, M. kansasii, M. tuberculosis (in earlier HIV infection), bacterial pneumonia (P. aeruginosa, N. asteroides, R. equi). Unusual: crypto, coccidioido, histo *(CID 22:671, 1996; CID 22:81, 1996)*. Definitive dx essential: BAL & transbronchial bx.

See page 70 for abbreviations and footnotes

TABLE 9A (30)

CLINICAL SYNDROME/MAJOR DIAGNOSTIC CONSIDERATIONS	DIAGNOSTIC CLUES/COMMENTS
Lung (continued)	
Hilar and/or mediastinal adenopathy 　Mycobacterium tuberculosis, Mycobacterium avium-intracellulare 　Fungal: Histoplasmosis, coccidioidomycosis, cryptococcosis, blastomycosis 　Lymphoma, Kaposi's sarcoma	See above
Pleural effusion 　Infections (66%): 　　Bacterial pneumonia　31% 　　P. carinii pneumonia　15% 　　M. tuberculosis　　　8% 　　Others (each <5%): Septic embolism, aspergillosis, C. neoformans, MAC 　Non-infectious (31%): 　　Hypoalbuminemia　　19% 　　Heart failure　　　　5% 　　Others: Kaposi's sarcoma (common in some series), atelectasis, uremia, 　　　ARDS	Incidence in 222 pts was 27% (AnIM 118:856, 1993). Large effusions associated with Kaposi's sarcoma, tuberculosis and lymphoma.
Pneumothorax 　P. carinii pneumonia (more common with aerosolized pentamidine)	Occurred in 2% of a large series of patients (AnIM 114:455, 1991). Has high mortality rate if associated with PCP (CID 23:624, 1996).
Pulmonary eosinophilia (Loeffler's syndrome)	Can be caused by drugs commonly used in HIV+ pts: sulfonamides, dapsone, penicillin (Ln 343:860, 1994).
Lymph Nodes (applies to lymphadenopathy without an obvious primary source)	
Generalized 　Etiologies: acute HIV infection, TBc, atypical mycobacteria, histoplasmosis, cocci-dioidomycosis, lymphoma, Kaposi's sarcoma, syphilis, Epstein-Barr virus, toxo-plasma, tularemia, sarcoid, CMV, and Castelman's disease (AIDS 10:61, 1996)	History and physical exam direct evaluation. If nodes fluctuant, aspirate and base rx on Gram and acid-fast stains. Pts receiving HAART may demonstrate fever and generalized lymphadenopathy from MAC infection (Ln 351:252, 1998) (Table 9B).
Lipomatosis 　Benign symmetric or "buffalo hump" associated with protease inhibition rx (Ln 350:1596, 1997)	Unusual accumulations of fat in cervical fat pad region, "horse collar" distribution, midsection ("protease paunch") and "moon facies" have been described in pts receiving protease inhibitor. No associated endocrin-opathies have been reported with these accumulations (5th Conf Retrovir & Ols 1998, Abst. 407, 408, 409, 412) (Table 5B).
Musculoskeletal System	
Pyomyositis (AIDS 7:1020, 1993) 　Staphylococcal; aerobic gram-negative bacilli (uncommon) (CID 22:372, 1996)	Clinical: may follow exercise, local trauma or injections. Swelling in muscular area, localized pain and fever. ESR usually ↑. Erythema often absent, can be indolent. WBC may be normal and blood cultures usually negative (AJM 90:595, 1991).
Osteomyelitis (Brit J Rheum 31:381, 1992) 　S. aureus, Strep. species, enterobacteriaceae, M. kansasii,　H. capsulatum, nocardia	Sinus tract cultures may give misleading results regarding etiology of osteomyelitis—bone biopsy necessary to establish dx.

TABLE 9A (31)

CLINICAL SYNDROME/MAJOR DIAGNOSTIC CONSIDERATIONS	DIAGNOSTIC CLUES/COMMENTS
Musculoskeletal System *(continued)*	

Arthritis, polyarticular
   Reiter's syndrome: urethritis or cervicitis, conjunctivitis, arthritis, and
   mucocutaneous lesions (circinate balanitis, keratoderma blennorrhagica)
	Clinical: Reiter's syndrome occurs in 0.5–10% of HIV+ patients, 75% are HLA B-27 positive *(Rheumatol Int 9:137, 1989)*. Typically, non-bacterial urethritis 7–14 days after sexual exposure. Asymmetric polyarticular arthritis involving large joints of legs, including toes, develops over several weeks. Mucocutaneous lesions include circinate balanitis and keratoderma blennorrhagica. Typically resolves in 3–4 months but ~50% have recurrences.
	Lab: Synovial fluid typically is translucent, 2000–100,000 cells/μl, >50% PMNs, culture negative, glucose <50 mg/dl lower than blood glucose.
	Rx: Since often associated with C. trachomatis, empirical rx for chlamydia *(see Table 12, page 77)* is appropriate. In non-HIV+ patients, methotrexate or folic acid antagonists have been used; they should not be used in HIV+ patients.

Psoriatic arthritis	Clinical: Psoriasis noted in 1–5% HIV+ population. Frequency of arthritis ↑ in HIV+ pts with psoriasis *(Rheum Dis Clin NA 17:59, 1991)*.
"Lightning pain" syndrome	Severely painful acute attack of arthralgia or myalgia, lasts a few hours to a few days. Often requires narcotics for relief. Clinical exam normal. Cause unknown, no sequelae *(Med J Aust 158:114, 1993)*.
Rheumatoid arthritis	Virtually never occurs in pts with HIV. Several pts with rheumatoid-factor positive RA have gone into remission after infection with HIV.
Arthritis, oligoarticular HIV-associated arthritis	Usually asymmetrical, lower limbs. HLA B27 negative. Synovial fluid: low WBC with PMNs *(Med J Aust 158:114, 1993)*.
Myopathy (progressive proximal muscle weakness)	
HIV-1 associated myopathy	Clinical: Proximal muscle weakness, ↑ creatinine kinase levels. Muscle biopsy: ½ had inflammatory infiltrates. ½ pts rx with and responded to prednisone *(AnIM 113:492, 1990)*.
Drug-associated: zidovudine (ZDV)	Clinical: Proximal muscle weakness and atrophy (legs >arms, "saggy butt" syndrome) occurred in 5/86 pts (6%) rx with ZDV >6 months (mean 45 weeks). Creatinine kinase ↑ (average 777 u/L). Muscle biopsy: "Ragged red fibers" on histology, abnormal mitochondria on EM. Improves with discontinuation of ZDV, recurs with rechallenge *(AnIM 113:492, 1990)*. ddC also causes a selective loss of mitochondrial DNA in vitro *(Ln 337:508, 1991)*.
Polymyositis	A dermatomyositis-like disease has been described in AIDS *(Rheum Dis Clin NA 17:117, 1991)*.

Pancreatitis
   (Hyperamylasemia with or without abdominal pain)
   44 cases: usual major causes—alcohol 39%, gallstones 2%; drugs: pentamidine 27%, ddI 9%, TMP/SMX 5%, 3TC esp. in children; opportunistic infections: CMV 5%, MAC 2%, other 9% *(AJM 98:243, 1995)*
	Clinical: Pancreatitis due to ddI can be fatal (0.35%). In pts with history of pancreatitis, 8/27 pts on ddI developed pancreatitis. Pancreatitis occurs in <1% on ddC. In patients with a history of pancreatitis on ddC, 3.2% developed pancreatitis or ↑ amylase. IV pentamidine is associated with pancreatic islet cell damage (hypoglycemia with later diabetes mellitus). It is rare but reported after long-term aerosolized pentamidine *(AJM 88:53N, 1990)*.

Peritoneal Disease	

Ascites, sudden onset
   Transudative ascitic fluid (<3 gm protein/100 ml)
      Concomitant hepatic cirrhosis (alcoholic), congestive heart failure, inferior vena cava obstruction, Budd-Chiari syndrome, hypoalbuminemia, vasculitis, hepatitis B or C
	Clinical: Symptoms and signs of underlying process.

See page 70 for abbreviations and footnotes

CLINICAL SYNDROME/MAJOR DIAGNOSTIC CONSIDERATIONS	DIAGNOSTIC CLUES/COMMENTS
Peritoneal Disease, Ascites *(continued)*	
Exudative ascitic fluid (>3 gm protein/100 ml) (>500 cells/mm suggests infection, neoplasm) Tuberculosis, lymphoma, cytomegalovirus	Clinical: Collect large volume (500–1000 ml), centrifuge; may reveal AFB on smear Biopsy: Etiology most often found on biopsy.
Renal Proteinuria and azotemia	
HIV-associated glomerulosclerosis	Clinical: 85% pts are black. Massive proteinuria of sudden onset, hypoalbuminemia, renal insufficiency rapidly progressing to endstage renal disease. Peripheral edema and hypertension minimal or absent. Renal biopsy: Focal glomerulosclerosis with mesangial deposits of C3, IgM. Course: Death in 3–6 months even with dialysis. Some reports suggest that ZDV may ↓ proteinuria and improve renal function *(AnIM 112:35, 1990)*. Corticosteroid rx ↓ serum creatinine, ↓ proteinuria in 4/4 pts *(AJM 97:145, 1994)*. Renal lesions associated with TGF-β expression and ↑ levels of HIV tat protein *(J Am Soc Neph 4:675, 1993)*.
HIV-associated IgA nephropathy	Clinical: Rarer than HIV glomerulosclerosis. All reported pts are white. Microscopic hematuria, minimal protein-uria. ↑ serum IgA. Progression of disease is slow. Thought to be immune complex disease *(NEJM 327:702, 1992)*.
Amyloidosis	Clinical: Very rare [1 case report with nephrotic syndrome *(CID 14:189, 1992)*].
Heroin nephropathy Nephrotoxic drugs: pentamidine, foscarnet, aminoglycosides, amphotericin B	
"Sepsis"/Bacteremia	
Disseminated pneumococcal disease	Clinical: 30–85% of pts with pneumococcal pneumonia have bacteremia. Rate of S. pneumoniae bacteremia is 100-fold ↑ in HIV+ patients. It often occurs in early stage HIV disease. 86% of serotypes are included in current vaccine *(Am J Epidem 138:909, 1993)*. Outcome of rx has been good, although rare relapsing infections reported *(CID 14:1050, 1992)*. In addition, S. pneumoniae may cause soft tissue infections *(JID 163:897, 1991)* *(See page 61)*.
Disseminated histoplasmosis may mimic sepsis syndrome	*CID 24:1195, 1997*
Haemophilus influenzae bacteremia	*See page 61*
Causes include those seen in the non-HIV+ patient, especially the febrile neutropenic patient: enterobacteriaceae, Pseudomonas sp., Staph. aureus, Staph. epidermidis	Nasopharyngeal carriage rates for Staph. aureus in HIV+ 44% vs 23% in hospital personnel; rates of Staph aureus bacteremia ↑ *(Europ J Clin Micro-ID 11:985, 1992)*.
Recurrent bacteremia Non-typhi salmonella, especially S. typhimurium (outside of U.S., Salmonella typhi)	In U.S., 20-fold ↑ in risk in HIV+ individuals *(Rev Inf Dis 9:925, 1987)*. With CD4 >200/mm³ clinical presentation and response to rx similar to HIV-negative individuals. With CD4 <200/mm³, diarrhea is a less prominent symptom. 1–16% relapse within several months *(ArIM 151:381, 1991)*. ZDV (≥400 mg/day) may be effective in preventing recurrences *(JID 163:415, 1991)*.
Mycobacterium avium-intracellulare (MAC)	*See page 64*
Bartonella henselae, quintana	*See pages 58 & 69*
Rhodococcus equi	*See page 64*

See page 70 for abbreviations and footnotes

TABLE 9A (33)

CLINICAL SYNDROME/MAJOR DIAGNOSTIC CONSIDERATIONS	DIAGNOSTIC CLUES/COMMENTS
Sinuses, paranasal Sinusitis: microbial flora similar to HIV-negative (S. pneumoniae, H. influenzae, M. catarrhalis) plus other Gram-positives (Staph. epidermidis, P. acnes), aerobic Gram-negatives (Pseudomonas aeruginosa), fungi [aspergillus, rhizopus (mucor), Alternaria alternata, H. capsulatum] (CID 24:1178, 1997). Rarely parasites (microsporidium, cryptosporidium, etc. (CID 25:267, 1997)	Clinical: Sinusitis occurs in ⅓ to ⅔ of adults with AIDS (Ear, Nose, Throat J 69:460, 1990). Sinusitis may be part of acquired atopy in AIDS (JID 167:283, 1993). ⅔ pts are symptomatic (fever, nasal congestion, discharge). X-ray: 79% had air fluid level, usually more than one sinus. Despite rx, 60% pts had recurrent or persistent infection (AJM 93:163, 1992). Antral puncture required for accurate cultures and indicated if rx against common pathogens fails (CID 16:404, 1993).
Skin/Hair[11]	
Eosinophilic folliculitis (resembles Ofuji's disease); marked pruritus, discrete, erythematous urticarial, follicular painless papules on trunk, head, neck, proximal extremities, 90% above the nipple line. ↑ eos, ↑ IgE. CD4 <250 in 10/13 pts (Mayo Clin Proc 67:1089, 1992). Astemizole controls symptoms. Itraconazole 200 mg po qd improves ~75% pts (fluconazole of no benefit) (Arch Derm 131:358, 1995). Isotretinoin 0.75–1.0 mg/kg/day may also benefit (Arch Derm 131:1047, 1995). Metronidazole 250 mg po tid for 3–4 weeks works in some pts (Arch Derm 131:1089, 1995).	
Maculopapular lesions	
Acute retroviral syndrome	Lesions 5–10 mm diameter, symmetrical, especially on face or trunk (may involve palms and soles), erythematous, non-pruritic. Stevens-Johnson syndrome (CID 19:798, 1994), see page 36. Constitutional "mono-like symptoms:" fever (87%), skin rash (68%). Mean duration of symptoms/signs 21 days (CID 17:59, 1993).
Molluscum contagiosum	Occurs in 8–15% AIDS pts. 2–5 mm pearly flesh-colored papules, often with **central umbilication** on face, anogenital region. Disseminated cryptococcosis, P. marneffei may mimic.
Syphilis, secondary	See Genital Tract, page 54
Candidiasis (47% of AIDS pts had mucocutaneous candidal infections in 1 series)	Children: diaper-rash type rash involving trunk and extremities. Adults: red, hemorrhagic maculopapular lesions.
Cryptococcosis	Common. Widespread skin-colored, dome-shaped translucent papules 1–4 mm in diameter. Resemble Molluscum contagiosum.
Histoplasmosis	Slightly pink 2–6 mm cutaneous papules to larger reddish plaques and multiple shallow crusted ulcerations.
Mycobacterial infections: M. tuberculosis, M. avium-intracellulare, M. kansasii, M. marinum, M. hemophilum	Vary from acneiform plaques, pustules or indurated verrucous plaques to ulcerative nodular lesions. See page 59. A case report of **painful** vesiculopustular rash secondary to hypersensitivity reaction to M. tbc antigen (tuberculide) (Ln 347:372, 1996).
Mycobacterium leprae	Clinical presentation of borderline leprosy similar in HIV+ and HIV−, but rx for neuritis less successful in HIV+ (Lep Rev 63:134, 1992).
Penicillium marneffei (See CID 23:125, 1996; 24:1080, 1997)	Clinically present with fever, weight loss, small umbilicated maculopapular skin lesions (2/3 pts), hepatosplenomegaly, adenopathy. Almost all pts lived or traveled in Southeast Asia (J AIDS 6:466, 1993; CID 15:744, 1992).
Cutaneous Pneumocystis carinii	Rare but reported with underlying PCP. More common if pt on aerosolized pentamidine. Typically verrucous translucent papules anywhere on body.
Human papillomavirus (warts, condyloma acuminatum)	Diffuse flat and filiform lesions, often in unusual sites. See GI and Genital Tract, above.
Drugs	HIV+ pts have ↑ frequency of skin reactions to most drugs.
Insect bites (scabies—axilla, groin, fingerweb; fleas—lower legs; mosquitoes—arms and legs)	Erythematous, urticarial papules.
Kaposi's sarcoma (CD4: mean 87/mm³, median 37/mm³)	Early lesions are round or irregular pinkish-red to violaceous macules to papules, usually non-tender. Often symmetrical along skin tension lines. (See below)
Nodular, verrucous, and/or ulcerative lesions	
Mycobacterial infections	See above

See page 70 for abbreviations and footnotes

CLINICAL SYNDROME/MAJOR DIAGNOSTIC CONSIDERATIONS	DIAGNOSTIC CLUES/COMMENTS
Skin/Hair, Nodular, verrucous, and/or ulcerative lesions *(continued)*	
Bacillary angiomatosis *(Reference: CID 22:794, 1996)*	Friable vascular papules, cellulitis, plaques and subcutaneous nodules, usually tender. May be confused with KS. Etiology: Bartonella henselae and B. quintana. May be isolated from blood (5–15 days incubation of lysis centrifugation cultures on blood agar, 5% CO_2) and identified with Warthin Stary stain. *See pages 58 & 69.*
Acanthamoeba, disseminated	Rare *(NEJM 331:85, 1994)*
Sporotrichosis	Uncommon, but reported
Cryptococcosis	*As above*
Histoplasmosis	*As above*
Kaposi's sarcoma: Kaposi-associated herpesvirus (KSHV) now called HHV 8 is found in biopsy samples and blood mononuclear cells of pts with AIDS-related or classical KS *(Ln 346:799, 1995).*	Skin usually 1st site of presentation. Lesions palpable, firm, non-tender nodules. Early lesions may resemble ecchymoses. Typically violaceous, hyperpigmented, involving head, neck. Later become confluent, form large tumor masses and occur throughout the body. Up to 40% GI involvement. Oral lesions may precede skin lesions.
Non-Hodgkin's lymphoma	Skin involved in 15% of pts with non-Hodgkin's lymphoma. Lesions are usually papules or nodules.
Mycobacterium avium-intracellulare (MAI/MAC)	Fever and extensive cutaneous nodules (granulomas or focal necroses) have been reported in pts infected with MAC who responded to HAART with immune reconstitution (↑ CD4 counts and ↓ viral load). Steroids may be useful rx *(5th Conf Retrovir & OI 1998, Abst. 726) (Table 9B).*
Vesicular bullous or pustular lesions	
Herpes simplex virus	Grouped vesicles on erythematous base, rapidly evolve into ulcerations or fissures. May persist as chronic large ulcerative lesions.
Varicella-zoster virus	Grouped vesicles on erythematous base. May be verrucous. In chronic form may persist as hyperkeratotic lesions. Dermatomal distribution.
Cytomegalovirus	Small reddish-purple macules that ulcerate. May present with non-healing perianal ulceration.
Staphylococcal impetigo	Erythematous crusted papules, may be pruritic on face, trunk, groin.
"Typical scabies"	Extremely pruritic, papular and vesicular lesions characterized by linear or serpentine burrows most commonly on hands, wrists, elbows, ankles. Average number of mites is 11.
Stevens-Johnson syndrome	Most often drug-related: TMP/SMX, fluconazole, ddl, anti-TBc drugs. 1 case reported with acute HIV infection *(CID 19:798, 1994).*
Porphyria cutanea tarda	Association with HIV described but the co-occurrence may reflect coexistence of risk factors, esp. alcohol use, Hep C, rather than causal association *(CID 20:348, 1995).* Lesions especially over sun-exposed areas.
Papulosquamous lesions	
Seborrheic dermatitis	Occurs in 20–80% HIV+ individuals, dandruff to patches and plaques of erythema with indistinct margins and yellowish scale on "hairy" areas. Malassezia furfur may be causative agent *(CID 22:S128, 1996).*
Xerotic eczema (dry-skin syndrome)	Occurs in 5–20% HIV+ individuals. Often severely pruritic and resistant to antihistamines.
Dermatophytosis (T. rubrum most common, then T. mentarophytes and E. floccosum)	Occurs in 20–35% HIV+ individuals. Widespread, often severe with scaly red pruritic papules and plaques.
Tinea versicolor	Patchy areas of fine scale and hypopigmentation. CD4 often >300/mm³. Usually resistant to topical agents.
Psoriasis	Occurs in 1.3–5% HIV+ individuals. Presents as (1) discrete plaques or (2) a diffuse dermatitis often associated with palmoplantar keratodermia. Distribution may be atypical: groin, axilla and scalp rather than elbows and knees. Common nail changes and psoriatic arthritis *(JRD 17:914, 1996).*

See page 70 for abbreviations and footnotes

CLINICAL SYNDROME/MAJOR DIAGNOSTIC CONSIDERATIONS	DIAGNOSTIC CLUES/COMMENTS
Skin/Hair, Papulosquamous lesions *(continued)*	
Crusted (Norwegian) scabies	**Highly contagious** to close contacts (health care workers). Characterized by erythema, hyperkeratosis and crusting. Pruritus is typically present but hyperkeratotic, crusted form may be absent. Burrows usually not seen. Gross nail thickening and subungual debris common. Alopecia, hyperpigmentation, pyoderma and eosinophilia may occur. Dx is based on demonstration of heavy mite burden (1000s) on scraping vs a few in typical scabies.
Folliculitis	
Staphylococcal folliculitis	An uncommon presentation is violaceous plaques (up to 10 cm) in groin, axilla and scalp.
Eosinophilic folliculitis	*See Skin, eosinophilic, folliculitis above*
Skin discoloration (reddish-brown, occ. black or bluish)	Seen in 75–100% of pts on clofazimine
Hair disease	
Diffuse thinning, premature graying, elongated eyelashes, peculiar straightening of previously curly hair has been observed in advanced HIV *(JRD 17:914, 1996)*	In African-Americans
Nail disease	
Onychomycosis	
Longitudinal pigmented nail bands	Seen in almost ½ pts on ZDV, more common in dark-skinned patients, occurs within 4–8 weeks of starting rx.
Systemic, wasting syndromes *(See Table 11, page 76)* "Slim" disease (enteropathic AIDS), rule out: Cryptosporidium and other causes of chronic diarrhea Mycobacterium avium-intracellulare complex (MAC) Mycobacterium tuberculosis Histoplasma capsulatum Kaposi's sarcoma Non-Hodgkin's lymphoma	Weight loss is common (29% in one series). Causes: opportunistic infections (47%), psychosocial factors (17%), drug-associated (7%), unexplained (29%) *(Int J STD 4:234, 1993)*. In Africa, most common symptom of AIDS is slim disease: weight loss (often >30% body weight), chronic fever, intermittent watery diarrhea without blood or mucus [¼–½ have parasites (cryptosporidium, I. belli)]. Many die without an apparent OI. Treatment unsuccessful. *See Table 11 for therapy.* Nutritional deficiencies were found in 86% of 125 HIV-infected IVDUs and could account for unexplained weight loss *(J AIDS & Human Retro 16:272, 1997)*. Rapid weight loss (>4 kg in <4 mos.) accompanied by anorexia is usually a sign of secondary infection, slower weight loss (>4 kg in >4 mos.) is often due to GI disease with diarrhea, less marked weight loss may be due to ↓ caloric intake *(NEJM 333:123, 1995)*.

Abbreviations: 2° = secondary; **abn** = abnormal; **AFB** = acid-fast bacilli; **AM/CL** = amoxicillin clavulanate; **ARDS** = adult respiratory distress syndrome; **ATS** = American Thoracic Society; **BAL** = bronchoalveolar lavage; **bc** = blood culture; **CD4** = T helper lymphocytes; **CHF** = congestive heart failure; **CNS** = central nervous system; **CPK** = serum creatinine phosphokinase; **CRAG** = cryptococcal antigen; **CSF** = cerebrospinal fluid; **CT** = computed tomographic scan; **CXR** = chest x-ray; **DIC** = disseminated intravascular coagulopathy; **DOE** = dyspnea on exertion; **DTR** = deep tendon reflex; **dx** = diagnosis; **Echo** = echocardiogram; **EIA** = enzyme immunoassay; **EMG** = electromyogram; **ERCP** = endoscopic retrograde cholangiopancreatography; **ESR** = erythrocyte sedimentation rate; **FTA/ABS** = fluorescent treponemal antibody-absorbed test; **hx** = history; **G6PD** = glucose-6-phosphate dehydrogenase; **HAART** = highly active antiretroviral therapy; **IDU** = injection drug user; **IL-2** = interleukin-2; **INH** = isoniazid; **ITP** = idiopathic thrombocytopenic purpura; **KOH** = potassium hydroxide; **LFTs** = liver function tests; **LP** = lumbar puncture; **LV** = left ventricular; **MAC** = Mycobacterium avium-intracellulare complex; **MHA-TP** = microhemagglutination-T. pallidum; **MRI** = magnetic resonance imaging; **M. tbc** = Mycobacterium tuberculosis; **NSAIDs** = non-steroidal anti-inflammatory drugs and salicylates; **PAS** = periodic acid Schiff stain; **PBMC** = peripheral blood mononuclear cells; **PCP** = Pneumocystis carinii pneumonia; **PCR** = polymerase chain reaction; **PI** = protease inhibitor; **PMN** = polymorphonuclear neutrophilic leucocytes; **RPR** = rapid plasma reagin test; **RTI** = reverse transcriptase inhibitor; **rx** = treatment; **SIADH** = syndrome of inappropriate antidiuretic hormone production; **TMP/SMX** = trimethoprim/sulfamethoxazole; **UTI** = urinary tract infection; **VDRL** = a reaginic antibody test (Venereal Disease Research Lab); **ZDV** = zidovudine

1. These summaries have extensively used the 6th Edition of THE MEDICAL MANAGEMENT OF AIDS, edited by Merle A. Sande and Paul A. Volberding, W.B. Saunders & Co., 1998. See Table 12 for details of treatment/disease entity; **2.** Adapted from R.W. Price and J.M. Worley, *ibid.;* **3.** Adapted from J.S. Greenspan, D. Greenspan, *ibid.;* **4.** Adapted from J.P. Cello, *ibid.;* **5.** Adapted from R.W. Goodgame, *AnIM 124:429, 1996;* J.G. Bartlett, et al., *CID 15:726, 1992;* J.P. Cello, MEDICAL MANAGEMENT OF AIDS, 5th Ed., 1996; **6.** Adapted from J. Hambleton, MEDICAL MANAGEMENT OF AIDS, 6th Ed. Eds: M.A. Sande, P.A. Volberding. W.B. Saunders & Co., 1998; J.P. Doweiko, *Blood Rev 7:121, 1993;* **7.** Adapted from P.C. Hopewell, *ibid.;* **8.** Adapted from P.C. Hopewell, H. Masur, *ibid.;* **9.** P. Goodman, *ibid.;* **10.** Adapted from L.O. Kaplan, *ibid.;* **11.** Adapted from T.C. Berger, MEDICAL MANAGEMENT OF AIDS, 5th Ed. Eds: M.A. Sande, P.A. Volberding. W.B. Saunders & Co., 1996; and M.J. Zalla, W.P. Daniel, Sr., & A.F. Fransway, *Mayo Clin Proc 67:1089, 1992.* Also ref.: *Ln 348:659, 1996.*

TABLE 9C (2)

SYNDROME	AGENT	STARTING DOSE	THERAPEUTIC DOSE	COMMENTS
Depression *(continued)*	Stimulants (especially good with despondency relating to medical illness)			
	Methylphenidate (Ritalin)	5 mg qAM	20–60 mg daily	Divide dosage tid
	Dextroamphetamine (Dexedrine)	5 mg qAM	5–40 mg daily	
	MAO inhibitors: Contraindicated			
AIDS Dementia	Zidovudine (Zovirax)	200 mg po tid		Higher dosage: 800–1200 mg may be necessary. *See Table 5B, page 16*
Anxiety	Anxiolytics			
	Clonazepam (Klonopin)	0.5 mg po q8h	0.5–2.0 mg q8h	Onset of action slow, long-acting (round the clock) (not FDA-approved for this indication)
	Lorazepam (Ativan)	0.5–1.0 mg q8h prn	0.5–2.0 mg q8h prn	Rapid onset of action
	Alprazolam (Xanax)	0.25–0.5 mg q8h prn	0.5–1.0 mg q8h prn	Rapid onset of action
	Buspirone (BuSpar)	5 mg po tid	10–15 mg po tid	Non-sedating, non-addictive. Suitable for chronic anxiety
Delirium	Haloperidol (Haldol) + Lorazepam (Ativan)	2–5 mg IM (some use low-dose IV) 2 mg IV		Correct specific cause if present
Mania	(Discontinue potential causative drugs)			
	Lithium	300 mg po tid	600 mg po tid	
	Carbamazepine (Tegretol)	200 mg po bid	400 mg po tid	Drug-drug interactions common, *Table 17*. Not FDA-approved for this indication.
	Valproic acid (Depakene)	250 mg po bid	250 mg po tid	Drug-drug interactions common, *Table 17*. Not FDA-approved for this indication.
Psychoses	Low potency			
	Chlorpromazine (Thorazine, Mellaril)	25–50 mg q8–12h po	50–800 mg qd	Very sedating, anticholinergic side-effects. Low risk extrapyramidal symptoms
	Mid potency			
	Perphenazine (Trilafon)	4 mg po q8h	8–16 mg qd (in divided doses)	Medium risk for sedation, anticholinergic side-effects
	High potency			
	Haloperidol (Haldol)	0.5–2.0 mg po bid or tid	2–100 mg po qd (in divided doses)	Low risk for sedation, anticholinergic side-effects. High risk extra-pyramidal symptoms. Case reports of neuroleptic malignant syndrome
Neuropathic pain (30–40% of pts), HIV sensory neuropathy, post-herpetic neuralgia, nucleoside toxicity	Carbamazepine or tricyclics as for depression, *above*			

TABLE 9D

PSYCHIATRIC AND NEUROLOGIC SIDE EFFECTS ASSOCIATED WITH ANTIRETROVIRAL DRUGS AND DRUGS USED TO TREAT HIV-ASSOCIATED OPPORTUNISTIC INFECTIONS OR MALIGNANCIES

DRUG	SIDE EFFECTS	FREQUENCY/SEVERITY	
Acyclovir	Long-term administration (2 years): confusion, dizziness, hallucinations, paresthesias (~1%), somnolence, visual abnormalities	~1%	+
Atovaquone	Headache, insomnia, dizziness (less than with TMP/SMX or pentamidine)	~10%	±
Azithromycin	Dizziness, headache (<1%), vertigo, somnolence, hypoacusis [on high dose or prolonged regimens (0.5 gm, 30–90 days, 14%)]	Rare	±
Bleomycin	None causally associated		
Ciprofloxacin	Dizziness, insomnia, nightmares, hallucinations, mania, irritability, tremor (↑ caffeine levels may exaggerate these side effects, *see Table 17, page 113*), ataxia, convulsions, lethargy, drowsiness, weakness, paresthesias, depersonalization, depression	0.4%	+
Clindamycin	? Neuro blockade in anesthesia (prolongation of apnea)	Rare	±
Clarithromycin	Headache (mild) 2%, hypoacusis (on high dose)	2%	±
Clofazimine	Dizziness, drowsiness, fatigue, headache, giddiness, taste disorder	<1%	±
Dapsone	Peripheral neuropathy (motor loss, usually reversible), vertigo, tinnitus, headache, insomnia	?	+
Didanosine (ddI)	Peripheral neuropathy 5–12% (major toxicity), headache 5%, seizure 3%, confusion 2%, insomnia 2%, anxiety 1%, nervousness 1%, dizziness 1%, abnormal thinking 1%, depression <1%, taste perversion <1%	5%	+ +
Doxorubicin	None causally associated		
Epoetin alfa	Headache, dizziness (occurred in equal frequency in placebo patients), seizures (10 cases reported, appear associated with underlying pathology)	15–20%	±
Ethambutol	Decreased visual acuity (optic neuritis, reversible) with 25 mg/kg/d, not with 15 mg/kg/d; headache, dizziness, mental confusion, possible hallucinations	?	+ +
Etoposide (VP16)	Transient cortical blindness	Rare	
Famciclovir	Headache (mild) 23%, paresthesias 3% (frequencies equal to placebo pts)	?	+
Filgrastim (G-CSF)	None causally associated		
Fluconazole	Headache 1.9%	~2%	±
Flucytosine	Ataxia, hearing loss, headache, paresthesias, Parkinsonism, vertigo, confusion, hallucinations, psychosis	<1%	±
Foscarnet	Seizures (10%, some related to underlying disease); >5% headache, paresthesias, dizziness, neuropathy	5–10%	+ +
Ganciclovir	Abnormal thoughts, ataxia, coma, confusion, dizziness, headache, nervousness, paresthesias, psychosis, somnolence, tremor	5%	+
Indinavir	Headache, insomnia, dizziness, taste perversion	~5%	±
Isoniazid	Peripheral neuropathy (↓ with pyridoxine, B6): convulsions, encephalopathy, optic neuritis, memory impairment, toxic psychosis	?	+
Itraconazole	Headache 4%, dizziness 2%	~3%	±
Lamivudine (3TC)	Headache 35%, neuropathy, dizziness, insomnia	~10%	±
Marinol	Confusion, anxiety, hallucinations, depression	?	±
Megestrol acetate (oral suspension)	Paresthesia, confusion, depression (frequencies equal to placebo)	1–3%	±
Ofloxacin	Dizziness, insomnia, hallucinations, paresthesias, seizures	1%	+
Pentamidine	Confusion (hallucinations 1.7%, dizziness 0.5%)	~2%	+
Primaquine	1 case report psychosis	?	
Pyrimethamine	Insomnia, light-headedness, depression, seizures	Rare	±
Rifabutin	Headache 3%, insomnia 1%	3%	±

TABLE 9D (2)

DRUG	SIDE EFFECTS	FREQUENCY/SEVERITY	
Rifampin	Headache, drowsiness, ataxia, dizziness, mental confusion, behavioral changes	?	±
Ritonavir	Drug interactions may potentiate CNS toxicity of other drugs		
Saquinavir	Headache, paresthesia	~1%	±
Sargramostim (GM-CSF)	None causally associated		
Stavudine (d4T)	Peripheral neuropathy, sleep disorders, mania	21%	+
TMP/SMX	Aseptic meningitis, convulsions, ataxia, vertigo, tinnitus, headache, hallucinations, apathy, depression, nervousness	<1%	+
Trimetrexate	None causally associated		
Valacyclovir	Same as acyclovir		
Vinblastine	Paresthesias, peripheral neuritis, depression, convulsions	Uncom.	+
Vincristine	Neuritic pain, sensory loss, paresthesias, ataxia, paralysis	Common	++
Zalcitabine (ddC)	Peripheral neuropathy (most frequent toxicity)	17–31%	++
Zidovudine (ZDV)	Headache, dizziness (at 500 mg/day, frequency equal to placebo patients). At higher doses: headache, dizziness, insomnia, paresthesias, somnolence	~5%	+

TABLE 10

BIOLOGICS IN TREATMENT OF HEMATOPENIAS: HIV AND DRUG-RELATED

DRUG NAME, GENERIC (TRADE) COST	COMMENTS ON USE, ADVERSE EFFECTS
Erythropoietin (Epogen, Procrit) 4000 units $48.00 Epoetin alfa	Not indicated unless erythropoietin (EPO) level ≤500 mU/ml after ensuring appropriate zidovudine dosage. 100 U/kg IV or SC 3x/week for 8 weeks. If no response, can increase dose 50–100 U/kg increments to a max. dose of 300 U/kg 3x/week. Follow retic. count and replace iron if necessary. Adverse effects similar in pts given placebo and those given EPO. Small increased frequency of fever in EPO patients.
Granulocyte-CSF or G-CSF, Filgrastim (Neupogen), 300 μg $161.30, and Granulocyte-monocyte-CSF or GM-CSF, Sargramostim (Leukine). 250 μg $126.04	Initial dose 5 μg/kg/d SC; if no response after 1 week, can increase to 7.5 μg/kg/d x7 days; if no response, max. dose 10 μg/kg x1 week. D/C if no response or when absolute PMN count >500/mm³ (AIDS Reader, Nov.-Dec., p. 185, 1996). Transient bone pain common (2° expanding marrow cell population). Viral-like prodrome with fever and myalgia much more common with GM-CSF than G-CSF. HIV replication activated by GM-CSF (Lancet 347:1123, 1996).
Intravenous immune serum globulin (IVIG) (Gamimune N, Gammar, and others). 100 ml $400 for 5% prep; $800 for 10% prep	IVIG has been given to AIDS pts with parvovirus B19 infection with resolution of viremia and improvement in red blood cell counts. Do not use saline as diluent, may use D5W. Dose for parvovirus: 400 mg/kg/d x10 days and then as necessary (NEJM 321:519, 1989). In children, IVIG dose for supportive therapy is 400 mg/kg monthly. In 70 adults, 200–400 mg/kg every 21 days for 31 weeks reduced frequency of infection and days of hospitalization vs 57 controls (Arch Int Med 156:2545, 1996). For immune thrombocytopenia 0.5–1.0 g/kg/d x3– 5 days; see Table 6D, page 26. Adverse reactions mild to moderate in severity and occur in 5% of infusions: chills, fever, nausea, vomiting, chest tightness, back or hip pain.
Rho (D) Immune Globulin, intravenous (human) (Winrho). 1500 IU $306.00	Effective in HIV thrombocytopenia (CID 21:415, 1995; CID 22:1129, 1996) at doses of 25–50 μg/kg/d x1 week (1500 IU = 300 μg); repeat infusions every 3 weeks. Advantages over IVIG: prepare in <5 min. and infuse over 3 min. Cost is 10% of IVIG. Adverse effects: occasional hypersensitivity and mild hemolysis. Rare cases of aseptic meningitis. Dapsone may work for HIV-associated thrombocytopenia (CID 221131, 1996).

TABLE 11
AGENTS FOR WASTING/WEIGHT LOSS
(Good References: *NEJM 333:83, 1995; Inf Agents Dis 4:76, 1995*)

Dronabinol (Marinol): FDA-approved as an appetite stimulant in AIDS patients with wasting. It is delta-9-THC, a major active substance in marijuana, a narcotic Schedule II controlled substance. Patients on 2.5 mg po bid (1 hr before lunch and dinner) have significant ↑ in appetite and weight gain over patients on placebo (139 pts in placebo-controlled study). Another two controlled trials failed to demonstrate significant weight gain (*J Pain Symptom Manag 10:89, 1995; Abst 386, 3rd CRV, 1996*). **Adverse effects:** CNS: dose-related "high" (elation, easy laughing) 8%, dizziness, confusion, paranoid reaction, somnolence (3–10%). GI: nausea, vomiting (2.5 mg cap $2.99)

Megestrol acetate (Megace): A synthetic oral progesterone approved for anorexia, cachexia or unexplained significant weight loss in AIDS patients. 800 mg po qd ↑ appetite and sense of well-being, 34/53 gained wt and 63% pts gained ≥ 5 lbs (*Ann Int Med 121:393, 1994*). In 2nd study, 34/44 pts gained weight, average 8 lbs (*Ann Int Med 121:400, 1994*). Most weight gain is fat but up to ⅓ may be lean body mass. A dose of 750 but not 250 mg/d for 12 weeks resulted in mean weight gain of 6 kg (*Abst 386, 3rd CRV, 1996*). **Usual dose** is 800 mg po qd x1 month, then 400 mg po qd x4 months. **Adverse effects:** Generally well tolerated; diarrhea, rash, impotence, edema, flatulence, weakness. Treatment results in ↓ testosterone levels, which may explain impotence and predominance of fat gain. Replacement testosterone (200 mg q2 weeks) should be considered, especially if plasma levels after 2–4 weeks are low. May produce menstrual irregularities in women and should not be given in pregnancy. For cost and convenience, oral suspension may have advantage over tablets: 40 mg tab $1.35 = $21.00/800 mg vs $8.65/800 mg oral suspension.

Anabolic Steroids

    Fluoxymesterone (Halotestin): Approved as an androgen replacement in men and for recurrent breast carcinoma in women. Placebo-controlled trial in progress (10 mg po bid) in AIDS wasting syndrome. (10 mg tab $1.69)

    Oxymetholone: Two recent studies (uncontrolled) demonstrated mean weight gain of 5.7–8.2 kg after 12–30 weeks with 50 mg tid (*Brit J Nut 75:126 & 247, 1996*).

    Nandrolone: Less virilizing than Halotestin and being studied in women. One study ↑ 2.3 kg after 16 wks (*AIDS 10:745, 1996*). Dose 100 mg biweekly (100 mg $14.05).

    Testosterone: 200–400 mg q2 weeks IM (100 mg $0.84). Reported in retrospective study to ↑ lean body mass by 2.6 lbs (*J AIDS 9:1178, 1995*). Another showed no ↑ weight (*AIDS 11:1347, 1997*).

    Oxandrolone (Oxandrin): 21 AIDS pts demonstrated ↑ weight gain (mean 16 lbs. at 120 days with 6.8 lbs of body cell mass although only 4 pts remained on rx) with 10 mg po bid (*IDSA Abstracts, 1996 & AIDS 10:1657, 1996*).

Recombinant Human Growth Hormone, mammalian cell-derived [rhGH(m), Serostim®] is approved for AIDS-related wasting syndrome. In Phase III, double-blind placebo-controlled trial rhGH (0.1 mg/kg/d x12 weeks, 90 pts): 1.6 kg ↑ weight, 3.0 kg ↑ in lean body mass, ↓ in fat mass, ↑ in treadmill work performance (*AnIM 125:873, 1996*). The 2nd Phase III study found significant ↑ in weight gain after 6 but not 8 weeks using 6 mg daily but no body composition studies were included. **Adverse effects:** joint stiffness, carpal tunnel syndrome, puffiness, paresthesias mild, responded to dose ↓; hyperglycemia. (Cost will be high and no effect on survival). Recommended dosages: >55 kg, 6 mg SC qd at bedtime; 45–55 kg, 5 mg SC qd; and 35–45 kg, 4 mg SC qd.

IGF-1: Insulin-like Growth Factor-1 use was associated with weight gain and nitrogen retention but produced hypoglycemia in highest dose (*J Clin Endo Metab 78:404, 1994; J Clin Endo Metab 81:3033, 1996*). Results in combination with human growth hormone disappointing (*AnIM 125:865, 1996*)

Fat Emulsions, intravenous: A Phase II open label clinical trial with Liposyn III in progress.

N-3 Fatty Acid Supplementation (Omega-3 fatty acids—fish oil): A trial of HIV-infected individuals without OIs received MaxEPA (R.P. Scherer, St. Petersburg, FL) and gained mean of 2.1 kg. These fatty acids may exert an anti-TNF or IL_1 effect (*J AIDS 11:258, 1996*).

Thalidomide is showing promise: 300 mg/d found to ↑ weight in wasted HIV and M. tuberculosis-infected individuals in Thailand more than those receiving anti-tuberculous rx alone (↑ 7% in 3 weeks) (*J AIDS 11:247, 1996*) and ↑ mean wt by 4.05 kg vs 1.3 kg in placebo in 28 pts with HIV & wasting over 12 wks (*AIDS 10:1501, 1996*). Makes pts very sleepy, so give at night. Also associated with **peripheral neuropathy** and well-known **teratogenicity**. Clinical trial in progress using 100–200 mg/d (for compassionate use, Celgene 1-800-801-8328).

TABLE 12
TREATMENT OF SPECIFIC INFECTIONS/MICROORGANISMS IN HIV+/AIDS PATIENTS

CAUSATIVE AGENT/DISEASE	MODIFYING CIRCUMSTANCES	SUGGESTED REGIMENS		COMMENTS
		PRIMARY	ALTERNATIVE	
Bacterial infections				
Bartonella				
Cat-scratch disease	B. henselae	Cat-scratch disease: efficacy of therapy not established. Most pts should receive symptomatic care, nodes resolve in 2–6 months. Antibiotics may benefit in severe disease (encephalopathy, retinitis): RIF, CIP, TMP/SMX, erythro, clarithro, azithro, or AM/CL *(PIDJ 11:474, 1992; Adv PID 11:1, 1996).*		
Bacillary angiomatosis; Peliosis hepatis	B. henselae, B. quintana	Erythro 500 mg qid po or doxycycline 100 mg bid po	Clarithro 500 mg bid or azithro 250 mg qd or CIP 500–750 mg bid, po	Most often an opportunistic infection in pts with AIDS. Diagnosis by biopsy of skin lesions. Lifelong suppression may be necessary. Clinical response in 3–4 days but requires up to 2 months to normalize lab parameters. Experience is more extensive with erythromycin than with doxycycline *(NEJM 330:1509, 1994).* May need 2 drugs for peliosis hepatis, osteomyelitis, or endocarditis; for 2nd drug, add rifampin or gentamicin. Good review: *NEJM 330:1509, 1994.*
Endocarditis *(AnIM 125:646, 1996)*	B. henselae, B. quintana	Erythro 500 mg qid po or IV. Bacteriostatic. Valve surgery in most reported pts.	Cidal but unproven drugs clinically: CIP, gentamicin, ceftriaxone	Hard to detect with automated blood culture systems. Need lysis-centrifugation and/or blind subculture onto chocolate agar at 7 & 14 days.
Trench fever	B. quintana	Doxycycline 100 mg bid po		
Suppression		Erythromycin 250–500 mg po qid (see Comments)	Clarithromycin, azithromycin, or ciprofloxacin in above doses	Life-long suppression likely to be required.
Campylobacter jejuni	CAUTION: *See Comment on quinolone resistance*	CIP 500 mg po or norflox 400 mg po q12h x5 d or azithro 500 mg po qd x3 d.	Erythromycin stearate 500 mg po qid x5 days	Reports of fluoroquinolone-resistant strains from many locations: Thailand, N. Africa, Spain & Mexico. 50% of Thai isolates CIP-resistant but responded to azithro *(CID 21:536 & 542, 1995).* Risk of Guillain-Barre syndrome: *NEJM 335:208, 1996 & 333:1374, 1995.*
Chlamydia trachomatis (non-gonococcal or post-gonococcal urethritis, cervicitis) *Reference: MMWR 47:RR-1, 1998*		Doxycycline 100 mg bid po x7 days or Azithromycin 1.0 gm po (single dose)	Erythromycin 500 mg qid po x7 days or Ofloxacin 300 mg bid po x7 days	Diagnosis: Lipase chain reaction (LCR) of voided urine sensitive/specific and non-invasive. Can detect antigen with EIA or culture. Treatment: If pregnant, do not use doxy or FQ; use erythromycin *[CID 20(Suppl.1):1, 1995]* or azithro. Azithro 1.0 gm po x1 is 98% effective *(JAMA 274:545, 1995).* Clarithromycin active in vitro vs C. trachomatis but not FDA-approved for STDs. Ofloxacin cure rate reported as 93% after 300 mg po bid x7 days *(AAC 36:1144, 1992).*
Clostridium difficile toxin-mediated diarrhea		Metronidazole 250 mg tid po x7–14 days	Vancomycin 125 mg qid po x7–14 days	Do not use cholestyramine with vancomycin. Avoid anti-motility agents. Relapse occurs in 10–20% of patients; vanco + rifampin x7–14 days.
Granuloma inguinale (Calymmatobacterium granulomatis)		Doxycycline 100 mg bid po x minimum of 3 weeks	Erythromycin 500 mg qid po x21 d (can be used in pregnancy) or TMP/SMX 1 DS tablet (160 mg TMP) bid po x21 d	Rare in U.S. Response to rx should be seen in 7 days; if none, dx questionable. Treatment failures and recurrences seen with doxycycline and TMP/SMX; if no response first few days of rx, add gentamicin 1 mg/kg q8h.

See page 96 for abbreviations.   NOTE: All dosage recommendations are for adults (unless otherwise indicated) and assume normal renal function.

CAUSATIVE AGENT/DISEASE	MODIFYING CIRCUMSTANCES	SUGGESTED REGIMENS		COMMENTS
		PRIMARY	ALTERNATIVE	
Bacterial infections *(continued)*				
Haemophilus ducreyi (chancroid)		Ceftriaxone 250 mg IM (single dose) or azithro 1.0 gm po single dose or erythro 500 mg qid po x7 d.	Ciprofloxacin 500 mg bid po x3 days	In HIV+ pts, failures reported with single dose azithro, may require usual regimen (0.5 gm po, then 250 mg po qd x4d).
Klebsiella/Enterobacter		P Ceph 3 or 4 or AP Pen or IMP or MER or BL/BLI or aztreonam or FQ. Use IV regimen[1]	Other fluoroquinolones, e.g., levofloxacin or trovafloxacin	Start treatment empirically. When in vitro susceptibility results available, select agent with narrowest spectrum of activity.
Listeriosis	Bacteremia, meningitis, focal infections	Ampicillin 50 mg/kg q6h IV	Trimethoprim/sulfamethoxazole 20 mg/-kg/d TMP (component) IV divided into q6h dosage	Some evidence suggests synergy with ampicillin + an aminoglycoside (gentamicin). Duration of rx 2–4 weeks. (Cephalosporins not active vs L. monocytogenes.) *(J AIDS 8:461, 1995)*
Lymphogranuloma venereum		Doxycycline 100 mg bid po x21 days	Erythromycin 500 mg qid po x21 days	Dx based on serology, biopsy contraindicated. Rectal LGV may require retreatment.
Mycobacterium tuberculosis Preventive treatment, infection without disease (positive tuberculin test)[2] or HIV+ pt with anergy and high risk for tuberculosis *(AnIM 119:185, 1993)*. Recent study suggests HIV+ pts with anergy need prophylaxis **only** if exposed to active tuberculosis *(NEJM 337:315, 1997)*. Therefore, the use of anergy testing in conjunction with PPD testing is no longer recommended for routine screening programs for TB among HIV-infected pts in U.S. *[MMWR 46(RR-15):1, 1997]*	Organisms likely to be INH-susceptible	INH 5 mg/kg/d (max. 300 mg/d) po + pyridoxine (B6) 25–50 mg po x 12 months *(See Comment)*. *For children, see Table 6, page 30*	If compliance problem: INH by DOT 15 mg/kg 2x/week x12 months. If INH not possible, no proven regimen, but reasonable options: RIF 600 mg po qd x12 mos.** OR ETB 15 mg/kg/d to a max. of 1.0 gm/d + RIF 600 mg/d po x9–12 months OR PZA 20 mg/kg/d to max. of 2.0 gm/d + RIF 600 mg/d po x2 months	For pts given ddC+ INH, suggest 50 mg pyridoxine/d. Duration of preventive rx unclear; recommendations range from 6–12 months. Recent study in Uganda suggests 6 mos. of INH or 3 mos. of INH + RIF also ↓ risk of TB *(NEJM 337:801, 1997)*. Resistant TBc occurred in HIV+ pts given INH + RIF by DOT—presumably due to malabsorption *(NEJM 332:336, 1995; AJM 127:289, 1997; CID 25:1044, 1997)*, although 1 recent study failed to detect **direct** effect on bioavailability of antimycobacterial drugs in pts with AIDS ± diarrhea *(CID 25:104, 1997)*. INH prophylaxis reported to ↓ progression of HIV *(Lancet 342:268, 1993)*.
	INH-resistant (or adverse reaction to INH), RIF-sensitive organisms likely	RIF 600 mg/d po x6–12 months** OR Rifabutin 300 mg po qd x12 mos.**	RIF 600 mg/d po** + ETB 15 mg/kg/d to max. of 1.0 gm x6–12 months OR PZA 20 mg/kg/d to max. of 2.0 gm/d + RIF 600 mg/d po** x2 months, then INH + RIF daily until sensitivities of index case (if available) known, then if INH-CR, dc INH and continue RIF for 9 mos.	IDSA guideline lists rifabutin in 600 mg/d dose as another alternative; however, current recommended max. dose of rifabutin is 300 mg/d.**
	INH- and RIF-resistant organisms likely	Efficacy of all regimens unproven. PZA 25–30 mg/kg/d to max. of 2 gm/d + ETB 15–25 mg/kg/d po x12 mos.	PZA 25–30 mg/kg/d to max. of 2.0 gm/d + ETB 15–25 mg/kg/d + CIP 750 mg bid or oflox 400 mg bid, all po, x6–12 months	If ETB used in dose above 15 mg/kg/d, monitor pt for retrobulbar neuritis. (Visual acuity and red/green color test, ≥ 10% loss considered significant.)

** See next page for options regarding concomitant use of protease inhibitors and RIF or rifabutin.

[1] *Dosages: P Ceph 3* (cefotaxime 2 gm q4–8h IV, ceftriaxone 2 gm qd IV), *AP Pen* (ticarcillin 3–4 gm q4–6h IV, piperacillin 3 gm q4h or 4 gm q6h IV), *IMP* 0.5 gm q6h IV, aztreonam 2 gm q8h IV, *CIP* 400 mg q12h IV, *P Ceph 4* (cefepime 2 gm q8h or q12h IV), *levofloxacin* 500 mg IV/day, *trovafloxacin* 300 mg IV x1, then 200 mg IV/day.

[2] Tuberculin test: The standard is the Mantoux test, 5 TU (intermediate) PPD in 0.1 ml diluent stabilized with Tween 80. Read at 48–72 hrs, measuring the maximum diameter of induration (not erythema). A reaction of ≥5 mm is defined as + in the HIV+ pt. For HIV+ pts who have received BCG ≥10 mm is cut-off for rx *(Brit Med J 304:1231, 1992)*.

See page 96 for abbreviations.   NOTE: All dosage recommendations are for adults (unless otherwise indicated) and assume normal renal function.

CAUSATIVE AGENT/DISEASE	MODIFYING CIRCUMSTANCES	SUGGESTED REGIMENS		COMMENTS
		PRIMARY	ALTERNATIVE	

Bacterial infections/Mycobacterium tuberculosis *(continued)*

Treatment, active tuberculosis

		INITIAL THERAPY	CONTINUATION PHASE OF THERAPY (in vitro susceptibility known)	

Isolation essential! *(See Table 9, page 59.)* Older observations on infectivity of susceptible and resistant M. tbc before and after rx *(Am Rev Resp Dis 85:511, 1962)* may not be applicable to MDR M. tbc or to the HIV+ individual. Extended isolation may be appropriate.

REFERENCE: *CID 22:683, 1996*

Treatment:
Active tuberculosis:

SEE COMMENTS FOR DOSAGE

Modifying circumstances	Initial therapy (Primary)	Continuation phase (Alternative)
• Rate of INH resistance known to be <4%	INH + RIF + PZA daily x2 months	INH + RIF daily x4 months (total 6 months)
	Authors add pyridoxine 25–50 mg po daily to regimens that include INH	
• Rate of INH resistance not known or ≥4% —Compliant pt	INH + RIF + PZA + either STM or ETB daily until susceptibility data available. Even if susceptible, INH + RIF + PZA for total of 2 months	INH + RIF daily to complete 6 months of therapy
—Non-compliant or unreliable pt	Directly observed therapy (DOT): 1. INH + RIF + PZA + either STM or ETB daily for 2 weeks and then 2–3x/week for 6 weeks OR 2. INH + RIF + PZA + either STM or ETB 3x/week for 6 months	INH + RIF 2–3x/week to complete 6 months of therapy
• Known resistance (or intolerance) to INH	—	DOT recommended for all drug-resistant tuberculosis: RIF + ETB + PZA
• Resistance (or intolerance) to RIF	—	INH + ETB + PZA daily x18 mos (≥12 months post-negative sputum cultures)
• Resistance to both INH and RIF. Multiple drug-resistant tuberculosis (MDR TB)	Want ≥3 drugs active vs MDR TB strains: INH + RIF + PZA + ETB or STM + additional second-line drug (AMK) + quinolone (CIP or sparfloxacin or levofloxacin)	Continue ≥3 drugs shown active in vitro vs patient's strain of MDR TB. Appropriate duration of therapy is not known.

Dose In mg/kg (max. daily dose)

Regimen*	INH	RIF	PZA	ETB	SM
Daily:					
Child	10–20 (300)	10–20 (600)	15–30 (2000)	15–25	20–40 (1000)
Adult	5 (300)	10 (600)	15–30 (2000)	15–25	15 (1000)
2x/wk (DOT):					
Child	20–40 (900)	10–20 (600)	50–70 (4000)	50	25–30 (1500)
Adult	15 (900)	10 (600)	50–70 (4000)	50	25–30 (1500)
3x/wk (DOT):					
Child	20–40 (900)	10–20 (600)	50–70 (3000)	25–30	25–30 (1500)
Adult	15 (900)	10 (600)	50–70 (3000)	25–30	25–3 (1500)

Second-line anti-TB agents can be dosed as follows to facilitate DOT:

Cycloserine 500–750 mg qd (5x/wk) po
Ethionamide 500–750 mg qd (5x/wk) po
Kanamycin or capreomycin 15 mg/kg qd (3–5x/wk) IM/IV
Ciprofloxacin 750 mg qd (5x/wk) po
Ofloxacin 600–800 mg qd (5x/wk) po
Levofloxacin 750 mg qd (5x/wk) po *(CID 21:1245, 1995)*

NOTE:
1. Clinical and microbiologic response same as in HIV-negative patient
2. Post-treatment long-term suppression not necessary for drug-susceptible strains

Concomitant protease inhibitor (PI) therapy	Option 1	Option 2	Option 3
Concomitant protease inhibitor (PI) therapy (3 options) *(Adapted from MMWR 45:921, 1996)*	Option 1 1. Hold or discontinue PI rx 2. INH 300 mg + RIF 600 mg + PZA 25 mg/kg + ETB 15 mg/kg daily for 2 mos, then INH + RIF for 4 mos. 3. Initiate PI at conclusion of rx for tuberculosis	Option 2 1. Hold or discontinue PI rx 2. INH 300 mg + RIF 600 mg + PZA 25 mg/kg + ETB 15 mg/kg daily for 2 mos (or until cultures for M. tbc neg.) 3. INH 15 mg/kg (not to exceed 900 mg) + ETB 50 mg/kg 2x/wk for 16 mos 4. Initiate PI during the 16-month continuation phase of anti-tuberculous rx	Option 3 1. Use nelfinavir 750 mg q8h or indinavir 800 mg q8h as the PI component of antiretroviral rx 2. INH 300 mg + rifabutin 150 mg + PZA 25 mg/kg + ETB 15 mg/kg daily for 2 mos, then INH + rifabutin for 7 mos

TABLE 12 (4)

CAUSATIVE AGENT/DISEASE	MODIFYING CIRCUMSTANCES	SUGGESTED REGIMENS		COMMENTS
		PRIMARY	**ALTERNATIVE**	
Bacterial infections (continued)				
Mycobacterium avium-intracellulare complex (MAC or MAI)	Primary prophylaxis—Pt's CD4 count 50–100/mm³	Clarithromycin 500 mg po bid OR Azithromycin 1200 mg po weekly	Rifabutin 300 mg po qd OR Azithromycin 1200 mg po weekly + RIF 300 mg po qd	Rifabutin reduces MAC infection rate by 55% (no survival benefit); clarithromycin by 68% (30% survival benefit); azithromycin by 59% (68% survival benefit) (CID 26:611, 1998). Azithromycin + rifabutin more effective than either alone but not as well tolerated (NEJM 335:392, 1996). Many drug-drug interactions, see Table 17, page 115. Rifabutin ↑ metabolism of ZDV with 32% ↓ in AUC. Clarithro ↑ blood levels of non-sedating antihistamines with attendant risk of arrhythmias. Need to be sure no active M. tbc; rifabutin used for prophylaxis may promote selection of rifamycin-resistant M. tbc.
	Treatment Either presumptive dx or after positive culture of blood, bone marrow, or other usually sterile body fluids, e.g., liver	[Clarithromycin 500 mg po bid or azithromycin 500 mg po qd] + Ethambutol 15–25 mg/kg/d + Rifabutin 300 mg po qd	Clarithromycin or azithromycin + ethambutol + rifabutin + one or more of: CIP 750 mg po bid Oflox 400 mg po bid Amikacin 7.5–15 mg/kg IV qd In pts receiving protease inhibitors can use [clarithromycin 500 mg bid (or azithromycin 600 mg qd) + ETB 15–25 mg/kg/d] if the pt has not had previous prophylaxis with a neomacrolide (Johns Hopkins AIDS Report 9:2, 1997).	Median time to negative blood culture: clarithromycin + ETB 4.4 weeks vs azithro + ETB 16 weeks. Adding clofazimine of no value (CID 25:621, 1997). One study suggests adding amikacin also of no value. Drug toxicity: With clarithro, 23% pts had to stop drug 2° to dose-limiting adverse reaction (AnIM 121:905, 1994). Combination of clarithro, ETB and rifabutin led to uveitis and pseudojaundice (NEJM 330:438, 1994); result is reduction in max. dose of rifabutin to 300 mg. Treatment failure rate is high. Reasons: drug toxicity, development of drug resistance, and inadequate serum levels. Serum levels of clarithro ↓ in pts also given RIF or rifabutin (JID 171: 747, 1995). If pt not responding to initial regimen after 2–4 weeks, add one or more drugs. Several anecdotal reports of pts not responding to usual primary regimen who gained weight and became afebrile with dexamethasone 2–4 mg/d po (AAC 38:2215, 1994; CID 26:682, 1998).
	Chronic post-treatment suppression—secondary prophylaxis	**Always necessary**. [Clarithro or azithro] + ETB (lower dose to 15 mg/kg/d (Dosage above)	Clarithro or azithro or rifabutin (dosage above)	Recurrences almost universal without chronic suppression. (This may change in pts with good response to HAART. See page 71.)
Mycobacterium celatum	Treatment	Easily confused with M. xenopi. Optimal regimen not defined. May be susceptible to clarithromycin, FQ (Clin Microbiol Inf 3:582, 1997).		Isolated from blood of patients with AIDS (CID 24:140 & 144, 1997). Usually resistant to INH, RIF, PZA, capreomycin (JCM 33:137, 1995).
Mycobacterium chelonae, ssp. abscessus, chelonae	Treatment	Clarithromycin (500 mg po bid x6 months effective in HIV– pts). M. chelonae sensitive in vitro to neomacrolides, generally resistant to fluoroquinolones.		M. abscessus susceptible in vitro to clarithromycin (100%), clofazimine, amikacin (70%) and cefoxitin (70%). M. chelonae susceptible in vitro to clarithromycin, tobramycin (100%), amikacin (80%) and IMP (60%) (AJRCCM 156:51, 1997).

See page 96 for abbreviations.

NOTE: All dosage recommendations are for adults (unless otherwise indicated) and assume normal renal function.

CAUSATIVE AGENT/DISEASE	MODIFYING CIRCUMSTANCES	SUGGESTED REGIMENS		COMMENTS
		PRIMARY	ALTERNATIVE	
Bacterial infections *(continued)*				
Mycobacterium fortuitum	Treatment	Optimal regimen not defined. Amikacin + cefoxitin + probenecid 2–6 weeks, then po TMP/SMX, or doxycycline 2–6 months *(J Inf Dis 152:50, 1985)*. Surgical excision of infected areas.		Resistant to all standard anti-TBc drugs. Sensitive in vitro to cefoxitin, imipenem, amikacin, TMP/SMX, CIP, oflox. Resistant to rifabutin, azithromycin, variably susceptible to clarithromycin *(JAC 39:567, 1997)*.
Mycobacterium genavense	Treatment	Regimens used include ≥2 drugs: ETB, RIF, clofazimine, ciprofloxacin, clarithromycin		Clinical: CD4 <50. Symptoms of fever, weight loss, diarrhea. Lab: growth in BACTEC vials slow (mean 42 days). Subcultures grow only on Middlebrook 7H11 agar containing 2 µg/ml mycobactin J—growth still insufficient for in vitro sensitivity testing *(Lancet 340:76, 1992; AnIM 117:586, 1992)*. Survival ↑ from 81 to 263 days in pts rx for at least 1 month with ≥2 drugs *(Arch Int Med 155:400, 1995)*.
Mycobacterium gordonae	Treatment	Regimen(s) not defined, but consider INH + RIF + ETB for 6 weeks with surgical excision.		In vitro: sensitive to ethambutol, rifampin, amikacin, ciprofloxacin, clarithromycin. Resistant to INH *(CID 14:1229, 1992)*. Surgical excision.
Mycobacterium haemophilum	Treatment	Regimen(s) not defined. In animal model, clarithro + rifabutin effective *(AAC 39:2316, 1995)*.		Clinical: Ulcerating skin lesions, synovitis, osteomyelitis. Lab: Requires supplemented media to isolate. Sensitive in vitro to: CIP, cycloserine, rifabutin. Over ½ resistant to: INH, RIF, ETB, PZA *(AnIM 120:118, 1994)*.
Mycobacterium kansasii	Treatment	RIF (600 mg po qd) + ETB (15 mg/kg/d po) + INH (300 mg po qd) for 15–18 months *(AnIM 120:945, 1994)*	In pts who do not respond, add sulfamethoxazole (or TMP/SMX) *(Rev Inf Dis 13:789, 1991)*	If organism resistant to (≥ 1 µg/ml) INH, discontinue INH (70–85% isolates are resistant). Almost all isolates resistant to PZA. Rx a minimum of 15 months after culture negative. M. kansasii sensitive in vitro to clarithro (MIC ≤ 2.0 µg/ml), erythromycin, amikacin.
Mycobacterium marinum	Treatment	(RIF + ETB) or minocycline or TMP/SMX or clarithromycin for at least 12 weeks *(Arch Int Med 147:817, 1986; AJRCCM 156:52, 1997)*. Surgical excision.		Sensitive in vitro to clarithromycin, reported effective in 2 pts (1 HIV+ who failed on other regimens) *(CID 18:664, 1994)*.
Mycobacterium scrofulaceum	Treatment	Although regimens not defined, clarithromycin + clofazimine with or without ethambutol. Surgical excision		In vitro resistant to INH, RIF, ethambutol, PZA, amikacin, CIP *(CID 20:549, 1995)*.
Mycobacterium simiae	Treatment	Regimen(s) not defined		In vitro: sensitive to sulfamethoxazole, ciprofloxacin. Resistant to INH, rifampin, ethambutol, kanamycin and clarithromycin *(CID 17:508, 1993)*
Mycobacterium xenopi	Treatment	Regimen(s) not defined *(CID 24:226 & 233, 1997)*. INH + RIF + ETB suggested but no clinical trials available *(Clin Chest Med 17:697, 1996)*. Not always susceptible to these agents in vitro *(CID 25:206, 1997)*.		In vitro: sensitive to clarithromycin *(Antimic Ag Chemo 36:2841, 1992)* and rifabutin *(JAC 39:567, 1997)*.

See page 96 for abbreviations.   NOTE: All dosage recommendations are for adults (unless otherwise indicated) and assume normal renal function.

CAUSATIVE AGENT/DISEASE	MODIFYING CIRCUMSTANCES	SUGGESTED REGIMENS		COMMENTS
		PRIMARY	ALTERNATIVE	
Bacterial infections (con't)				

Neisseria gonorrhoeae (gonococcus)
Reference: MMWR 47: RR-1, 1998
	Gonorrhea; urethritis, conjunctivitis, proctitis; mucopurulent cervicitis; epididymoorchitis (sexually acquired)	Ceftriaxone 125 mg IM x1 dose
		OR
		cipro 500 mg po x1 dose
		OR
		ofloxacin 400 mg po x1 dose
		PLUS—for chlamydia:
		EITHER azithro 1.0 gm po x1 dose
		OR
		doxycycline 100 mg po bid x7 days
		------------------------------ 	
		Another option: trovafloxacin 200 mg po/d x5 days
			Alternatives for ceftriaxone (all **single dose**):
			  Cefixime 400 mg po,
			  ceftizoxime 500 mg IM,
			  cefotaxime 500 mg IM,
			  cefotetan 1 gm IM,
			  cefoxitin 2 gm IM + 1 gm probenecid po.
			Quinolone, **single dose** alternatives:
			  Enoxacin 400 mg po,
			  lomefloxacin 400 mg po,
			  norfloxacin 800 mg po,
			  trovafloxacin 100 mg po.
			Spectinomycin 2 gm IM x1
				50% of patients have concomitant C. trachomatis, treatment regimens should include rx for C. trachomatis. Ciprofloxacin or ofloxacin should not be used in pregnant women or in children. Spectinomycin not effective in gonococcal pharyngitis; for pharyngeal infection use ceftriaxone or ciprofloxacin. Strains with MICs to FQ of 1–2 μg/ml reported in SE Asia and Australia, may not respond to recommended po FQ doses (*MMWR 43:227, 1994; Sex Trans Dis 23:103, 1996*)). Preliminary report suggests that rx of gonorrhea ↓ HIV virus titers in semen.
				Single 2.0 gm dose of azithromycin yields high (99–100%) cure rate for gonococcal urethritis (and genital chlamydial infections) but has high rate of GI side-effects.

Pelvic inflammatory disease (PID), salpingitis, tuboovarian abscess. Etiology polymicrobic: gonococcus, C. trachomatis, bacteroides, enterobacteriaceae, streptococci, mycoplasma *Reference: MMWR R47:RR-1, 1998*	Outpatient (limit to pts with temp <38°C, WBC <11,000/ mm³, minimal evidence of peritonitis, active bowel sounds & able to tolerate oral nourishment	[Ceftriaxone 250 mg IM single dose + doxycycline 100 mg bid po x14 days] or [(Ofloxacin 400 mg bid po x14 days) + either clindamycin 450 mg qid po or metronidazole 500 mg bid po x14 days]	[Cefoxitin 2.0 gm IM single dose + probenecid 1.0 gm concurrently + doxycycline] OR Trovafloxacin 200 mg po once daily x14 days	Indications to hospitalize: compliance as an outpatient unlikely, pregnant, peritonitis, suspected pelvic abscess, temp >38°C, need for laparoscopy to clarify diagnosis, failure to respond as outpatient in 72 hours, diagnosis uncertain. If patient should be hospitalized but cannot be, add metronidazole 0.5 gm bid po. 15/16 pts with tuboovarian abscess successfully rx with antibiotics + CT-directed needle drainage (*Radiol 182:399, 1992; Hosp Pract 30:61, 1995*). PID incidence reduced when high-risk pts screened and treated for chlamydial infection (*NEJM 334:1362, 1996*).
	Hospitalized	[Cefotetan 2 gm IV q12h or cefoxitin 2.0 gm q6h IV] + doxycycline 0.1 gm IV or po q12h. Rx at least 4 days and afebrile for 48 hrs. After IV rx, doxy 0.1 gm bid po or clinda 0.45 gm qid po to complete 14 days	Clindamycin 900 mg q8h IV + gentamicin (2.0 mg/kg initial dose then 1.5 mg/kg q8h IV) (can be given in same IV). Rx as with cefoxitin. Follow with oral agent (doxycycline or clindamycin) to complete 14 days.	IV clinda effective vs C. trachomatis, effectiveness of po clinda not determined (*CID 19:720, 1994*). Other alternative combinations: (1) AM/SB + doxy or (2) oflox + either clinda or metro or (3) cipro 200 mg IV q12h + doxy 100 mg IV/po q12h + metronidazole 500 mg IV q8h
Prostatitis, acute Etiologies: N. gonorrhoeae, C. trachomatis. In homosexual men, can be E. coli	Age usually ≤ 35 years	Treat as gonorrhea: ceftriaxone followed by doxycycline or azithromycin *(see above)*		Each of the fluoroquinolones is active vs N. gonorrhoeae. Ofloxacin is active vs C. trachomatis and approved for rx. Ciprofloxacin is marginal, not approved. Norfloxacin is not active. If it cannot be determined whether N. gonorrhoeae, C. trachomatis or enterobacteriaceae is involved, ofloxacin provides the broadest coverage. Overall cure rates vs enterobacteriaceae ~80%. Although azithro has some in vitro activity vs E. coli, it is not appropriate for monotherapy. In AIDS patients, the prostate may be a focus of Cryptococcus neoformans despite fluconazole suppression (*AnIM 115:285, 1991*).

See page 96 for abbreviations.

NOTE: All dosage recommendations are for adults (unless otherwise indicated) and assume normal renal function.

CAUSATIVE AGENT/DISEASE	MODIFYING CIRCUMSTANCES	SUGGESTED REGIMENS		COMMENTS
		PRIMARY	ALTERNATIVE	
Bacterial infections/Prostatitis, acute *(continued)*				
Enterobacteriaceae	Age usually >35 years	(Norfloxacin 400 mg bid po) or (Ciprofloxacin 500 mg bid po) or (Ofloxacin 300 mg bid po) for 3–4 wks	TMP/SMX 1 ds bid po for 3–4 weeks. If chronic, rx for 3 months. Another alternative: trovafloxacin 200 mg po qd x28 days	
Rhodococcus equi (Corynebacterium equi)	Pulmonary	Vancomycin 1.0 gm IV q12h + erythromycin 0.5 gm IV q6h ± RIF 600 mg po qd for at least 2–6 months or until afebrile and then oral suppressive regimen *(see Comments)*	[Erythromycin (0.5 gm IV q6h) or imipenem (0.5 gm IV q6h)] + rifampin 600 mg po qd for at least 2 weeks or [ciprofloxacin 750 mg bid po ≥2 weeks]	3/4 pts have positive blood cultures *(Medicine 73:119, 1994)*. Prolonged oral suppressive therapy (macrolide + rifampin) indicated since relapses are frequent. Optimal therapeutic regimen not known.
Salmonella sp.	Bacteremia, recurrent	Ciprofloxacin (CIP) 750 mg po bid x14 days. If relapse occurs, CIP 500 mg po bid indefinitely	If isolates sensitive, ampicillin or trimethoprim/sulfamethoxazole	Norfloxacin, ofloxacin, lomefloxacin, and ceftriaxone are effective in vitro but not approved by FDA for rx of GI infections. Ciprofloxacin-resistant strains of S. typhi have been reported (5% of strains submitted to National Reference Labs UK, 1996).
Shigellosis	Treatment Acute	Ciprofloxacin 500 mg po bid x5–7 days	(TMP/SMX-DS bid po x3 days) or (azithro 500 mg po x1, then 250 mg/d x4 d.)	Norfloxacin, ofloxacin and lomefloxacin are effective in vitro but not approved by FDA for rx of GI infections.
	Recurrent	Ciprofloxacin 500 mg po bid (perhaps 750 mg po qd) indefinitely		
Staphylococcus aureus	Treatment: Folliculitis/furunculosis	Dicloxacillin 500 mg po qid for 7–14 days. If refractory/ recurrent, add rifampin 600 mg po qd	Erythromycin 500 mg po qid for 7–14 days or Mupirocin (Bactroban), apply to affected area tid for 5 days (if infection not disseminated)	
	Bacteremia and/or endocarditis	PRSP [(nafcillin or oxacillin 2.0 gm IV q4h x4 wks) + gentamicin 1.0 mg/kg q8h IV or IM x3–5 days)]	[(Cephalothin 2.0 gm q4h IV or cefazolin 2.0 gm q8h IV) + gentamicin]	In IDUs with right-sided endocarditis, 2 weeks rx with nafcillin/gentamicin is usually adequate *(AnIM 109:619, 1988)*.
	Suppression: Recurrent infections (most likely pt is a nasal carrier)	Mupirocin (Bactroban), apply to nasal vestibule tid x10 days	Dicloxacillin 500 mg qid po + rifampin 600 mg po qd x10 days	Culture nasal vestibule to determine if nasal carrier. Effective vs both MSSA and MRSA.

TABLE 12 (8)

CAUSATIVE AGENT/DISEASE	MODIFYING CIRCUMSTANCES	SUGGESTED REGIMENS		COMMENTS
		PRIMARY	ALTERNATIVE	
Bacterial infections (continued)				
Streptococcus pneumoniae				

Pneumonia—culture and in vitro susceptibility results available	Susceptible or intermediate resistance to pen G in vitro	Ceftriaxone:
		    Over age 50—1 gm IV q24h
		    Under age 50—2 gm IV q24h
		OR
		Penicillin G: 2 million units IV q4h
			Erythromycin 500 mg IV q6h
			OR
			azithromycin 500 mg IV/day
			OR
			clindamycin 600 mg IV q8h
				The prevalence of high-level pen G-resistant S. pneumo continues to increase, with 1997 percentages ranging up to 15%. Resistant strains are often cross-resistant to erythromycin, azithromycin, clarithromycin and cephalosporins. U.S. isolates may or may not be clindamycin-susceptible. β-lactam/β-lactamase inhibitor combinations are not effective, as mechanism of resistance is target change, not β-lactamase production.

	High-level resistance to pen G in vitro	Vancomycin 1.0 gm IV q12h OR levofloxacin 500 mg IV q24h	Trovafloxacin 200 mg IV q24h OR (Grepafloxacin 600 mg **po** q24h or sparfloxacin 200 mg **po** q24h—NOTE: no IV preparations currently available)	Case report of 18-mo.-old with high-level pen G resistant S. pneumo pneumonia developing meningitis during rx with full dose cefotaxime and then cefuroxime; responded to vanco + rifampin (*J Peds 132:174, 1998*).
Meningitis—culture and in vitro susceptibility results available	Susceptible to pen G in vitro	Aq. pen G 4 million units IV q4h OR ceftriaxone 2.0 gm IV q24h STEROIDS ?—*see Comment*	For severe penicillin allergy (IgE-mediated anaphylaxis, angioneurotic edema): Chloramphenicol 12.5 mg/kg q6h IV	**Adjunctive dexamethasone**, 0.4 mg/kg IV q12h x2 days optional: (1) In children, steroids do **not** reduce CSF penetration of vanco. (2) In adults, unclear if steroids ↓ vanco CSF penetration. If steroids used, add rifampin 600 mg/day IV or po.
	Intermediate or high-level resistance to pen G in vitro	Vancomycin 15 mg/kg IV q6–12h (*see Comment*) + ceftriaxone 2.0 gm IV q12h STEROIDS ?—*see Comment*	Meropenem may work—1.0 gm IV q8h. Trovafloxacin under evaluation. Severe penicillin allergy: Vanco + rifampin 600 mg po/IV per day	**Vanco dosage**: Due to low/erratic CSF penetration, recommended dosage in children of 15 mg/kg q6h is double usual dose; little data in adults but reasonable if S. pneumo highly resistant (*PIDJ 16:895, 1997*).

Syphilis (Treponema pallidum)
Reference: MMWR 47:RR-1, 1998
	Primary (chancre), secondary (rash, mucositis, lymphadenopathy), and early latent (<1 year)	Benzathine penicillin G 2.4 mu IM x1. Dose for children: 50,000 units/kg IM up to max. of 2.4 mu	Doxycycline 100 mg po bid x14 days
			or
			Tetracycline 500 mg po qid x14 days.
			
			For failures of initial rx, re-treat with benzathine penicillin G 2.4 mu IM weekly x3.
				If early latent, do CSF VDRL to exclude neurosyphilis.
				  For all stages, penicillin best drug. If penicillin allergy, skin test if available or desensitize and treat with penicillin. Erythromycin not acceptable alternative agent (*CID 20:387, 1995*); use doxycycline if unable to desensitize.
				  Limited data on efficacy of alternative regimens. Need baseline titered VDRL (RPR) and repeat titered serology at 3, 6, 12, 24 months. Repeat rx if (1) persistent clinical signs, (2) titer increases 4-fold or fails to decrease 4-fold after 3–6 months. Even with recommended rx, serologic relapse frequent (*Am J Med 99:55, 1995*).

	Late latent: >1 year duration and negative CSF exam	Benzathine penicillin G 2.4 mu IM q weekly x3 weeks	Doxycycline 100 mg po bid x28 days or Tetracycline 500 mg po qid x28 days	CSF exam mandatory in late latent stage in HIV+ patients.
	Neurosyphilis or optic neuritis	Aqueous penicillin G 18–24 mu IV/day x10–14 days	Procaine pen G 2.4 mu IM qd + probenecid 500 mg po qid x14 days	Again, pen G is best drug. If penicillin allergic, attempt to desensitize and treat. Chloramphenicol should be efficacious but no data. Follow serology titers as above.

See page 96 for abbreviations.   NOTE: All dosage recommendations are for adults (unless otherwise indicated) and assume normal renal function.

TABLE 12 (9)

CAUSATIVE AGENT/DISEASE	MODIFYING CIRCUMSTANCES	SUGGESTED REGIMENS		COMMENTS
		PRIMARY	ALTERNATIVE	
Bacterial infections (*continued*)				
Bacterial vaginosis		Metronidazole 0.5 gm bid po x7 days or metronidazole 2.0 gm po as single dose or metronidazole vaginal gel[1] (0.75%) 1 applicator (5 gm) intravaginally bid x5 days	Clindamycin 0.3 gm bid po x7 days or clindamycin cream (2%) 1 applicator (5 gm) intravaginally hs x7 days	Metronidazole: avoid in 1st trimester of pregnancy. Based on recent analysis, metronidazole 2.0 gm po single dose may be as effective as 5–7 day course (*JAMA 268:92, 1992*). NOTE: Product labeling gives dosage as q6h but CDC 1993 STD Guidelines recommend bid dosage.
Fungal infections				
Aspergillosis	Sinusitis and/or pneumonia	Standard ampho B: rapid ↑ to 1.0–1.5 mg/kg qd IV. No standard total dose. If response, chronic suppression probably necessary: 1.0 mg/kg IV 3x/week	*See footnote[2]* Ampho B lipid complex (ABLC) (Abelcet) or Ampho B cholesteryl complex (Amphotec) or Liposomal ampho B (AmBisome) or Amphotericin colloidal dispersion (ABCD)	No proven regimen in AIDS pts. Itraconazole reported to fail in 16/16 AIDS pts (*Am J Med 97:135, 1994*). Voriconazole 200 mg q12h po showing promise in clinical trials (Pfizer).
Blastomycosis		Amphotericin B 0.5–1.0 mg/kg IV until evidence of response, then itraconazole 200 mg/d po with breakfast or if pt not severely ill, start with itraconazole 200 mg/day po with breakfast	Limited data with lipid preparations of ampho B	In HIV– pt, itraconazole is drug of choice (*Am J Med 93:489, 1992*). Experience in HIV+ pts is limited, hence more traditional regimen is recommended. Should give itra with food or acidic cola to increase absorption.
Candidiasis (Good general review: CID 26:259, 1998)	Primary prophylaxis	*See Table 8, page 35*		
	Candidemia, hepatosplenic candidiasis, endocarditis	Ampho B 0.6–1.0 mg/kg/d IV x7 days followed by 0.8–1.2 mg/kg qod IV until definite evidence of resolution. Most pts should receive 0.5–1.0 gm total dose (*CTID 14:S106, 1992*).	Fluconazole (not for endophthalmitis) 400 mg IV x7 d., then po x14 d. after last positive blood culture. Another flucon regimen: 600–800 mg IV x3 d., then 400 mg po x14 d. [*CID 22(S2):S95, 1996*].	Ampho B lipid complex successful in pts who failed standard ampho B: 5 mg/kg/d (up to total 1.1 gm) (*CID 21:1184, 1995*). Some failure pts treated with combination of ampho B + fluconazole (*AAC 39:1907, 1995*). Ampho B colloidal dispersion (ABCD) effective in non-AIDS immunocompromised pts. (*CID 26:461, 1998*).
	Esophagitis—fluconazole-sensitive	Fluconazole 200 mg po x1, then 100 mg qd x ≥3 weeks (or 2 weeks after symptoms resolve) OR Itraconazole oral solution 100 mg po qd x ≥3 weeks	Ampho B 0.3–0.5 mg/kg/d IV. Lipid preparations of ampho B should work but no data in AIDS.	Chronic suppression pros and cons discussed under post-treatment chronic suppression. Clinical failure may be due to unrecognized concomitant H. simplex esophagitis. Flu had similar results to itra in 2 studies (*JID 176:227, 1997; CID 24:1204, 1997*).
	Esophagitis—fluconazole-resistant	Ampho B 0.3 mg/kg/d IV	Can try itraconazole oral solution 100–200 mg po daily or Lipid preparation of ampho B	Fluconazole use likely a factor in emergence of resistant candida and ↑ in non-albicans species resistant to azoles but issue still debated (*CID 24:1129, 1997*).

[1] Each 5 gm of gel contains 37.5 mg of metronidazole

[2] May be as effective and less nephrotoxic than standard ampho B **but much more expensive**. Dosages: ABLC 5.0 mg/kg/d IV over 2 hrs; Ampho B cholesteryl complex 3–4 mg/kg/d IV given as 1 mg/kg/hr; Liposomal ampho B 3–5 mg/kg/d IV given over 1–2 hrs; ABCD 2–4 mg/kg/d IV [doses up to 8 mg/kg/d have been given to bone marrow transplant recipients (*CID 24:636, 1997*)

See page 96 for abbreviations.   NOTE: All dosage recommendations are for adults (unless otherwise indicated) and assume normal renal function.

TABLE 12 (10)

CAUSATIVE AGENT/DISEASE	MODIFYING CIRCUMSTANCES	SUGGESTED REGIMENS		COMMENTS
		PRIMARY	ALTERNATIVE	
Fungal infections (continued)				
Candidiasis (continued)	Stomatitis—fluconazole-sensitive (if initial infection, assume sensitive)	Fluconazole 200 mg 1st dose and then 100 mg po qd x14 days or Itraconazole oral solution 200 mg po qd or 100 mg po bid for 7–14 days Then consider chronic suppression (see Comment)	Nystatin solution or tablets (vaginal pastilles) 500,000 to 1,000,000 u po 3–5x/day for 3–5 days or Clotrimazole troches 10 mg po 5x/day for 3–5 days Then consider chronic suppression	With flucon, symptoms ↓ in several days, rx longer to ↓ relapse. Advantage of chronic suppression with fluconazole is prevention of cryptococcal disease, esophageal candidiasis, and perhaps other fluconazole-susceptible fungal infections. Concern with chronic suppression is promoting fluconazole-resistant Candida species. See below for chronic suppression regimen. Flu had similar results to itra in 3 studies (JID 176:227, 1997; CID 24:1204, 1997; AJM 104:33, 1998)). Itra oral solution superior to tablets in controlled study (J Clin Path 50:477, 1997). Fluconazole 100 mg po qd superior to liquid nystatin (500,000 u 4x/day in controlled study (CID 24:1204, 1997).
	Stomatitis—fluconazole-resistant Usually C. albicans with acquired resistance. C. krusei, C. (Torulopsis) glabrata intrinsically resistant	Itraconazole oral solution 100 mg bid (approx. 55% response). For failures— 1. Nystatin pastilles 1–2 po 4x/d. or 2. Ampho B oral suspension, 100 mg po qid	Can try vaginal nystatin tablets, 100,000 units each. Dissolve in mouth tid or Unresponsive cases may require IV ampho B.	Fluconazole resistance ↑ with multiple episodes, lower CD4, longer duration of rx, use of systemic azoles (JID 173:219, 1996). Also ↑ with weekly vs daily doses (3rd CRV, 1996). Some fluconazole-resistant strains are susceptible to itra or keto. Fluconazole-resistant C. glabrata & C. krusei in 19% of AIDS pts (J Clin Micro 32:2092, 1994). 1 report documents clinical failure with emergence of resistance to fluconazole, itra, flucytosine and amphotericin associated with extensive use of all 4 drugs (CID 26:183, 1998). Nystatin pastilles have bitter taste.
	Vaginitis—fluconazole-sensitive	Fluconazole 150 mg po x1 dose (Some authorities recommend 200 mg po 1st day, then 100 mg po qd until improvement, 3–5 days)	Miconazole vaginal tablets 1 qd hs x3 days or cream (2%) qd hs x7 days or Clotrimazole cream (1%) qd hs x7 d. or 100 mg vaginal tablet, 2 tabs qd hs x3 d.	Miconazole and clotrimazole cream and 100 mg troches available without prescription. Relapse common. See Stomatitis, above, for pros and cons of chronic suppression. Chronic suppression regimen below. (See NEJM 337:1896, 1997)
	Vaginitis—fluconazole-resistant	Ampho B 0.3–0.5 mg/kg/d IV. Ampho B lipid complex should work—no data	None at present. Can try itraconazole or ketoconazole but most strains cross-resistant.	Reference: CID 22:726, 1991
	Post-treatment chronic suppression (secondary prophylaxis) for oral, esophageal, vaginal infection)	Fluconazole: Recommendations vary from 100 mg po qd to 100–150 mg po q week to rx of only clinically significant disease.	If fluconazole-resistant, i.e., failed flu suppression, may be forced to continue ampho B (0.3 mg/kg IV qd or 1 mg/kg IV q week)	Advantages: Prolonged chronic suppression of candida and reduced risk of cryptococcal infection (NEJM 332:700, 1995). Disadvantages: Theoretic concern of enhanced risk of emergence of fluconazole (azole)-resistant Candida species.
Coccidioidomycosis	Primary prophylaxis	Not recommended for most pts, consider for pts from endemic area with CD4 <50/μl. Primary fluconazole 200 mg po qd, alternative itraconazole 200 mg po qd. Risk in HIV+ ↑ (Am J Med 94:235, 1993) (Table 8).		

See page 96 for abbreviations.　　　　NOTE: All dosage recommendations are for adults (unless otherwise indicated) and assume normal renal function.

TABLE 12 (11)

CAUSATIVE AGENT/DISEASE	MODIFYING CIRCUMSTANCES	SUGGESTED REGIMENS		COMMENTS
		PRIMARY	ALTERNATIVE	
Fungal infections/Coccidioidomycosis *(continued)*				
Pulmonary and extra-pulmonary (not meningitis)	Treatment	Approaches to rx vary: Fluconazole 400–800 mg po qd for ≥9 months OR Itraconazole 200 mg bid po OR Ampho B 0.5–1.0 mg/kg/d IV x7 d., then 0.8 mg/kg IV qod. Total dose ≥2.5 gm. No data on lipid ampho B preps, but they should be efficacious.		Lung infection in 80% of pts. Despite rx with ampho B ± subsequent po azole, mortality reported as 60% *(CID 23: 563, 1996)*. ↑ number of cases in Arizona since 1990 (250 cases), 600 cases in 1995 *(MMWR 45:1069, 1997)*. Relapses in roughly 25% of pts. *See post-rx suppression, below.*
Meningitis	Treatment	Fluconazole 400–800 mg qd po OR [IV amphotericin B as for pulmonary + 0.1–0.3 mg daily intrathecal (intra-ventricular via reservoir device)]	Lipid ampho B preps should substitute for standard IV ampho B but no data	*CID 13:S100, 1992.*
	Suppression	Fluconazole 400 mg/day po as single dose or 200 mg po bid	Amphotericin B 1.0 mg/kg once/week IV or itraconazole 200 mg bid po (not for meningitis; does not penetrate CSF) *(AnIM 120:932, 1994)*	Relapses are common in both HIV+ and HIV– pts *(AnIM 124:305, 1996)*. Lifelong suppression indicated.
Cryptococcosis	Primary prophylaxis	Authors do not recommend primary prophylaxis. If fluconazole used for primary prophylaxis or chronic suppression of candida, risk of cryptococcosis reduced *(NEJM 332:700, 1995) (Table 8)*.		
Cryptococcemia* and/or Meningitis * Cryptococci in blood may be manifest by positive blood culture or positive test of serum for cryptococcal antigen	Treatment	Amphotericin B (initial rx) with flucon-azole completion rx.: • Ampho B: 0.7–1.0 mg/kg/d IV until afebrile, headache, nausea and vomiting gone. • Then dc ampho B, start flucon 400 mg po qd to complete 8–10 week course. • Then maintain on flucon 200 mg po qd indefinitely. If ampho B only, total dose 2.5 gm. *(NEJM 337:15, 1997)*	Fluconazole 400 mg po qd x6–10 weeks, then suppressive rx or Some authorities would use ampho B + flucytosine[1] 25 mg/kg q6h po until patient afebrile and cultures negative (~6 wks). or Ampho B lipid complex 5 mg/kg/d x2 wks and then 3x/wk x4 wks *(CID 22:315, 1996)*. Role of other lipid preps under evaluation *(AIDS 11:1463, 1997)*.	If normal mental status, >20 cells/mm³ CSF, and CSF crypto antigen <1:1024, fluconazole alone is reasonable *(CID 22:322, 1996)*. Serum cryptococcal antigen useful in dx (95% sens.); no help in monitoring therapy. If ↑ CSF pressure, lower with CSF removal. Lumbar drains or V-P shunts have been used to control persistent ↑ CSF pressure *(see Table 9A)*. No data on steroids. Must monitor 5-FC levels: peak 70–80 mg/L, trough 30–40 mg/L. No itraconazole. Does not penetrate CSF. *(Recent reference: CID 22:329, 1996)*
			Fluconazole 400 mg po qd + flucytosine 37.5 mg/kg q6h po x10 weeks	At 10 weeks, clinical success with flucon + flucyt 63% (median time to sterile cultures 23 d.) vs ~35% fluconazole or ~40% ampho B alone *(CID 19:741, 1994)*. With lower dose (200 mg tid) ZDV, flucytosine hematotoxicity is less of a problem than with higher dosages.
	Suppression	Fluconazole 200 mg/d po indefinitely (lifetime)	Ampho B 0.5–1.0 mg/kg IV 1x/week	Itraconazole probably not as effective as fluconazole. ACTG 159 trial discontinued itraconazole.
Fusariosis		Amphotericin B (dosage as in coccidioidomycosis)		Clinical: Focal, sometimes blackened skin lesions, fungemia. Ampho B occasionally effective, but mortality ~75%.
Histoplasmosis	Primary prophylaxis	Not recommended for most pts, consider for pts from endemic area with CD4 <50/µl. If used: primary itraconazole 200 mg po qd, alternative fluconazole 200 mg po qd *(Table 8B)*..		

[1] Flucytosine = 5-FC

See page 96 for abbreviations.

NOTE: All dosage recommendations are for adults (unless otherwise indicated) and assume normal renal function.

TABLE 12 (12)

CAUSATIVE AGENT/DISEASE	MODIFYING CIRCUMSTANCES	SUGGESTED REGIMENS		COMMENTS
		PRIMARY	ALTERNATIVE	
Fungal infections (continued)				
Histoplasmosis (continued)	Treatment (see Comment)	Amphotericin B 0.5–1.0 mg/kg/d IV x7 d., then 0.8 mg/kg qod (or 3x/wk) IV to total dose of 10–15 mg/kg and then suppressive rx	• Itraconazole: 300 mg po bid x3 d, then 200 mg po bid for 12 weeks or 400 mg qd x12 wks (85–90% response) and then chronic suppression. • Fluconazole: 800 mg qd (400 mg bid) for 12 wks (36/49 or 74% with mild to moderate disease responded (AJM 103:223, 1997) (3rd best)	Ampho B for severe infection; itra for less severe cases. Do not use itra in pts with meningitis; itra does not achieve adequate CSF concentrations. Don't need food or acidic cola for itra if new oral solution used instead of capsules. See drug-drug interactions with azole antifungals, especially rifamycins, Table 17.
	Suppression	Itraconazole 200 mg po qd indefinitely	Amphotericin B 1.0 mg/kg IV weekly or biweekly indefinitely (lifetime)	10–20% relapses with ampho B, 60% with ketoconazole. Itraconazole: 2/42 (5%) pts relapsed with median follow-up 2 yrs (AnIM 118:610, 1993) & 2/46 with median follow-up 87 wks (J AIDS & HR 16:100, 1997).
Penicillium marneffei	Treatment	Ampho B 0.5–1.0 mg/kg/d x2 wks, then itra 200–400 mg/d x6 wks and then chronic itra suppression at 200 mg/d	Itraconazole 200 mg po tid x3 days, then 200 mg bid po x12 weeks, then 200 mg po qd	16 of 21 pts responded to ampho B, 6 of 7 to itra (J AIDS 6:466, 1993). Resistance to ampho B, flucon, sensitivity to itra reported (CID 15:744, 1992; AAC 37:2407, 1993). Prolonged suppressive rx probably required (CID 23:125, 1996—review of 155 pts).
Sporotrichosis—Extracutaneous	Treatment	Amphotericin B 0.5–0.6 mg/kg qd IV x2 weeks, then 0.8 mg/kg qod. Total dose 1.5 gm	Itraconazole 300 mg po bid x6 months; then 200 mg po bid (CID 17:210, 1993)	It is not clear whether or not post-treatment suppressive rx is needed.
Trichosporon beigelii, Scedosporium inflatum	Treatment	Not defined; usually resistant to ampho B and azoles. Case reports responding to ampho B + flucytosine or itra. Surgical excision if possible.		
Parasitic infections				
Protozoan—Intestinal				
Blastocystis hominis	Role as pathogen controversial. No controlled rx trials.	Can eliminate with TMP/SMX (Ln 339:428, 1992) or iodoquinol 650 mg po tid x20 d. (Adv Parasit 32:2, 1993). Metronidazole also suggested, 750 mg po tid x10 days.		
Cryptosporidium parvum	No therapy proven efficacious. Self-limited in immunocompetent pts. Chronic diarrhea in AIDS pts. EID 3:51, 1997	Can try paromomycin 500–750 mg tid or qid. Others suggest 1.0 gm po bid.1.0 gm po bid Modify paromomycin as required	Azithro 1200 mg po bid x1 d. then 1200 mg/d x27 d. then 600 mg/d suppressive. For lactose-free azithro, contact Pfizer: (203) 441-6148.	Nitrazoxamide under investigation (Unimed Pharmaceuticals). Supplemental benefit from Imodium, diphenoxylate, or tincture of opium (may need in combination). Octreotide (Sandostatin) may help, but expensive.
Cyclospora cayetanesis		Immunocompetent pts: TMP/SMX-DS tab 1 po bid x7 d.	AIDS pts: TMP/SMX-DS 1 po qid x10 d.; then tab 1 po 3x/wk.	Refs.: Ln 345:691, 1995; AnIM 121:654, 1994
Entamoeba histolytica	Asymptomatic cyst passer	Paromomycin (aminosidine in U.K.) 500 mg po tid x7 d. OR iodoquinol (Yodoxin) 650 mg po tid x20 d.	Diloxanide furoate[NUS] (Furosemide) 500 mg po tid x10 d.	Metronidazole not effective vs cysts.

See page 96 for abbreviations.

NOTE: All dosage recommendations are for adults (unless otherwise indicated) and assume normal renal function.

TABLE 12 (13)

CAUSATIVE AGENT/DISEASE	MODIFYING CIRCUMSTANCES	SUGGESTED REGIMENS		COMMENTS
		PRIMARY	ALTERNATIVE	
Parasitic infections — Protozoan infections — intestinal *(continued)*				
Entamoeba histolytica *(continued)*	Patient with diarrhea/dysentery	Metronidazole 750 mg po tid x10 d followed by: Either [iodoquinol (was diiodohydroxyquin) 650 mg po tid x20 d.] or [paromomycin 500 mg po tid x7 d.]	(Tinidazole[NUS] 1.0 gm po q12h x3 d.) or (ornidazole[NUS] 500 mg po q12h x5 d.) followed by:	Drug side-effects in Table 13, page 102. Colitis can mimic ulcerative colitis; ameboma can mimic adenocarcinoma of colon. Dx: trophs or cysts in stool. Watch out for non-pathogenic but morphologically identical E. dispar *(CID 20:1453, 1995)*.
	Extraintestinal infection, e.g., hepatic abscess	Metronidazole 750 mg IV/po tid x10 d. followed by iodoquinol 650 mg po tid x20 d. Outside U.S., may substitute tinidazole (600 mg bid or 800 mg tid) po x5 d. for metro.		Serology positive with extraintestinal disease
Giardia lamblia *Ref.: CID 25:545, 1997*		Metronidazole 250 mg po tid x5 d. OR albendazole 400 mg po qd x5 d.	(Tinidazole[NUS] 2.0 gm po x1) OR (quinacrine[NUS] 100 mg po tid after meals x5 d.)	Treat asymptomatic cyst passers. Dx: detect antigen in stool.
Isospora belli		TMP/SMX-DS tab 1 po qid x10 d., then bid x3 weeks	(Pyrimethamine 75 mg/d po + folinic acid 10 mg/d po) x14 d.	Chronic suppression in AIDS pts; either 1 TMP/SMX-DS tab 3x/wk OR (pyrimethamine 25 mg/d po + folinic acid 5 mg/d po)
Microsporidia (5 species, pathogenic)		There is no standard treatment. Suggestions for therapy derived from in vitro data and reported clinical experience with small numbers of patients.		Can be detected by light microscopy in stool specimens with modified trichrome stain *(NEJM 326:161, 1992)*. Metronidazole (500 mg po bid) diarrhea ↓ in 10/19 pts, 0 cleared.
Enterocytozoon bieneusi and Encephalitozoon (Septata) intestinalis	Treatment	Albendazole 400 mg po bid *(CID 21:70, 1995)* and then chronic suppression	Atovaquone 750 mg tid *(AIDS 10:619, 1996)* and then chronic suppression	Of 10 pts rx with albendazole: 3 rapid response, 4 no response. Nutritional therapy (low-fat, low-residue diet with simple carbohydrates), 8/9 pts had ↓ stool volume and frequency *(CID 18: 819, 1994; J Inf Dis 169:178, 1994)*. Atovaquone: 8/8 improved, stools ↓ from 10 to 3/d, weight gain avg. 9.5 lbs, but organisms not eradicated.
Encephalitozoon hellum	Treatment	Not established—see *Comments*	Albendazole, itraconazole, fluconazole reported to have efficacy in single case reports *(J Infect 27:229, 1993)*. Ocular lesions have responded to fumagillin eye-drops *(Am J. Ophth 115:293, 1993; ID Clin NA 8:483, 1994)*.	
Parasitic Infections – Protozoan – Extraintestinal				
Babesiosis (B. microti) *Ref.: CID 22:611, 1996*	Treatment	Clindamycin 600 mg po tid x7 d. + quinine 650 mg po tid x7 d.. Exchange transfusion if >10% parasitemia and hemolysis.	Pentamidine effective in hamsters, no human data.	Long-term suppressive rx probably indicated: clindamycin + doxycycline + azithromycin (2.0 gm po qd) has been used *(CID 22:809, 1996)*.
Pneumocystis carinii pneumonia (PCP)	**Not acutely ill,** able to take po meds. PaO₂ >70 mmHg	(Dapsone 100 mg po qd + TMP 5 mg/kg po tid x21 d.) OR (TMP/SMX-DS, 2 tabs po q8h x21 d.) NOTE: Concomitant use of corticosteroids usually reserved for sicker pts with PaO₂ <70 *(see below)*	[(Clindamycin (600 mg IV or 300–450 mg po) q8h + primaquine 15 mg base po qd] x21 d. OR atovaquone suspension 750 mg po bid with food x21 d.	DAP/TMP, TMP/SMX, clinda/prima regimens equally effective. Rash/fever 10% with DAP/TMP, 19% with TMP/SMX, 21% with clinda/prima. **After 21 days, chronic suppression in AIDS pts (see below)**.

See page 96 for abbreviations.   NOTE: All dosage recommendations are for adults (unless otherwise indicated) and assume normal renal function.

TABLE 12 (14)

CAUSATIVE AGENT/DISEASE	MODIFYING CIRCUMSTANCES	SUGGESTED REGIMENS		COMMENTS
		PRIMARY	ALTERNATIVE	
Parasitic Infections – Protozoan – Extraintestinal *(continued)*				
Pneumocystis carinii pneumonia (PCP) *(con't)*	**Acutely ill,** po rx not possible. PaO₂ <70 mmHg	[Prednisone 15–30 min. before TMP/SMX—start with 40 mg po bid x5 d., then 40 mg qd x5 d., then 20 mg po qd x11 d.] + [TMP/SMX (15 mg of TMP component/kg/d) IV div. q6–8h x21 d.]	Prednisone as in primary rx PLUS [(Clinda 900 mg IV q8h) + (primaquine 15 mg base po qd)] x21 d. OR Pentamidine 4 mg/kg/d IV x21 d.	**Trimetrexate another alternative:** 45 mg/M² IV (over 60–90 min) qd x21 days + leucovorin (folinic acid) 20 mg/M² IV q6h x24 days (continue 3 days after trimetrexate). After 21 days, chronic suppression *(see below)*. PCP can occur in absence of HIV infection and steroids *(CID 25:215 & 219, 1997)*.
		Can substitute IV prednisolone (reduce dose 25%) for po prednisone		
	Primary prophylaxis and post-treatment suppression *Ref.: CID 25(Suppl.3): S299, 1997*	(TMP/SMX-DS, 1 tab po qd or 3x/wk) OR (dapsone 100 mg po qd) OR (TMP/SMX-SS, 1 tab po qd)	(Pentamidine 300 mg in 6 ml sterile water by aerosol q4 wks) OR (dapsone 200 mg po + pyrimethamine 75 mg po + folinic acid 25 mg po—all once a week)	TMP/SMX-DS regimen also provides cross-protection vs toxo and other bacterial infections. Dapsone + pyrimethamine protects vs toxo. Atovaquone suspension 1500 mg once daily also appears effective.
Toxoplasma gondii (Reference: Remington and McLeod in Infectious Diseases, Gorbach et al., Eds., 2nd Ed., 1997, pp 1620–40)				
Immunologically normal patients *(For pediatric doses, see reference)*				
	Acute illness with lymphadenopathy	No specific rx unless severe/persistent symptoms or evidence of vital organ damage		
	Acquired via transfusion (lab accident)	Treat as for active chorioretinitis		
	Active chorioretinitis; meningitis; lowered resistance due to steroids or cytotoxic drugs	[Pyrimethamine (pyri) 50–100 mg po bid on 1st day, then 25 mg qd] + [sulfadiazine (see footnote[1]) 1–1.5 gm po qid] + leucovorin (folinic acid) 10 mg or more/day]—see *Comment*. Treat 1–2 wks beyond resolution of signs/symptoms; continue leucovorin 1 wk after stopping pyri.		For congenital toxo, toxo meningitis in adults, and chorioretinitis, add prednisone 1 mg/kg/d in 2 div. doses until CSF protein conc. falls or vision-threatening inflammation has subsided. Adjust folinic acid dose by following CBC results.
	Pregnancy—1st 18 weeks of gestation, or to term if fetus not infected	Spiramycin [From FDA, call (301) 443-5680] 1.0 gm po q8h		For fetal infection after week 17 or late maternal infection—*see reference for details.*
Acquired immunodeficiency syndrome (AIDS)				
	Cerebral toxoplasmosis *Ref.: See Remington & McLeod ref., above*	Pyrimethamine (pyri) 200 mg x1 po, then 75–100 mg/d po] + (sulfadiazine 1–1.5 gm po q6h) + (folinic acid 10–15 mg/d po) x3–6 wks and then suppressive rx *(see below)*	[Pyri + folinic acid (as in primary regimen)] + 1 of the following: (1) Clinda 600 mg po/IV q6h or (2) clarithro 1.0 gm po bid or (3) azithro 1.2–1.5 gm po qd or (4) dapsone 100 mg po qd. Treat 3–6 wks, then suppression	Use alternative regimen for pts with severe sulfa allergy. If multiple ring-enhancing brain lesions (CT or MRI), >85% of pts respond to 7–10 days of empiric rx; if no response, suggest brain biopsy. IgG toxo antibody positive in approx. 84% *(NEJM 327: 1643, 1992)*.
	Primary prophylaxis, AIDS pts—IgG toxo antibody + CD4 count <100/μl	(TMP/SMX-DS, 1 tab po qd) or (TMP/SMX-SS, 1 tab po qd)	(Dapsone 50 mg po qd) + (pyri 50 mg po q week) + (folinic acid 25 mg po q week)	Prophylaxis for pneumocystis also effective vs toxo. Refs.: *CID 25(Suppl.3):S299, 1997; Amer Fam Phys 56:1387, 1997)*
	Suppression after rx of cerebral toxo	(Sulfadiazine 500–1000 mg po 4x/d) + (pyri 25–50 mg po qd) + (folinic acid 10–25 mg po qd)	(Clinda 300–450 mg po q6–8h) + (pyri 25–75 mg po qd) + (folinic acid 10–25 mg po qd)	(Pyri + sulfa) prevents PCP and toxo; (clinda + pyri) prevents toxo only.

[1] Sulfonamides for toxo. Sulfadiazine now commercially available. Sulfapyrazine, sulfamethazine, and sulfamerazine about as effective as sulfadiazine; other sulfas tested (sulfathiazole, sulfapyridine, sulfadimetine, and sulfisoxazole) much less effective.

See page 96 for abbreviations.   NOTE: All dosage recommendations are for adults (unless otherwise indicated) and assume normal renal function.

CAUSATIVE AGENT/DISEASE	MODIFYING CIRCUMSTANCES	SUGGESTED REGIMENS		COMMENTS
		PRIMARY	ALTERNATIVE	
Parasitic Infections—Protozoan—Extraintestinal (continued)				
Vaginitis—*MMWR 47:RR-1, 1998*				
Candidiasis, vulvo-vaginal Pruritus, thick cheesy discharge, pH <4.5	Candida sp.	Fluconazole 150 mg single dose po or intravaginal: miconazole or clotri-mazole or butoconazole or tiocona-zole or terconazole	Nystatin, intravaginal	Intravaginal azoles available both OTC and by prescription; duration of rx ranges from single dose to 1, 3, or 7 days. Uncomplicated disease in normal host responds well to any azoles. Complicated candidiasis in abnormal host (diabetes, AIDS, resistant candida), treat for 10–14 days. *Also see pages 85 & 86.*
Trichomoniasis Copious foamy dis-charge, pH >4.5	Trichomonas vaginalis	Metronidazole (2.0 gm as single dose) (contraindicated in 1st trimester of pregnancy)	Metronidazole 500 mg bid po x7 days	Treat male sexual partners (2.0 gm as single dose). Repeat-ed failure: metro 2.0 gm single dose po qd x5 d. Resistance to metronidazole/tinidazole rare but occurs (*Ln 346:1110, 1995*). Case report of successful rx of resistant trich. with 250 mg of paromomycin in cream intravaginally once daily x14 d. (*Ln 346:1110, 1995*).
Nematode infections				
Strongyloides sterco-ralis (strongyloidiasis)		Ivermectin 200 μg/kg po qd x1–2 d. or Albendazole 400 mg po qd x3 days	Thiabendazole (Mintezol) 25 mg/kg (maximum 1.5 gm) po q12h x2 d. or 7–10 d. for hyperinfection syndrome	Retreatment often required. Failures occur with standard thiabendazole (*Chest 104:119, 1993*). Albendazole is better tolerated than thiabendazole. Long-term suppressive rx likely to be necessary. Response to ivermectin in 7/7 with remissions ≥7 months (*CID 17:900, 1993*).
Ectoparasites				
Pediculus humanus corporis (body lice)		Treat the clothing. Organism lives in, deposits eggs in seams of clothing. Discard clothing; if not possible, treat clothing with 1% malathion powder or 10% DDT powder.	Body louse leaves clothing only for blood meal. Nits in clothing viable for 1 month. Ref.: *Med Lett 38:6, 1997.*	
P. humanus var. capitis (head louse, nits) **Phthirus pubis (crabs)**		Permethrin, 5% prescription strength (ELIMITE) or 1% non-prescription (Nix). Wash hair, apply lotion for 10 min., then rinse off, comb; 2nd treatment 7–10 days after 1st to kill newly hatched lice (all products). Lindane (Kwell) 1%, less effective (use only if failed other therapy). Seizures can occur from coverage of broad areas or ingestion. Pyrethrin (RID) over-the-counter.	Benefit of residual permethrin on hair reduced by shampoos or vinegar. No residual effect with lindane or pyrethrin products. Nit removal important adjunct. Use nit comb ± enzymatic egg remover (CLEAR is one example). Treat sex partners if body or pubic lice. Cost: Permethrin 60 gm $18.10; lindane 60 ml $2.60–10.50; pyrethrin 60 ml $6.11.	
Sarcoptes scabiei (scabies, mites)	Immunocompetent patients	Primary: Permethrin 5% cream (Elimite). Apply to entire skin from chin to toes. Leave on 8–10 hrs. repeat in 1 week. Alternative: Lindane 1% lotion. Apply as for permethrin OR ivermectin 200 μg/kg po x1 (*NEJM 333:26, 1995*)	Trim fingernails. Reapply to hands after handwashing. Pruritus may persist x2 wks after mites gone. Do not use lindane in pregnancy or in young children—absorbed through skin; can use 6–10% precipitated sulfur in petrolatum daily x3 d.	
	AIDS patients, CD4 <150/mm³ (Norwegian scabies—*see Comments*)	For Norwegian scabies: Permethrin as above on day 1, then 6% sulfur in petrolatum daily on days 2–7, then repeat x several weeks.	Norwegian scabies in AIDS pts: Extensive, crusted. Can mimic psoriasis. Not pruritic. ELIMITE: 60 gm $18.10; lindane 60 ml $2.60–10.50. **Highly contagious—isolate!**	

See page 96 for abbreviations.   NOTE: All dosage recommendations are for adults (unless otherwise indicated) and assume normal renal function.

TABLE 12 (16)

CAUSATIVE AGENT/DISEASE	MODIFYING CIRCUMSTANCES	SUGGESTED REGIMENS		COMMENTS
		PRIMARY	ALTERNATIVE	
Viral infections				
Cytomegalovirus (CMV) Marked ↓ in CMV infections with Highly Active Antiretroviral Rx *(5th CRV, Abst 184)*	Primary prophylaxis (CD4 <50 or CD4 <100 + previous OI) (IDSA recommends "for consideration" in all pts *(Table 8)*	None—see *Comment*	Ganciclovir (GCV) 1.0 gm po tid with food (fatty). (Syntex 1654 study showed 49% ↓ CMV retinitis *(NEJM 334:1491, 1997)* but CPCRA 023 did not find significant reduction but did show 25% neutropenia). See *Comment*	Authors do not recommend primary prophylaxis with po GCV because: (1) Initial retinitis peripheral and rarely sight-threatening, (2) low serum levels may promote GCV resistance, (3) expense (~$16,000/yr), (4) limited data on efficacy as prophylactic drug [less cost effective than other prevention strategies in HIV *(J AIDS & HR 16:15, 1997)*]. CMV encephalitis may occur in pts on oral GCV treatment.
Colitis, esophagitis	Treatment	Foscarnet: *see retinitis for dosage* Ganciclovir: *see retinitis for dosage*		If renal disease, prefer GCV; if bone marrow suppression, prefer FOS. bid foscarnet 90 mg IV effective in 9/10 with GI CMV infections *(AAC 41:1226, 1997)*. Value of chronic suppression documented only for retinitis but reasonable for esophagitis, colitis, hepatitis, neuritis/encephalitis—should also serve to ↓ risk of retinitis.
Encephalitis and ventriculoencephalitis	Treatment	Not defined. May occur in pts on GCV suppression. A combination of foscarnet 90 mg IV bid and ganciclovir 5 mg IV bid was effective in stabilizing or improving symptoms in 74% of cases *(5th CRV, Abst. 263)*.		
Hepatitis		Efficacy of agents not established		
Lumbosacral polyradiculopathy/myelitis	Treatment	Ganciclovir *(as with retinitis)*	Foscarnet, but clinical data lacking	Reports on 21 rx pts, neurologic stabilization or functional improvement in ½. Improvement sometimes delayed (several months) *(CID 20:747, 1995)*.
Mononeuritis multiplex	Treatment	Not defined		Due to necrotizing vasculitis of epineural arteries *(Ann Neurol 29:139, 1991)*, hence may not respond to rx.
Pneumonia (+ lung biopsy) *(See Table 9, page 64)*	Treatment—See *Comment for criteria for diagnosis*	If CMV diagnosis firm: Use induction doses of IV ganciclovir or IV foscarnet as used for CMV retinitis.		Criteria for diagnosis: CMV isolated from bronchial brush or BAL, histopathology consistent with CMV. Most pts have CD4 <60 and documented extrapulmonary CMV (e.g., retinitis). Blood and urine CMV cultures not helpful *(CID 23:76, 1996)*. In transplant pts with CMV, success reported with combination of GCV + IV immune globulin *(NEJM 324:1005,1991)*. 11/16 with AIDS showed initial improvement with either ganciclovir or foscarnet but disease eventually progressed despite maintenance *(CID 23:76, 1996)*.

See page 96 for abbreviations.   NOTE: All dosage recommendations are for adults (unless otherwise indicated) and assume normal renal function.

TABLE 12 (17)

CAUSATIVE AGENT/DISEASE	MODIFYING CIRCUMSTANCES	SUGGESTED REGIMENS		COMMENTS
		PRIMARY	ALTERNATIVE	
Iral infections/Cytomegalovirus *(continued)*				
Retinitis While vast majority of pts have <50 CD4/mm^3 several pts now reported who developed recurrent retinitis when CD4 rose to >200 following response to HAART	Treatment: Induction therapy *For chronic suppression (maintenance therapy), see below*	Ganciclovir (GCV): 5.0 mg/kg IV (at constant rate over 1 hr) q12h x14–21 days OR Foscarnet (FOS): 60 mg/kg (adjusted for renal function) IV at constant rate (requires infusion pump) over minimum of 1 hr q8h (or 90 mg/kg q12h) x14–21 days OR Combination of intraocular ganciclovir (GCV) implant (delivers 1–2 μg/hr x6–7 mos.) + (either concomitant IV GCV as above or oral GCV 1.0 gm tid)	Cidofovir 5 mg/kg IV q week x2 wks with probenecid (2 gm po 3 hrs before cidofovir dose, 1 gm 2 hrs immediately after dose, and 1 gm 8 hrs after dose) and 1 liter of normal saline IV 1 hr before cidofovir infusion *(AnIM 126:257 & 264, 1997)* OR For pts who fail monotherapy with GCV or FOS, consider combination therapy with both: (GCV 5 mg/kg q12h IV) and (FOS as either 60 mg/kg q8h or 90 mg/kg q12h)	Comprehensive reviews of many important clinical issues: *J AIDS & HR 14(Suppl. 1), 1997* and *Arch Ophthal 114:863, 1996.* 4 pts reported who developed retinal inflammatory response to HAART (2–16 weeks after ↑ CD4 >200) including painless vitreitis and macular edema associated with vision loss. Corticosteroid rx ↓ inflammatory reaction without reactivation of CMV retinitis *(5th CRV, Abst. 751) (Table 9B).* Differential dx: HIV retinopathy, herpes simplex retinitis *(Arch Ophthal 114:834, 1996),* varicella-zoster retinitis (rare, hard to diagnose). Cannot use GCV ocular implant alone as approx. 50% risk of CMV retinitis other eye at 6 mos. & 31% risk visceral disease *(Arch Ophthal 12:153, 1994).* Risk ↓ with systemic rx *(CID 24:620, 1997; NEJM 337:83, 1997).* Watch for retinal detachments; 50–60% within 1 yr of dx of retinitis. Equal efficacy of IV GCV and FOS. FOS rx takes more time due to saline hydration. GCV avoids nephrotoxicity of FOS; FOS avoids bone marrow suppression of GCV.
	Suppression (maintenance therapy). May be indefinite but with immune reconstitution (response to HAART) some authorities now discontinuing suppression	GCV 5 mg/kg IV qd or 6 mg/kg IV qd 5 days/week OR FOS 90–120 mg/kg/day IV with hydration and dose adjusted for renal function (NOTE: oral and IV hydration found equally effective: 1700 ml/day. *Abst 298 from 4th Conf. on Retroviruses, 1997)*	Combination of GCV intraocular implant q6 mos. + oral GCV as under induction therapy OR Cidofovir 5 mg/kg IV q2 wks + probenecid and hydration (as above under induction therapy)	Potential emergence of resistant CMV, approx. 10% pts. treated ≥3 months developed urine culture CMV isolates resistant to GCV *(JID 163:716, 1991),* hence may be reason for clinical failure. Treatment options: reinduction with same drug IV, switch to 2nd drug, or add (combine) with local rx. Local rx includes GCV implants or experimental intravitreal rx: (1) GCV 2x/wk or q wk *(CID 23:76, 1996);* (2) FOS q wk or less often *(Am J Ophth 114:742, 1992);* (3) Cidofovir 20 μg q6 wks *(AnIM 125:98, 1996).*
Hairy leukoplakia (Epstein Barr virus, EBV)		Usually asymptomatic and no treatment indicated	Acyclovir (800 mg po 5x/d) or topical podophyllin resin (one application) (not currently FDA-approved for this indication)	Patients usually asymptomatic, lesions respond to rx but recur.
Hepatitis B	Concomitant HIV infection	Lamivudine (3TC) 150 mg po bid + zidovudine 300 mg po bid ± a protease inhibitor (flares of Hep B reported when 3TC stopped)	Interferon use in dual infections not defined	Report of ↓ in plasma HBV DNA concentrations in pts with dual HIV and HBV infection *(AnIM 125:705, 1996; AJM 125:705, 1996).* Reports of 3TC-resistant HBV after months of rx in non-HIV infected liver transplant recipients *(Hepatol 24:714, 1996; Ln 349:20, 1997).*
Hepatitis C	Concomitant HIV infection	Interferon alfa-2b 5 mu 3x/wk subcutaneously x3 mos., then 3 mu subcutaneously 3x/wk x9 mos. *(see SANFORD GUIDE TO ANTIMICROBIAL THERAPY 1998 for specifics)*	Recommendation: rx of Hep C in HIV+ stable pts with interferon indicated while on antiretroviral rx	In multicenter, prospective, open, nonrandomized study of pts with dual HIV and HCV infection, sera became neg. for HCV RNA in 33% pts by 12 mos.; relapses occurred in 31%. More frequent response in pts with CD4 count >500 and HCV plasma burden <10^7 copies/ml *(CID 23:585, 1996).*

See page 96 for abbreviations.　　　NOTE: All dosage recommendations are for adults (unless otherwise indicated) and assume normal renal function.

TABLE 12 (18)

CAUSATIVE AGENT/DISEASE	MODIFYING CIRCUMSTANCES	SUGGESTED REGIMENS		COMMENTS
		PRIMARY	ALTERNATIVE	
Viral infections *(continued)*				
Herpes simplex virus (HSV)	Mucocutaneous (oral, anal, genital, skin) Treatment Mild	Acyclovir 400 mg po tid x5–10 days	Famciclovir 250 mg po tid x5–10 days OR Valacyclovir 1.0 gm po bid x5–10 days	Famciclovir and valacyclovir not FDA-approved for this indication but should work *(Abst 13, 3rd CRV, 1996)*. Chronic suppression indicated if frequent recurrences and/or extensive disease. 1% foscarnet cream applied 5x/d in acyclovir-unresponsive ulcers had 90% partial to complete response *(Abst 167, 3rd CRV, 1996)*. Cidofovir 0.3 or 1% topical gel was effective in >50% of ulcers that had failed acyclovir *(JID 176:892, 1997)*.
	Severe—extensive disease, systemic toxicity	Acyclovir 5.0 mg/kg q8h IV x5–10 d. For encephalitis, ↑ to 10 mg/kg IV q8h x10 days	Foscarnet 40 mg/kg q8h IV x21 days OR Ganciclovir 5 mg/kg IV q12h x5–10 days	Severe disease not responding to acyclovir may represent resistant virus. Options for resistance: IV foscarnet or for accessible lesions, topical ophthalmic solution of trifluridine q8h *(J AIDS 12:147, 1996)*.
	Suppression, post-treatment, only if recurrences are frequent or severe	Acyclovir 400 mg po bid or 200 mg po tid indefinitely. [Higher doses 800 mg 4x/d. more effective in 1 study *(5th CRV, Abst. 499)*]	Foscarnet 40 mg/kg IV qd indefinitely OR Famciclovir 250 mg po bid OR Valacyclovir 500 mg po qd	NOTE: For pts taking acyclovir for chronic suppression who then develop CMV retinitis, stop acyclovir when ganciclovir started— GCV active vs H. simplex.
Human herpesvirus 8 (Kaposi's sarcoma-associated herpesvirus)		*See Table 19, Treatment of HIV-Associated Malignancies*		
Human papillomavirus (HPV) Progression of disease correlates with ↑ HIV RNA in plasma *(5th CRV, Abst. 258)*	Condyloma acuminatum (CA) (anogenital warts)	Podofilox or 25% podophyllin in tincture of benzoin apply topically, wash after 1–4 hours. Apply weekly x4. If not effective, use alternative rx.	Interferon alfa-2b or alfa-n3 1.0 million units (0.1 ml) into lesions 3x/week x3 weeks. (Only 10 million units/1.0 ml vial is satisfactory. Other concentrations are hypertonic.)	Do not rx cervical warts until results of Pap smear known. Avoid podophyllin and podofilox in pregnant women. Alternatives: cryotherapy with liquid nitrogen, electrocautery. IV 5-fluorouracil may be effective in severe CA. Reference: *MMWR 42(RR-14):1, 1993*. Cidofovir topical gel under study.
Molluscum contagiosum virus	Treatment	Usually rx with destructive modalities: cryotherapy with liquid nitrogen, light electrocautery, or curettage.	Reports of spontaneous regression, occ. with transient suppuration, in pts responding to HAART. 3 pts also responded to either IV or topical cidofovir *(5th CRV, Abst. 504)*.	Interferon alfa is not effective. Spontaneous resolution observed in pts with good response to combination antiretroviral therapy.
	Suppression	Retinoic acid (Retin A) applied once nightly to face may ↓ rate of appearance but does not affect established lesions.		Retinoic acid cannot be used on eyelids or genitalia. Lesions in disseminated cryptococcosis, histoplasmosis may resemble molluscum contagiosum.
Parvovirus B-19	"Pure red cell aplasia"	Immunoglobulin G 0.4 gm/kg IV qd x5–10 days. Repeat if relapse occurs		Persistent parvovirus B-19 infection is a cause of anemia in HIV+ pts. Found in ⅓ HIV+ pts *(J Invest Med 45:65A, 1997)*. Rx with IVIG resulted in cure or remission enabling full ZDV dosage *(AnIM 113:926, 1990)*.

See page 96 for abbreviations.

NOTE: All dosage recommendations are for adults (unless otherwise indicated) and assume normal renal function.

TABLE 12 (19)

CAUSATIVE AGENT/DISEASE	MODIFYING CIRCUMSTANCES	SUGGESTED REGIMENS		COMMENTS
		PRIMARY	ALTERNATIVE	
Viral infections *(continued)*				
Progressive multifocal leukoencephalopathy		No effective therapy. No improvement with cytarabine in 13 pts *(CID 23:1066, 1996)*. However, both resolution of clinical and neuroimaging abnormalities and prolongation of survival (72 to 273 days) have been observed after effective HAART *(5th CRV, Abst. 463 & 464)*.		
Varicella zoster virus (VZV) ↑ frequency of zoster reported within 2 mos. of starting HAART (7% of 193 pts) *(5th CRV, Abst. 501)*	Herpes zoster (shingles) Severe: >1 dermatome, trigeminal nerve, or disseminated	Acyclovir (Zovirax) 10–12 mg/kg IV (infuse over 1 hr) q8h x7–14 days	Foscarnet 40 mg/kg IV (infuse over 2 hrs) q8h or 60 mg IV q12h for 14–26 days. *See Comments*	Treatment must be begun within 72 hours of onset of vesicles. Chronic post-treatment suppression not required. Acyclovir: adjust dose if renal function ↓. Acyclovir-resistant VZV occurs in HIV pts previously rx with acyclovir. Foscarnet: 4 of 5 pts rx responded, although 2 relapsed within 14 days *(AnIM 115:19, 1991; J AIDS 7:254, 1994)*. Famciclovir not evaluated in HIV+ pts. IV preparation not available. Valacyclovir, an ester of acyclovir, well absorbed, bioavailability ↑ 3–5x.
	Not severe	Acyclovir 800 mg po 5 x/day OR Famciclovir 500 mg po tid OR Valacyclovir 1.0 gm po tid All for 7 days		
	Varicella (chickenpox)	Acyclovir 10–12 mg/kg IV (infuse over 1 hr) q8h x7 days		Adjust dosage if renal function ↓.
Miscellaneous conditions				
Aphthous ulcers, recurrent (RAU)		Thalidomide 200 mg po qd x14–28 days (investigational)		In one series 16/29 pts responded vs 2/28 placebo. Side effects: somnolence (7/29) and rash (6/29) *(NEJM 336:1487, 1997)*. For compassionate use of thalidomide, contact Celgene, 1-800-801-8328.
Gingivitis (periodontitis/ stomatitis) *(See Table 9, page 47)*		* Topical Betadine and chlorhexidine gluconate (Peridex) mouthwash + antibiotics effective vs anaerobes (metronidazole, clindamycin or amoxicillin/clavulanate). Often requires curettage debridement.		
Psoriasis	Mild to moderate	Topical steroids + tar		Methotrexate rx has been associated with rapid immune suppression and death *(AnIM 106:19, 1987)*.
	Severe	Skin lesions may improve with ZDV		
Seborrheic dermatitis	Scalp, mild-moderate	Regular use of dandruff shampoo containing selenium sulfide (Selsun), zinc pyrithione (Head & Shoulders, Danex, Zincon) or sulfur and salicylic acid (Vanseb, Sebulex) + medium potency steroid solution (triamcinolone 0.1%), ketoconazole shampoo (2%).		Extremely common in HIV+ patients. Involves hairy areas of scalp, face, chest, back and groin.

NOTE: All dosage recommendations are for adults (unless otherwise indicated) and assume normal renal function.

TABLE 12 (20)

CAUSATIVE AGENT/DISEASE	MODIFYING CIRCUMSTANCES	SUGGESTED REGIMENS		COMMENTS
		PRIMARY	ALTERNATIVE	
Miscellaneous conditions *(continued*				
Seborrheic dermatitis *(continued)*	Facial, trunk, and/or groin	Topical imidazole cream (ketoconazole 2%, clotrimazole 1%) + low potency topical steroid (hydrocortisone 1–2.5%, desonide 0.05%) applied 2x daily	For refractory trunk lesions, ↑ strength of topical steroid. For severe disease, ketoconazole 200–400 mg po qd x2–4 weeks	

* This is the regimen used by J.S. Greenspan, *Medical Management of AIDS*, 5th Edition. Eds.: M.A. Sande, P.A. Volberding, W.B. Saunders & Co., 1996

Abbreviations: AM/SB = ampicillin/sulbactam, **AP Pen** = antipseudomonal penicillin; **AUC** = area under the curve (blood concentration vs time), **BL/BLI** = β-lactam/β-lactamase inhibitors, **CIP** = ciprofloxacin; **5th CRV** = 5th Conference on Retroviruses & Opportunistic Infections 1998; **ddC** = zalcitabine, **DOT** = directly observed therapy, **DRSP** = drug-resistant S. pneumoniae, **ETB** = ethambutol, **IDSA** = Infectious Diseases Society of America, **IDU** = injection drug users, **IMP** = imipenem cilastatin; **INH** = isoniazid, **INH-CR** = complete INH resistance, **itra** = itraconazole; **keto** = ketoconazole; **MER** = meropenem, **MRSA** = methicillin-resistant Staph. aureus, **MSSA** = methicillin-sensitive Staph. aureus, **neomacrolides** = azithromycin, clarithromycin, roxithromycin, **NUS** = not available in the U.S., **oflox** = ofloxacin, **OTC** = over the counter, **P Ceph 3** = parenteral 3rd generation cephalosporin; **P Ceph 4** = parenteral 4th generation cephalosporin (cefepime, cefpirome[NUS]); **PRSP** = penicillinase-resistant synthetic penicillins, **PZA** = pyrazinamide, **RIF** = rifampin, **STM** = streptomycin, **TMP** = trimethoprim, **TMP/SMX** = trimethoprim/sulfamethoxazole, **VDRL (RPR)** = nontreponemal serologic tests for syphilis (in contrast to FTA/ABS test, **ZDV** = zidovudine

NOTE: All dosage recommendations are for adults (unless otherwise indicated) and assume normal renal function

TABLE 13

DRUGS USED IN TREATMENT AND/OR CHRONIC SUPPRESSION OF AIDS-RELATED INFECTIONS:
ADVERSE EFFECTS, COMMENTS, COST

DRUG NAME, GENERIC (TRADE)/ USUAL DOSAGE/COST*	ADVERSE EFFECTS/COMMENTS
Antifungal Drugs	

Non-lipid amphotericin B (Fungizone): 0.3–1 mg/kg/d as single infusion
100 mg $34.58
	Non-lipid amphotericin B (Fungizone):
	Admin.: Commercial ampho B is a colloidal suspension that must be prepared in electrolyte-free D5W at 0.1 mg/ml to avoid precipitation. No need to protect drug suspensions from light. Ampho B infusions often cause chills/fever, myalgia, anorexia, nausea, rarely hemodynamic collapse/hypotension. Postulated due to release of proinflammatory cytokines; hypersensitivity reaction cannot be excluded. Manufacturer recommends a test dose of 1 mg, but often not done (1st few ml of 1st dose is a test dose). Duration of infusion usually 4 or more hrs. No difference found in 1- vs 4-hr infusions (*AAC 34:1402, 1992; AJM 93:123, 1992*) except chills/fever occurred sooner with 1-hr. infusion. Frequency and severity of febrile reactions decrease with repeated doses.
	  Severe rigors respond to meperidine (25–50 mg IV). Premedication with acetaminophen, diphenhydramine, hydrocortisone (25–50 mg) and heparin (1000 units) had no influence on rigors/fever (*CID 70:755, 1995*). If cytokine postulate correct, NSAIDs or high-dose steroids may prove efficacious but their use may risk worsening infection under rx or increased risk of nephrotoxicity (i.e., NSAIDs). Clinical side effects ↓ with ↑ age (*CID 26:334, 1998*).
	Toxicity: Major concern is nephrotoxicity (15% of 102 pts surveyed, *CID 26:334, 1998*). Manifest initially by kaliuresis and hypokalemia, then fall in serum bicarbonate (may proceed to renal tubular acidosis), ↓ in renal erythropoietin and anemia, and rising BUN/serum creatinine. Hypomagnesemia may occur.
	  Can reduce risk of renal injury by (a) pre- and post-infusion hydration with 500 ml saline (if clinical status will allow salt load), (b) avoidance of other nephrotoxins, e.g., radiocontrast, aminoglycosides, cis-platinum, (c) perhaps use of lipid prep of ampho B.

Lipid ampho B products: Amphotericin B lipid complex (ABLC) (Abelcet): 5 mg/kg/d as single infusion 100 mg IV $173.33	**Ampho B lipid complex (ABLC) (Abelcet):** **Admin.:** Indicated for rx of invasive fungal infections in pts refractory or intolerant to non-lipid ampho B. Consists of ampho B complexed with 2 lipids. Compared to standard ampho B, larger volume of distribution, rapid blood clearance and high tissue concentrations (liver, spleen, lung). Dosage: 5 mg/kg once daily; infuse at 2.5 mg/kg/hr; adult and ped. dose the same. Do NOT use an in-line filter. Do not dilute with saline solution or mix with other drugs or electrolytes. **Toxicity:** Fever and chills in 14–18%; nausea 9%, vomiting 8%; serum creatinine ↑ in 11%; renal failure 5%; anemia 4%; ↓ K 5%; rash 4%.
Amphotericin B cholesteryl complex (Amphotec): 3–4 mg/kg/d as single infusion 100 mg $160.00	**Ampho B cholesteryl complex (Amphotec):** **Admin.:** Approved for rx of aspergillosis in pts who either failed or are intolerant to standard ampho B. Consists of ampho B deoxycholate stabilized with cholesteryl sulfate resulting in a disc-shaped colloidal complex. Compared to standard ampho B, larger volume of distribution, rapid blood clearance, high tissue concentrations. Dosage: Initial dose for adults & children: 3–4 mg/kg/day. If necessary, can ↑ to 6 mg/kg/day. Dilute in D5W & infuse at 1 mg/kg/hr. Do NOT use in-line filter. **Toxicity:** Chills 50%, fever 33%, ↑ serum creatinine 12–20%; ↓ Ca 6%, ↓ K 17%.
Liposomal amphotericin B (AmBisome): 3–5 mg/kg/d as single infusion 100 mg $376.00	**Liposomal amphotericin B (AmBisome):** **Admin.:** Approved for empirical rx for presumed fungal infections in febrile neutropenic pts; rx of pts with aspergillus, candida and/or cryptococcus infections refractory to conventional ampho B, or in pts where renal impairment or unacceptable toxicity precludes the use of conventional ampho B; and rx of visceral leishmaniasis. Dosage: 3–5 mg/kg/d IV as single dose infused over a period of approx. 120 min. If infusion is well tolerated, infusion time can be reduced to 60 min. **Major toxicity:** Generally less than ampho B. Nephrotoxicity 18.7% vs 33.7% for ampho B, chills 47% vs 75%, nausea 39.7% vs 38.7%, vomiting 31.8% vs 43.9%, rash 24% for both, ↓ Ca 18.4% vs 20.9%, ↓ K 20.4% vs 25.6%, ↓ Mg 20.4% vs 25.6%.
Amphotericin B colloidal dispersion (ABCD) (Amphocil) (I) (*JID 173:1208, 1996*)	
Ampho B oral suspension available (Fungizone): Dose: 100 mg (1 ml) po 4x/d 100 mg $1.50	

* From 1997 Red Book, Medical Economics Data. Price is average wholesale price (AWP).
All dosage recommendations are for adults (unless otherwise indicated) and assume normal renal function

DRUG NAME, GENERIC (TRADE)/ USUAL DOSAGE/COST*	ADVERSE EFFECTS/COMMENTS
Fluconazole (Diflucan) 100 mg tabs $6.88 200 mg tabs $11.25 400 mg IV $118.75 Oral suspension: 350 or 800 mg bottles	Maximum tolerated dose: 2000 mg/d. **Pharmacology:** absorbed po, water solubility enables IV. Peak serum levels (see Table 15, page 107). t/2 22 hrs. 12% protein bound. CSF levels 50–60% of serum in normals, ↑ in meningitis. Up to 85% of plasma concentrations have been found in breast milk (PIDJ 14: 235, 1995). No effect on mammalian steroid metabolism. **Drug-drug interactions common,** see Table 17. Side-effects overall 16% [more common in HIV+ pts (21%)]. Nausea 3.7%, headache 1.9%, skin rash 1.8%, abdominal pain 1.7%, vomiting 1.7%, diarrhea 1.5%, ↑ SGOT 20%. Alopecia (scalp, pubic crest) in 12–20% pts on ≥400 mg po qd after median of 3 months (reversible in approx. 6 mos.) (AnIM 123:354, 1995). Rare: severe hepatotoxicity, exfoliative dermatitis. Anaphylaxis (CID 13:81, 1993), thrombocytopenia, leucopenia. Good reference: NEJM 330:263, 1994. ? congenital anomalies (CID 22:336, 1996).
Flucytosine (Ancobon) 500 mg $1.99	AEs: Overall 30%. GI 6% (diarrhea, anorexia, nausea, vomiting); hematologic 22% [leucopenia, thrombocytopenia, when serum level > 100 µg/ml (esp. in azotemic pts)]; hepatotoxicity (asymptomatic ↑ SGOT, reversible); skin rash 7%; aplastic anemia (rare--2 or 3 cases). False ↑ in serum creatinine on EKTACHEM analyzer.
Griseofulvin (Fulvicin, Grifulvin, Grisactin) 500 mg $1.36	Photosensitivity, urticaria, GI upset, fatigue, leucopenia (rare). Interferes with warfarin drugs. Increases blood and urine porphyrins, should not be used in patients with porphyria. Minor disulfiram-like reactions. Exacerbation of systemic lupus erythematosus.
Imidazoles, topical: for vaginal and/or skin use	Not recommended in 1st trimester of pregnancy. Local reactions: 0.5-1.5%: dyspareunia, mild vaginal or vulvar erythema, burning, pruritus, urticaria, rash. Rarely similar symptoms in sexual partner. Expense of treating vaginitis topically: Butoconazole x3 d $20.16, clotrimazole x7 d $14.71, miconazole x3 d $24.36, terconazole x3 d $23.34, tioconazole x1 dose $24.20.
Itraconazole (Sporanox) 100 mg tabs $6.04 (with cola or food) 10 mg/ml oral solution (fasting state) 100 mg of oral solution $6.53	Itraconazole now available in tablet and solution forms—the 2 are not interchangeable. To obtain the highest plasma concentration, the tablet is given with food and acidic drinks (e.g., cola) while the solution is taken in the fasted state; under these conditions, the peak conc. of the capsule is approx. 30 mg/ 100 ml and of the solution 54 mg/100 ml. Peak levels are reached faster (2.2 vs 5 hrs) with the solution. Protein-binding for both preparations is over 99%; the latter explains the virtual absence of penetration into the CSF (do not use to treat meningitis). Oral solutions more desirable if taste and increased expense are acceptable. Most common adverse effects are dose-related nausea 10% and abdominal discomfort 5.7%. Allergic rash 8.6%, edema 3.5%, and hepatitis 2.7% reported. ↑ doses may produce hypokalemia 2% and ↑ blood pressure 3.2%. Thrombocytopenia and leucopenia reported (AnIM 125:157, 1996). Other concern, as with fluconazole and ketoconazole, is **drug-drug interactions; see Table 17. WARNING: Co-administration with terfenadine, astemizole, cisapride, oral triazolam and oral midazolam contraindicated. Itra will ↑ serum levels of these drugs and life-threatening arrhythmias have resulted.**
Ketoconazole (Nizoral) 100 mg $3.06	Gastric acid required for absorption—cimetidine, omeprazole, antacids block absorption. In achlorhydria, dissolve tablet in 4 ml 0.2N HCl, drink with a straw. Coca-Cola ↑ absorption by 65% (AAC 39:1671, 1995). CSF levels "none". **Drug-drug interactions important, see Table 17. Some interactions can be life-threatening.** Liver toxicity of hepatocellular type reported in about 1:10,000 exposed pts—usually after several days to weeks of exposure. At doses of ≥800 mg/d serum testosterone and plasma cortisol levels fall. With high doses, adrenal (Addisonian) crisis reported.
Miconazole (Monistat IV) 200 mg—not available in U.S.	IV miconazole indicated in patient critically ill with Pseudallescheria boydii. Used in some centers as prophylaxis or in initial rx regimens in febrile neutropenic pts (AJM 83:1103, 1987; J Clin Onc 8:280, 1990). Very toxic due to vehicle needed to get drug into solution.
Nystatin (Mycostatin) 30 gm cream $27.51, 500,000 u oral tab $0.60	Topical: virtually no adverse effects. Less effective than imidazoles and triazoles. PO: large doses give occasional GI distress and diarrhea.
Terbinafine (Lamisil) 250 mg tabs $6.22	Rare cases of symptomatic cholestatic hepatitis reported. In controlled trials, changes in ocular lens and retina reported—clinical significance unknown. Major drug-drug interaction is 100% ↑ in rate of clearance by rifampin. AEs: All mild, transient and rarely caused discontinuation of rx. % with AE, terbinafine vs placebo: nausea/diarrhea 2.6–5.6 vs 2.9; rash 5.6 vs 2.2; taste abnormality 2.8 vs 0.7.

* From 1997 Red Book, Medical Economics Data. Price is average wholesale price (AWP).
All dosage recommendations are for adults (unless otherwise indicated) and assume normal renal function

TABLE 13 (3)

DRUG NAME, GENERIC (TRADE)/ USUAL DOSAGE/COST*	ADVERSE EFFECTS/COMMENTS
Antimycobacterial Drugs:	
FIRST LINE DRUGS	
Isoniazid (INH) (Nydrazid, Laniazid, Teebaconin) 300 mg/d po 300 mg tab $0.05 100 mg/ml in 10 ml vials (IM) (Nydrazid, Apothecon) $15.85	**Adverse effects:** Overall ~1%. **Peripheral neuropathy** (<1.0%); pyridoxine 25 mg daily will ↓ incidence; other neurologic sequelae, convulsions, optic neuritis, toxic encephalopathy, psychosis, muscle twitching, dizziness and alterations of sensorium, coma (all rare); allergic skin rashes, lymphadenopathy and vasculitis (SLE-like syndrome), fever, minor disulfiram-like reaction, flushing after Swiss cheese, constipation, **hepatitis** (children 10% mild ↑ SGOT, normalizes with continued rx, age <20 yrs rare, 20–34 yrs 0.3%, 35–40 yrs 1.2%, ≥50 yrs 2.3%) (also ↑ with daily alcohol); acute liver failure (fatal or requiring transplantation (*Lancet 345:555, 1995*); blood dyscrasias (rare); + antinuclear antibody 20%.
Rifampin (Rifadin, Rimactane, Rifocin) 600 mg/d po 300 mg cap $2.11 (IV available, Hoechst Marion, 600 mg $79.38)	**Adverse effects:** Produces an orange-brown discoloration of urine, tears (can stain contact lens), semen, and sweat. Can falsely elevate lab measurements of bilirubin. **Drug-drug interactions:** Many *(see Table 17)*: induces liver cytochrome P450 system (CYP3A) to ↑ drug metabolism, e.g., ↑ Coumadin requirement, ↑ steroid dosage in pts with Addison's disease or asthmatics, ↓ effectiveness of oral contraceptives (uterine bleeding, pregnancies), methadone less effective, reduced levels of azole antifungals, e.g., fluconazole. "Flu syndrome": Manifest as fever/chills, headache, bone pain, dyspnea if rifampin ingestion irregular. Hepatotoxicity: 16 deaths reported in 500,000 recipients. Minor enzyme changes common and resolve while continuing the drug. Alcoholics with preexisting liver disease prone to rifampin-induced toxicity. Interstitial nephritis reported.
Ethambutol (Myambutol) 15–25 mg/kg/d po 400 mg tab $1.78	**Adverse effects: Optic neuritis** with decreased visual acuity, central scotomata, and loss of green and red perception at 25 mg/kg/d, not at 15 mg/kg/d; peripheral neuropathy and headache (~1%), rashes (rare), arthralgia (rare), hyperuricemia (rare). Monthly evaluation of visual acuity (>10% loss considered significant), red/green color discrimination; usually reversible if drug discontinued. Anaphylactoid reaction. **Comment:** Disrupts outer cell membrane in M. avium with ↑ activity of other drugs.
Pyrazinamide (PZA) 25 mg/kg d po 500 mg tab $1.12	**Adverse effects: Arthralgia; hyperuricemia** (with or without symptoms); hepatitis (not over 2% if recommended dose not exceeded); gastric irritation; photosensitivity (rare). Serum uric acid if symptomatic gouty attack occurs. **Comment:** Maximum dose 2.0 gm/d.
Streptomycin 0.75–1.0 gm/d IM (or IV) 1.0 gm $0.30	**Adverse effects:** Overall 8%. **Ototoxicity,** vestibular dysfunction (vertigo); paresthesias; dizziness and nausea (all less in pts receiving 2–3 doses/week); tinnitus and high frequency loss 1%; nephrotoxicity (rare); peripheral neuropathy (rare); allergic skin rashes 4–5%; drug fever. Available from Pfizer/Roerig 1-800-254-4445. Reference for IV use: *CID 19:1150, 1994.*
Rifamate® *(see Comment for content)* 2 tablets single dose po qd (1 hr before meal). 1 tab $2.43	**Adverse effects:** Same as individual components. **Comments:** 1 tablet contains 150 mg INH, 300 mg RIF
Rifater® *(See Comment for content)* If pt not >55 kg: 6 tablets single dose po qd (1 hr before meal). 1 tab $1.80	**Adverse effects:** Same as individual components. **Comments:** 1 tablet contains 50 mg INH, 120 mg RIF, 300 mg PZA. Used in 1st 2 months of rx (PZA 25 mg/kg). Purpose is convenience in dosing, ↑ compliance *(AnIM 122:951, 1995)* but costs 1.5x more.
SECOND LINE DRUGS Para-aminosalicylic acid (PAS) (Na+ or K+ salt) (Paser) 4–6 gm po bid (200 mg/kg/d) 450 mg tab $0.08	**Adverse effects: Gastrointestinal irritation** 10–15%; goitrogenic action (rare); depressed prothrombin activity (rare); G6PD-mediated hemolytic anemia (rare), drug fever, rashes, hepatitis, myalgia, arthralgia. Retards hepatic enzyme induction, may ↓ INH hepatotoxicity. Available from Jacobus Pharm. Co. (609) 921-7447; CDC (404) 639-3670.

* From 1997 Red Book, Medical Economics Data. Price is average wholesale price (AWP).
All dosage recommendations are for adults (unless otherwise indicated) and assume normal renal function

DRUG NAME, GENERIC (TRADE)/ USUAL DOSAGE/COST*	ADVERSE EFFECTS/COMMENTS
Antimycobacterial Drugs/SECOND LINE DRUGS *(continued)*	
Ethionamide (Trecator-SC) 500–1000 mg/d (10–15 mg/kg/d) po as 1–3 doses. 250 mg tab $1.70	**Adverse effects: Gastrointestinal irritation** (up to 50% on large dose); goiter; peripheral neuropathy (rare); convulsions (rare); changes in affect (rare); difficulty in diabetes control; rashes; hepatitis; purpura; stomatitis; gynecomastia; menstrual irregularity. Give drug with meals or antacids; 50–100 mg pyridoxine per day concomitantly; SGOT monthly. Possibly teratogenic.
Cycloserine (Seromycin) 750–1000 mg/d (15 mg/kg/d) po as 2–4 doses. 250 mg cap $3.83	**Adverse effects:** Convulsions, **psychoses** (5–10% of those receiving 1.0 gm/day); headache; somnolence; hyperreflexia; increased CSF protein and pressure, peripheral neuropathy; contraindicated in epileptics and active alcoholics; 50 mg pyridoxine for every 250 mg cycloserine should be given concomitantly.
Amikacin (Amikin) 7.5–10 mg/kg/d IV or IM 500 mg vial $32.89	**Adverse effects:** Nephrotoxicity; **ototoxicity** [usually high frequency loss—especially with larger total dose (>10 gm), longer duration (>10 days), prior aminoglycosides, pos. family history, assoc. renal impairment and rising trough level (>10 µg/ml). All aminoglycosides may cause or ↑ neuromuscular blockade. Use with caution in pts with myasthenia gravis, Parkinsonism, botulism, with neuromuscular blocking drugs *(Table 17)*, or with massive transfusion of citrated blood. Avoid concurrent use with ethacrynic acid, furosemide or methoxyflurane. ↑ risk of nephrotoxicity with cis platinum, vancomycin, radiocontrast agents. **Comments:** With edema, ascites, and/or obesity, base calculation of est. creatinine clearance on lean body mass and ideal body weight. For dosing with renal impairment, *see Table 16.*
Capreomycin sulfate (Capastat sulfate) 1.0 gm/d (15 mg/kg/d) as 1 dose IM 1.0 gm $24.33	**Adverse effects: Nephrotoxicity** 36%, **ototoxicity** (auditory 11%), eosinophilia, leucopenia, skin rash, fever, hypokalemia, neuromuscular blockade. Abnormal liver function tests, ? related. Capreomycin is an aminoglycoside and shares group side-effects of nephrotoxicity, ototoxicity, and potential neuromuscular blockade.
Amithiozone (Thioacetazone, Tibione, Thioparamizone) (NOT MARKETED IN U.S.) 150 mg/d po	**Adverse effects:** Common: nausea, vomiting, skin rash, dizziness. Uncommon: bone marrow depression, jaundice 0.2%, and renal toxicity. Marked differences in frequency of side effects between racial groups noted, Asia > Africa. Total incidence 21–38%, ½ in 1st 4 weeks, ½ lasted 6 days or less, ½ mild. **Comments: Skin reactions** reported in 20% of HIV+ pts. Felt to be responsible for a 3% **mortality** *(Lancet 1:627, 1991).* In trial comparing RIF/INH/PZA (RHZ) with SM/thiacetazone/INH (STH), relative risk of death with STH 1.6, drug reactions 11.7 and sputum negative at 2 months RHZ 74% vs 37% in STH *(Lancet 344:323, 1994; ibid., 345:62, 1995).*
Clofazimine (Lamprene) 50 mg/d po (with meals) 50 mg $0.13	**Adverse effects:** Skin: **pigmentation (pink-brownish black)** 75–100%, dryness 20%, pruritus 5%. GI: abdominal pain 50% (rarely severe leading to exploratory laparoscopy), splenic infarction (very rare), bowel obstruction (very rare), GI bleeding (very rare). Eye: conjunctival irritation, retinal crystal deposition.
Rifabutin (Mycobutin) 300 mg/d po (prophylaxis or treatment) 150 mg $3.96	**Adverse effects:** In an anti-MAI trial, rifabutin-related adverse effects occurred in 77% of pts receiving 600 mg (high dose) rifabutin with either clarithro or azithro. Most common was a fall in WBC, then nausea/vomiting/diarrhea in 42%, diffuse polyarthralgia in 19%, and anterior uveitis in 8% *(CID 21:594, 1995).* Uveitis responds to topical steroids and cycloplegics *[CID 22(Suppl. 1):S43, 1996].* Subsequently, max. dose of rifabutin reduced to 300 mg. Other adverse effects similar to rifampin: skin rash 11%, orange-tan to brown skin pigmentation *(CID 21:1515, 1995).* Discolored (reddish) urine 30%. Lab: ↑ SGOT/SGPT 8%.
Fluoroquinolones	Review drug/drug interactions before prescribing. Serious, rarely fatal anaphylactic reactions, some with 1st dose reported. All FQs are GABA inhibitors, may account for CNS toxicities. Fatal hepatic failure (very rare) reported with FQ *(Lancet 343:378, 1994).* Achilles tendinitis and rupture reported *(NEJM 332:193,1995).* In U.S., FQs not approved for use in children <14 yrs. In Europe there are published data on FQ use in >1000 prepubertal children, including MRI studies in some with no evidence of cartilage damage *(JAC 30:414, 1992).* A consensus report of Intl. Soc. of Chemotherapy states: "Caution: use of FQs is justified when alternative safe therapy is not available" *Ped IDJ 14:1, 1995).* In the HIV+ child, such might include MDR-tuberculosis and recurrent salmonella bacteremia.

* From 1997 Red Book, Medical Economics Data. Price is average wholesale price (AWP).
All dosage recommendations are for adults (unless otherwise indicated) and assume normal renal function

DRUG NAME, GENERIC (TRADE)/ USUAL DOSAGE/COST*	ADVERSE EFFECTS/COMMENTS
Antimycobacterial Drugs/SECOND LINE DRUGS/Fluoroquinolones *(continued)*	
Ciprofloxacin (Cipro) 750 mg bid po 750 mg tab $3.62 400 mg IV $28.81	**Adverse effects:** Overall 16.5%, 3.5% discontinued secondary to side effects. GI 1.5%: nausea, diarrhea, vomiting, abdominal pain. **CNS** 0.4%: headache, restlessness, insomnia, nightmares, toxic psychosis (very rare). Skin 0.6%: rash, angioedema. Other more rare (<1%) include arthralgia, interstitial nephritis. Lab: ↑ SGOT 1.7%, ↑ alk p'tase 0.8%, ↓ WBC 0.4%, ↑ creatinine 1.1%. Safety in children, pregnant women not established, in animal models at 5–16x human dosage, cartilage erosion and arthropathy occurred. **Comment:** This is not an FDA-approved indication, i.e., use in mycobacterial rx is investigational.
Ofloxacin (Floxin) 400 mg bid po 400 mg tab $4.34 400 mg IV $26.40	**Adverse effects:** Overall 11%, 4% discontinued secondary to side effects. GI: nausea 3%, diarrhea 1%. **CNS:** insomnia 3%, headache 1%, dizziness 1%. Other uncommon (<1%) include arthralgia, skin rash, Stevens-Johnson syndrome. Lab: eosinophilia, ↑ SGPT, hematuria. Arthropathy in animal models as above. **Comment:** This is not an FDA-approved indication, i.e., use in mycobacterial rx is investigational.
Sparfloxacin (Zagam) 400 mg loading dose, then 200 mg po qd 200 mg tab $6.68	The most active of the fluoroquinolones against M. tuberculosis and MAC. Adverse effects (in HIV– pts): GI distress, photosensitivity. Has been used in limited compassionate use protocol for multidrug-resistant TB [Dr. Bender (313) 996-7297] but not FDA-approved for TB or MAI.
Clarithromycin (Biaxin) 500 mg bid po 500 mg $3.45 *(FDA approved for MAC; investigational for other atypical mycobacteria, not effective vs M. tuberculosis)*	**Adverse effects:** Overall ~13%, ~3% discontinued drug secondary to side effects. GI ~13%: diarrhea 3%, nausea 3%, abnormal taste 3%, abdominal pain 2%, dyspepsia 2%. 1 case report of corneal opacities *(JAC 34:605, 1994)*. CNS: headache 2%. Lab (each <1%): ↑ SGOT, alk p'tase, ↓ WBC, ↑ prothrombin time 1%, ↑ BUN 4%, ↑ creatinine <1%. Should not be used in pregnant women, has demonstrated adverse effects in animals at blood levels 2–17x higher than achieved in humans.
Azithromycin (Zithromax) 250–500 mg/d po, 1200 mg/week po 250 mg $6.22 *(Investigational in T. gondii, not effective vs M. tuberculosis)*	**Adverse effects:** Overall 12%, 0.7% discontinued drug secondary to side effects. GI 12.8%: diarrhea 4%, nausea 3%, abdominal pain 2%, vomiting 1%. CNS 1%, ototoxicity (3/21 pts 30–90 days after 500 mg/d, *Lancet 343:241, 1994*). Lab: ↑ SGOT 1.5%, WBC ↓ or ↑ 1%, others <1%. Has not been studied in pregnant women. In rats no embryopathy at dose of 60x human total dose.
Imipenem-cilastatin (Primaxin) 500 mg q6h IV 500 mg $26.99	Active in vitro vs M. tuberculosis. Being used in some trials. **Adverse effects:** Local: phlebitis 3%. Hypersensitivity 2.5%: rash, pruritus, eosinophilia <1%. Blood: + Coombs <1%, neutropenia <1%. Renal: oliguria <0.2%. Hepatic: ↑ SGOT, SGPT, alk p'tase <1%. CNS (0.2%): confusion, seizures (with 0.5 gm q6h 0.5–1.0% but with 1.0 gm q6h ~10%). GI: nausea 2%, vomiting 2% especially with too rapid IV, diarrhea 3%. **Comment:** This is not an FDA-approved indication, i.e., use is investigational.
Antiparasitic Drugs	
Albendazole (Albenza) Doses vary with indication, 200–400 mg bid po 200 mg tab $0.88	**Adverse effects:** Teratogenic, Pregnancy Cat. C. Give after negative pregnancy test. Abdominal pain, nausea/vomiting, alopecia, ↑ serum transaminase. Rare reports of bone marrow suppression.

* From 1997 Red Book, Medical Economics Data. Price is average wholesale price (AWP).
All dosage recommendations are for adults (unless otherwise indicated) and assume normal renal function

TABLE 13 (6)

DRUG NAME, GENERIC (TRADE)/ USUAL DOSAGE/COST*	ADVERSE EFFECTS/COMMENTS
Antiparasitic Drugs *(continued)*	
Atovaquone (Mepron) 750 mg bid po x21 days 750 mg/5 ml suspension $12.50	**Adverse effects:** Discontinuation rate 9%. Skin rash 23%, only 4% required discontinuation of rx, pruritus 5%. GI: nausea 21%, diarrhea 19%, vomiting 14%, abdominal pain 4%. CNS: headache 16%, insomnia 10%, dizziness 3%. General: fever 14%. Lab: anemia (Hgb <8.0 gm/dl, 6%), neutropenia (<750/mm³, 3%), ↑ AST 4%, ↑ amylase 7%. **Comments:** Has not been evaluated in anti-PCP prophylaxis or severe PCP. Better absorbed with meals. Plasma concentration 3x higher when taken with fatty (>23 gm) meal *(J AIDS 8:247, 1995)*. May have clinical use vs microsporidia.
Clindamycin (Cleocin) 600 mg q6h po or IV 150 mg cap $0.70 (generic) 600 mg IV $13.86	**Adverse effects:** Diarrhea ± C. difficile toxin, nausea, rash, neutropenia, eosinophilia
Dapsone (Dapsone USP) 100 mg qd or 2x weekly po 100 mg $0.18	**Adverse effects:** Nausea, vomiting, rash, and oral lesions *(CID 18:630, 1994)*. Hemolytic anemia if G6PD deficient, methemoglobinemia (usually asymptomatic but if pt has dyspnea, O_2 saturation disproportionately low to pO_2; check for methemoglobinemia—if >10–15%, discontinue dapsone). Peripheral neuropathy (rare). **Comment:** Usually tolerated even if rash after TMP/SMX.
Iodoquinol (Yodoxin) 650 mg tid po 650 mg $0.38	**Adverse effects:** Nausea, abdominal cramps, rash, acne, increase in thyroid size and PBI. Optic atrophy risk if daily dose over 2 gm.
Ivermectin (Stromectol) Strongyloidiasis: 200 µg/kg x1 dose po Onchocerciasis: 150 µg/kg x1 po Scabies: 200 µg/kg x1 po 6 mg tabs $9.38	**Adverse effects:** Mild side-effects—fever, pruritus, rash
Metronidazole (Flagyl) 500–750 mg bid–tid po 250 mg $0.03	**Adverse effects:** GI: nausea, vomiting, metallic taste. Neuro: headache, paresthesias, avoid alcohol during & 48 hours post-rx (disulfiram-like reaction). Dark urine, tears, sweat (harmless).
Paromomycin (Humatin) 500 mg tid or qid po 250 mg $2.00	**Adverse effects:** GI: doses of >3 gm, nausea, abdominal cramps, diarrhea. CNS: vertigo, headache. Skin: rash. **Comment:** This is an aminoglycoside similar to neomycin ("non-absorbed", ~3% of dose is absorbed). Discontinue promptly if patient complains of tinnitus, ↓ in hearing, or vertigo.
Pentamidine isethionate (IV)(Pentam 300) 4 mg/kg/d IV 300 mg $113.00	**Adverse effects:** Hypotension with rapid IV administration, rash, nausea, vomiting, nephrotoxicity, cardiac arrhythmia (ventricular tachycardias including torsade de pointes), neutropenia (15%), thrombocytopenia, pancreatitis, hypocalcemia, hypoglycemia followed by hyperglycemia. Sterile abscesses after IM administration. **Comments:** Pentamidine inhibits distal nephron absorption of Na⁺ with resultant hyperkalemia similar to K-sparing diuretics *(AnIM 122:103, 1995)*.
Pentamidine (aerosol) (NebuPent) 300 mg/month (prophylaxis) 300 mg $113.00	**Adverse effects:** Cough may respond to bronchodilator, upper lobe pneumocystis may occur if given with patient sitting. **Comment:** Risk of extrapulmonary pneumocystis and pneumothorax greater than with systemic prophylaxis. Use aerosol only in patients intolerant of oral drugs.

TABLE 13 (7)

DRUG NAME, GENERIC (TRADE)/ USUAL DOSAGE/COST*	ADVERSE EFFECTS/COMMENTS
Antiparasitic Drugs (*continued*)	
Primaquine 15 mg (base) qd po 26.3 mg $0.76	**Adverse effects:** Hemolytic anemia if G6PD deficient; may cause clinically significant methemoglobinemia; nausea/abdominal pain if taken on empty stomach.
Pyrimethamine (Daraprim, Malocide) 50–75 mg qd po 25 mg $0.40 (Leucovorin, tablet 25 mg $21.02—*see Comments*)	**Adverse effects:** Rash, vomiting, diarrhea, xerostomia, megaloblastic anemia, neutropenia, thrombocytopenia. Rarely: headache, insomnia, seizures. **Comments:** Folinic acid (leucovorin) used to reduce pyrimethamine-induced bone marrow suppression. In vitro and in mice, ZDV antagonizes pyrimethamine.
Sulfadiazine 1.0–1.5 gm q6h po 500 mg tablet $0.34	**Adverse effects:** Compared to non-HIV pts, dramatic ↑ in incidence of pruritus, rash, Stevens-Johnson syndrome, myalgia/arthralgia. Traditionally thought on hypersensitivity basis. New data support postulate of dose-dependent accumulation of toxic sulfonamide metabolites that fail to clear due to concomitant glutathione deficiency in the AIDS pt *(Brit J Pharm 39:621, 1995; JAC 34:1, 1994)*. In addition, can cause hemolytic anemia in G6PD-def. pts. All sulfonamides can cause crystalluria. Do not use in newborns or late stages of pregnancy.
Trimethoprim (Proloprim) 5 mg/kg q6h po 200 mg $1.58	**Adverse effects:** Rash, pruritus, marrow suppression rare. Rare cases of aseptic meningitis [fever, headache, CSF ↑ cells (monos), ↑ protein] reported *(CID 19:431, 1994)*. **Comment:** Fewer reactions than TMP/SMX.
Trimethoprim (TMP)- sulfamethoxazole (SMX) (Cotrim, Bactrim, Septra) (Dosage depends on indication) 1 double-strength tab (160 TMP/800 mg SMX) $0.09; 160/800 mg IV $16.00	**Adverse effects:** Compared to non-AIDS pts, dramatic dose-dependent ↑ in pruritus, skin rash, Stevens-Johnson syndrome. In pts given TMP/SMX + steroids for PCP, % skin reactions ↓ from 47 to 13 *(CID 18:319, 1994)*. Initially thought hypersensitivity was reason; accumulating data support hypothesis of dose-dependent accumulation of toxic sulfonamide metabolites (hydroxylamine). Clearance of metabolites requires glutathione and AIDS pts are deficient *(Brit J Pharm 39:621, 1995; JAC 34:1, 1994)*. May explain ability 2/3 of time to rx through rash *(Arch Derm 130:1383, 1994)*. Beware progressive exanthem—some pts progress to exfoliation and/or Stevens-Johnson syndrome. Tremors associated with high dose *(CID 22:598, 1996)*. TMP competes with creatinine for tubular secretion and can ↑ serum creatinine (reversible); TMP also blocks distal renal tubular reabsorption of Na⁺ & secretion of K⁺. ↑ serum K⁺ in 21% of pts *(AnIM 124:316, 1996)*.
Trimetrexate (Neutrexin) 45 mg/M² qd IV + leucovorin 20 mg/M² q6h IV 25 mg $52.80	**Adverse effects:** Overall discontinuation rate 10% vs 29% with TMP/SMX. Skin rash 6%, fever 8%, nausea/vomiting 5%, confusion 3%, neutropenia 30%, thrombocytopenia 10%, anemia 7%, ↑ liver function tests 14%, hyponatremia 5%, hypocalcemia 2% (overall side-effects rate 53%).

* From 1997 Red Book, Medical Economics Data. Price is average wholesale price (AWP).
All dosage recommendations are for adults (unless otherwise indicated) and assume normal renal function

TABLE 13 (8)

DRUG NAME(S) GENERIC (TRADE)	DOSAGE/ROUTE/COST*	COMMENTS/ADVERSE EFFECTS
Antiviral Drugs (other than antiretroviral)		
Cytomegalovirus		
Cidofovir (Vistide)	5 mg/kg IV q week x2, then q2 weeks. (375 mg $727) Properly timed IV prehydration with normal saline and oral probenecid **must be used with each cidofovir infusion** (*see pkg insert for details*). Renal function (serum creatinine and urine protein) must be monitored prior to each dose (*see pkg insert for details*).	**Adverse effects: Nephrotoxicity**; dose-dependent proximal tubular injury (Fanconi-like syndrome): proteinuria, glycosuria, bicarbonaturia, phosphaturia, polyuria (nephrogenic diabetic insipidus now reported, *Ln 350:413, 1997*), ↑ creatinine. Concomitant saline prehydration, probenecid, extended dosing intervals allowed use. Recurrent iritis with IV administration has been reported (*CID 25:337, 1997*). Other toxicities: nausea 48%, fever 31%, alopecia 16%, myalgia 16%, probenecid hypersensitivity 16%, neutropenia 29%. No effect on hematocrit, platelets, LFTs. 25% of pts dc IV cidofovir due to toxicity. **Comment:** Recommended dosage, frequency or infusion rate of cidofovir must not be exceeded. Dose must be reduced or discontinued if changes in renal function occur during rx. For ↑ of 0.3–0.4 mg/dl in serum creatinine, cidofovir dose must be ↓ from 5 to 3 mg/kg; discontinue cidofovir if ↑ of 0.5 mg/dl above baseline or 3+ proteinuria develops (for 2+ proteinuria, observe pts carefully and consider discontinuation).
Cidofovir gel (Forvade)		Available for topical rx of acyclovir-resistant mucocutaneous HSV in AIDS pts through "expanded access" from Gilead, 1-800-GILEAD5.
Foscarnet (Foscavir)	60 mg/kg q8h IV (6 gm $73.27)	**Adverse effects: Major clinical toxicity is renal impairment (⅓ of patients)**—↑ creatinine, proteinuria, nephrogenic diabetes insipidus, ↓ K+, ↓ Ca++, ↓ Mg++ (may be prolonged, *CID 25:933, 1997*). Toxicity ↑ with other nephrotoxic drugs [amphotericin B, aminoglycosides or pentamidine (especially severe ↓ Ca++)]. Adequate hydration may ↓ toxicity. Other: headache, mild (100%); fatigue (100%); nausea (80%), fever (25%). CNS: seizures. Hematol.: ↓ WBC, ↓ Hgb. Hepatic: liver function tests ↑. Neuropathy. Penile ulcers.
Ganciclovir (Cytovene)	IV: 5 mg/kg q12h x14 days (induction) 5 mg/kg IV qd or 6 mg/kg 5x/wk (suspension) (500 mg IV $34.80)	**Adverse effects:** Granulocytopenia 25%, thrombocytopenia 21%, anemia 6%. Fever 48%. GI 50%: nausea, vomiting, diarrhea, abdominal pain 19%, rash 10%. Retinal detachment 11% (relationship to ganciclovir ?). Confusion, headache, psychiatric disturbances (*NEJM 335:1397, 1996*) and seizures. Neutropenia may respond to granulocyte colony stimulating factor (G-CSF or GM-CSF). Severe myelosuppression may be ↑ with coadministration of zidovudine or azathioprine. **Comment:** Drug should be reconstituted immediately before use and unused portion discarded. Reconstituted solution should not be refrigerated.
	Oral: 1.0 gm tid with food (fatty meal) (250 mg cap $3.90)	**Adverse effects:** Hematologic less frequent than with IV. Granulocytopenia 18%, anemia 12%, thrombocytopenia 6%. GI, skin same as with IV. Retinal detachment 8%.
	Intraocular implant (Vitrasert) (~$4000/device + cost of surgery)	**Adverse effects:** Late retinal detachment (7/30 eyes). Does not prevent CMV retinitis in good eye or visceral dissemination. **Comment:** Replacement every 6 months recommended (*NEJM 337:83, 1997*).
Herpesvirus (non-CMV)		
Acyclovir (Zovirax or generic)	200 mg po tab $1.14 400 mg po tab $2.22 800 mg po tab $4.31 500 mg IV $59.51	**po:** Generally well-tolerated with occ. diarrhea, vertigo, arthralgia. Less frequent rash, fatigue, insomnia, fever, menstrual abnormalities, acne, sore throat, muscle cramps, lymphadenopathy **IV:** Phlebitis, caustic with vesicular lesions with IV infiltration, CNS (1%): lethargy, tremors, confusion, hallucinations, delirium, seizures, coma (*CID 21:435, 1995*). Improve 1–2 weeks after rx stopped. Renal 5%): ↑ creatinine, hematuria. With high doses may crystallize in renal tubules → obstructive uropathy (rapid infusion, dehydration, renal insufficiency and ↑ dose ↑ risk). Hepatic: ↑ ALT, AST. Uncommon: neutropenia (*CID 20:1557, 1995*), rash, diaphoresis, hypotension, headache, nausea.
Famciclovir (Famvir)	250 mg cap $3.18 500 mg cap $6.39	Metabolized to penciclovir. Side-effects similar to acyclovir, included headache, nausea, diarrhea, and dizziness but incidence did not differ from placebo (*JAMA 276:47, 1996*).

* From 1997 Red Book, Medical Economics Data. Price is average wholesale price (AWP).
All dosage recommendations are for adults (unless otherwise indicated) and assume normal renal function

TABLE 13 (9)

DRUG NAME(S) GENERIC (TRADE)	DOSAGE/ROUTE/COST*	COMMENTS/ADVERSE EFFECTS
Penciclovir (Denavir)	Topical 1% cream: apply to area of recurrence of herpes labialis with start of sx and q2h x4 d.	Adverse effects: Well tolerated.
Trifluridine (Viroptic)	1 drop 1% solution q2h (max. 9 drops/d.) for max. of 21 d. (7.5 ml 1% solution $66.66)	Mild burning (5%), palpebral edema (3%), punctate keratopathy, stromal edema
Valacyclovir (Valtrex)	500 mg cap $2.82	An ester of acyclovir that is well-absorbed, bioavailability 3–5x greater than acyclovir. Side-effects similar to acyclovir. Thrombotic thrombocytopenic purpura/hemolytic uremic syndrome reported in pts with advanced HIV disease and transplant recipients participating in clinical trials of valacyclovir at doses of 8 gm/day.

Hepatitis

DRUG NAME(S) GENERIC (TRADE)	DOSAGE/ROUTE/COST*	COMMENTS/ADVERSE EFFECTS
Interferon alfa is available as alfa-2a (Roferon-A), alfa-2b Intron-A)	3 million units: Roferon $33.94, Intron $33.92; Infergen 9 μg $35.28	**Adverse effects (IV dosage):** Flu-like syndrome is common, esp. during 1st week of rx: fever 98%, fatigue 89%, myalgia 73%, headache 71%. GI: anorexia 46%, diarrhea 29%. CNS: dizziness 21%. Rash 18%, later profound fatigue & psychiatric symptoms (depression, anxiety, emotional lability and agitation), alopecia, ↑ TSH, autoimmune thyroid disorders with hypo- or hyperthyroidism. Hematol.: ↓ WBC 49%, ↓ Hgb 27%, ↓ platelets 35%. Acute reversible hearing loss and/or tinnitus in up to ⅓ (Ln 343:1134, 1994). Side-effects ↑ with ↑ doses and dose reduction necessary in up to 46% receiving chronic rx for HSV.
Lamivudine (3TC) (Epivir)	See Table 5B, page 16	

Influenza A

DRUG NAME(S) GENERIC (TRADE)	DOSAGE/ROUTE/COST*	COMMENTS/ADVERSE EFFECTS
Amantadine (Symmetrel, Intuition) or Rimantadine (Flumadine HCl)	Amantadine and rimantadine doses are the same (rimantadine approved only for prophylaxis in children, not treatment). Adult dose: 100 mg bid. Amantadine 100 mg of syrup $1.81 Rimantadine 100 mg tab $1.61	**Side-effects/toxicity:** CNS (nervousness, anxiety, difficulty concentrating, and lightheadedness). Symptoms occurred in 6% on rimantadine vs 14% on amantadine. They usually ↓ after 1st week and disappear when drug dc. GI (nausea, anorexia). Some serious side-effects—delirium, hallucinations, and seizures—are associated with high plasma drug levels resulting from renal insufficiency, esp. in older pts, those with prior seizure disorders, or psychiatric disorders. In pts with impaired renal function, dosage of both drugs should be reduced (amantadine: creatinine clearance <50 ml/min, rimantadine: CrCl <10 ml/min); see package inserts and Table 15. Both drugs teratogenic in animals and contraindicated during pregnancy (Med Lett 39:72, 1997).

Respiratory Syncytial Virus (RSV) and other

DRUG NAME(S) GENERIC (TRADE)	DOSAGE/ROUTE/COST*	COMMENTS/ADVERSE EFFECTS
Ribavirin (Virazole) Aerosol	1.1 gm/day (6 gm vial for inhalation $1319.85)	**Ribavirin side-effects:** Anemia, rash, conjunctivitis: Read package insert. Avoid procedures that lead to drug precipitation in ventilator tubing with subsequent dysfunction. Significant teratogenicity in animals. Pregnant health care workers should avoid direct care of pts receiving aerosolized ribavirin. Neither oral nor IV ribavirin is marketed in U.S.
IV immunoglobulin (RespiGam)	FDA approval January 1996 (50 ml $599.21)	RespiGam side-effects rare: fatal anaphylaxis, pruritus, rash, wheezing, fever, joint pain.

Warts

DRUG NAME(S) GENERIC (TRADE)	DOSAGE/ROUTE/COST*	COMMENTS/ADVERSE EFFECTS
Interferon alfa-2b or alpha-n3	1 million units (0.1 ml) into lesion	**Side-effects:** Have to use vials containing 10 million units/1.0 ml. Cost: 0.1 ml $10.50
Podofilox (Condylox)	3.5 ml for topical application, $62.30	**Side-effects:** Local reactions—pain, burning, inflammation in 50%. No systemic effects.
Imiquimod (Aldara)	Cream applied 3x/week to maximum of 16 weeks. 250 mg packets $9 each	Mild erythema, erosions, itching and burning

* From 1997 Red Book, Medical Economics Data. Price is average wholesale price (AWP).
All dosage recommendations are for adults (unless otherwise indicated) and assume normal renal function

TABLE 14A
METHODS FOR PENICILLIN DESENSITIZATION

Perform in ICU setting. Discontinue all β-adrenergic antagonists. Have IV line, ECG and spirometer *(Curr Clin Topics Inf Dis 13:131, 1993)*. Once desensitized, rx must not lapse or risk of allergic reactions ↑. A history of Stevens-Johnson syndrome, exfoliative dermatitis, erythroderma are nearly absolute contraindications to desensitization (use only as an approach to IgE sensitivity).

Oral Route: If oral prep available and pt has functional GI tract, oral route is preferred. 1/3 pts will develop transient reaction during desensitization or treatment, usually mild.

Step *	1	2	3	4	5	6	7	8	9	10	11	12	13	14
Drug (mg/ml)	0.5	0.5	0.5	0.5	0.5	0.5	0.5	5.0	5.0	5.0	50	50	50	50
Amount (ml)	0.1	0.2	0.4	0.8	1.6	3.2	6.4	1.2	2.4	4.8	1.0	2.0	4.0	8.0

* Interval between doses: 15 min. After Step 14, observe for 30 minutes, then 1.0 gm IV

Parenteral Route:

Step **	1	2	3	4	5	6	7	8	9	10	11	12	13	14	15	16	17
Drug (mg/ml)	0.1	0.1	0.1	0.1	1.0	1.0	1.0	10	10	10	100	100	100	100	1000	1000	1000
Amount (ml)	0.1	0.2	0.4	0.8	0.16	0.32	0.64	0.12	0.24	0.48	0.1	0.2	0.4	0.8	0.16	0.32	0.64

** Interval between doses: 15 min. After Step 17, observe for 30 minutes, then 1.0 gm IV

[Adapted from Sullivan, TJ, in Allergy: Principles and Practice, Middleton, E., et al, Eds. C.V. Mosby, 1993, p. 1726, with permission]

TABLE 14B
PROTOCOL FOR RAPID ORAL TMP/SMX DESENSITIZATION

Hour	Dose TMP/SMX*
0	0.004/0.02 mg
1	0.04/0.2 mg
2	0.4/2 mg
3	4/20 mg
4	40/200 mg
5	160/800 mg

* Perform in office or hospital. Use oral suspension [40 mg TMP/ 200 mg SMX/5 ml (tsp.)]. Take 6 oz. water after each dose. Corticosteroids, antihistaminics not used. 19/22 patients were successful. Failures: chills and/or vomiting *(CID 20:849, 1995)* *(Other ref.: AIDS 5:311, 1991)*.

Note: Although rare, life-threatening reactions (including hypotension) can occur in patients being desensitized, especially within several months of a preceding severe reaction *(CID 23:1313, 1996; CID 25:754, 1997)*.

ALTERNATE SLOW DOSE ESCALATION PROTOCOL

Day	Dose TMP/SMX**
1	10/50
2	20/100
3	30/150
4	40/200
5	60/300
6	80/400 (suspension or tablet)

** Perform in office or hospital. Use oral suspension as above. 79% of patients on this regimen still on TMP/SMX after 6 months vs 59% in group receiving direct rechallenge [but total side effects and severity (low grade) of side effects similar in both groups *(Inf in Med 14[Suppl.B]:33, 1997)*].

TABLE 15: PHARMACOKINETICS OF ANTIRETROVIRAL DRUGS AND DRUGS USED IN TREATMENT OF HIV-ASSOCIATED INFECTIONS IN ADULTS

DRUG	ORAL ABSORPTION (%)	SERUM HALF-LIFE (t/2)(hr)	PEAK SERUM LEVELS[1] (μg/ml)	PROTEIN BINDING (%)	AVG. CSF PENETRATION (%)	RENAL EXCRETION (%)
Antiretroviral Agents:[2]						
Delavirdine	85	5.8	19 ± 11	98	0.4	<5
Didanosine (ddI)	37[3]	1.5	0.6–2.9[5]	<5	19–21	20
Indinavir	Good (~80)	1.8	12617 nM	60		10
Lamivudine (3TC)	86	3.7	3.3	<36	15	71
Nelfinavir	80	3.5–5	3–4	>98		<2
Nevirapine	>90	25–30	2	60	45	81
Ritonavir	Good (~65)	3.2	7.8	90		
Saquinavir softgel	approx. 12[6]	ND	2.5	98	negligible	~1%
Stavudine (d4T)	85	1.1	1.2	"not"	9	55
Zalcitabine (ddC)	>80	1.2–1.8	4–11 ng/ml[5]	<4	20	62–75
Zidovudine	42–95	0.6–1.7	1.2[5]	35	15–20	63–95[4]
Antiparasitic Agents:						
Albendazole	poor (↑ by fat)	8–12	0.5–1.6	70	low	<1
Atovaquone (suspension)	47 (↑ with fatty food)	67	11.5	>99.9	<1	<1
Clindamycin	75	2.4	7.7	85–94	None	10–15
Dapsone	86–100	28	2.3	70–90	+	70–85
Ivermectin	ND	16	0.05	ND	ND	<1
Metronidazole	90	6–14	20–25 (IV)	20	16–43	<20
Pentamidine IV	None	9.4	0.6 (IV)	69	None	80
Pyrimethamine	+	95–118	0.13–0.4	87	13–26	Low
Sulfadiazine	Good	17	100–150 (IV)	45	High	Most
Trimethoprim	Good	11	2.0	44	30 (I)	50–60
TMP/SMX	Good	10/11	1/40 (O) 9/106 (IV)	44/70	50/40	67/84
Trimetrexate	None	11		95		10–30
Antifungal Agents:						
Amphotericin B	None	24	0.5–2.0	>90	<2.5	40
Fluconazole	85	20–30	4–8	11	80	65
Flucytosine	78–89	2.4–4.8	70–80	3–4	High	90
Itraconazole soln	55–99	20–30	1.9	99	<10	<1
Ketoconazole	75[4]	8	3.5	99	<10	2
Antiviral Agents:						
Acyclovir	15–30	2.5	0.5–1.0 (O)	9–33	50 (I)	15
Cidofovir	None	3–4	~15			>90
Famciclovir	77	2.0	3.0–4.0	<20	94	73
Foscarnet	None	0.5–6	445–579 μM/L	14–17	43	80–82
Ganciclovir	<7	2.9	9.5[5]	1–2	25–70	90
Valacyclovir	55	2.5–3.3	3.3	15	50	45
Antimycobacterial Agents:						
Amikacin	None	2	21	0–11	10–24	98
Azithromycin	37	40	0.4	12–50	<1	5
Ciprofloxacin	70	4	4.3	20–40	5–19	40–50
Clarithromycin	50	5–7	2–3	65–70		30
Ethambutol	77	3–4	2–4	40	50 (I)	80
Isoniazid	90	1	1–5	Low	90	50–70
Ofloxacin	98	7	3.5–5.3	32	8–20	70–80
Pyrazinamide	Good	9–10	30–50		>90	70
Rifabutin	20	45	0.2–1.0	72–85	50	<10
Rifampin	90–95	2–3	7	80	10–20	3–30
Sparfloxacin	92	16–30	1.3	45	ND	10
Streptomycin	None	3	20–30	Low	±	60–90

Abbreviations: **μM** = micromolar, **NA** = not applicable, **(IV)** = after IV dosing, **(IM)** = after IM dosing, **(I)** = inflamed meninges, **(O)** = after oral dosing, **ND** = no data
[1] Levels following "usual dose", Tables 5, 12; [2] Intracellular half-life may be more important; [3] In children 2–89%; chewable tablets absorption ↑ 20–25%; [4] Requires gastric acid for absorption; [5] ZDV 1 μg/ml = 3.74 μM/L, ddI 1 μg/ml = 5.0 μM/L; ddC 1 ng/ml = 4.76 nmol/L, ganciclovir 1 μg/ml = 3.92 μM/L; [6] based on ↑ area under concentration curve (AUC) data

TABLE 16
DOSAGE OF ANTIMICROBIAL DRUGS IN ADULT PATIENTS WITH RENAL IMPAIRMENT

Adapted from DRUG PRESCRIBING IN RENAL FAILURE, 4th Ed., Aronoff et al (Eds.), American College of Physicians (in press) and Berns et al, Renal Aspects of Antimicrobial Therapy for HIV Infection. In: P. Kenimel & J. Berns, Eds., HIV INFECTION AND THE KIDNEY, Churchill-Livingstone, 1995, pp 195–236. UNLESS STATED, ADJUSTED DOSES ARE % OF DOSE FOR NORMAL RENAL FUNCTION.

Drug adjustments are based on the patient's estimated endogenous creatinine clearance, which can be calculated as:

$$\frac{(140-age)(ideal\ body\ weight\ in\ kg)}{(72)(serum\ creatinine,\ mg/dL)}$$ for men (x 0.85 for women)

Ideal body weight for men: 50.0 kg + 2.3 kg per inch over 5 feet
Ideal body weight for women: 45.5 kg + 2.3 kg per inch over 5 feet

NOTE: For the following drugs, there is no need for adjustment of dosage in patients with renal impairment: **azithromycin, ceftriaxone, chloramphenicol, clindamycin, delavirdine, dirithromycin, doxycycline, grepafloxacin, minocycline, nafcillin, pyrimethamine, rifabutin, trovafloxacin**.

The following is a selected list of drugs commonly used in the care of HIV-infected patients. For data on additional antimicrobials, see Table 17 of the 1998 SANFORD GUIDE TO ANTIMICROBIAL THERAPY.

ANTIMICROBIAL	HALF-LIFE (NORMAL/ESRD) hr	DOSE FOR NORMAL RENAL FUNCTION[§]	METHOD* (see footnote)	ADJUSTMENT FOR RENAL FAILURE Estimated creatinine clearance (CrCl), ml/min			HEMODIALYSIS, CAPD	COMMENTS
				>50–90	10–50	<10		
ANTIBACTERIAL ANTIBIOTICS **Aminoglycoside Antibiotics**:			**Traditional multiple daily doses—adjustment for renal disease**					
Amikacin	1.4–2.3/17–150	7.5 mg/kg q12h	D&I	60–90% q12h	30–70% q12–18h **Dose for CAVH[1]**	20–30% q24–48h	HEMO: ⅔ normal dose AD[2] CAPD: 15–20 mg lost/L dialysate/day¶ (see Comment)	High flux hemodialysis membranes lead to unpredictable aminoglycoside clearance, measure post-dialysis drug levels for efficacy and toxicity. With CAPD, pharmacokinetics highly variable— check serum levels. ¶Usual method for CAPD: 2 liters of dialysis fluid placed qid or 8 liters/day (give 8Lx20 mg lost/L = 160 mg of amikacin supplement IV per day) Adjust dosing weight for obesity: [ideal body weight + 0.4(actual body weight – ideal body weight)] (CID 25:112, 1997).
Gentamicin, Tobramycin	2–3/20–60	1.7 mg/kg q8h	D&I	60–90% q8–12h	30–70% q12h **Dose for CAVH[1]**	20–30% q24–48h	HEMO: ⅔ normal dose AD[2] CAPD: 3–4 mg lost/L dialysate/day	
Netilmicin	2–3/35–72	2.0 mg/kg q8h	D&I	50–90% q8–12h	20–60% q12h **Dose for CAVH[1]**	10–20% q24–48h	HEMO: ⅔ normal dose AD[2] CAPD: 3–4 mg lost/L dialysate/day	
Streptomycin	2–3/30–80	15 mg/kg (max. of 1.0 gm) q24h	I	50% q24h	q24–72h **Dose for CAVH[1]**	q72–96h	HEMO: ½ normal dose AD[2] CAPD: 20–40 mg lost/L dialysate/day	

ONCE-DAILY AMINOGLYCOSIDE THERAPY: ADJUSTMENT IN RENAL INSUFFICIENCY

Creatinine Clearance (ml/min.) Drug	>80 Dose q24h (mg/kg)	60–80	40–60	30–40	20–30 Dose q48h (mg/kg)	10–20	<10
Gentamicin/Tobramycin	5.1	4	3.5	2.5		3	2
Amikacin/kanamycin/streptomycin	15	12	7.5	4	7.5	4	3
Isepamicin[NUS]	8	8	8	8 q48h	8	8 q72h	8 q96h
Netilmicin	6.5	5	4	2	3	2.5	2.0

Cephalosporins; Penicillins; Beta-lactam/beta-lactamase inhibitors; Carbapenems—see Table 17, SANFORD GUIDE TO ANTIMICROBIAL THERAPY 1998

Fluoroquinolone Antibiotics: adjust dosage of grepafloxacin and trovafloxacin in patients with hepatic insufficiency (see package inserts)

Ciprofloxacin	4/6–9	500–750 mg po (or 400 mg IV) q12h	D	100%	50–75%	50%	HEMO: 250 mg po or 200 mg IV q12h CAPD: 250 mg po or 200 mg IV q8h	CAVH: 200 mg IV q12h

[1] **CAVH** = continuous arteriovenous hemofiltration (NEJM 336:1303, 1997); [2] **AD** = after dialysis. See page 111 for other footnotes and abbreviations.

TABLE 16 (2)

ANTIMICROBIAL	HALF-LIFE (NORMAL/ESRD) hr	DOSE FOR NORMAL RENAL FUNCTION⁵	METHOD* (see footnote)	ADJUSTMENT FOR RENAL FAILURE Estimated creatinine clearance (CrCl), ml/min >50–90	10–50	<10	HEMODIALYSIS, CAPD	COMMENTS
Fluoroquinolone Antibiotics (continued)								
Levofloxacin	4–8/76	500 mg qd IV, PO	D[1]	100%	50%	25–50%	HEMO/CAPD: Dose for CrCl <10	CAVH: No data
Ofloxacin	7.0/28–37	400 mg po/IV q12h	I	100%	50%	25–50%	HEMO: 100 mg bid CAPD: Dose for CrCl <10	CAVH: 300 mg/d
Sparfloxacin	15–20/38.5	400 mg day 1, then 200 mg qd	D&I	100%	50–75%	50% q48h	HEMO: Dose for CrCl <10 CAPD/CAVH: No data	
Macrolide Antibiotics: adjust dose of azithromycin in patients with hepatic insufficiency (see package insert)								
Clarithromycin	5–7/22	0.5–1.0 gm q12h	D	100%	75%	50–75%	HEMO: Dose AD CAPD: None	ESRD dosing recommendations based on extrapolation
Erythromycin	1.4/5–6	250–500 mg q6h	D	100%	100%	50–75%	HEMO/CAPD/CAVH: None	Ototoxicity with high doses in ESRD. Vol. of distribution increases in ESRD.
Tetracycline Antibiotics								
Tetracycline	6–10/57–108	250–500 mg qid	I	q8–12h	q12–24h	q24h	HEMO/CAPD/CAVH: None	Avoid in ESRD
Miscellaneous Antibacterial Antibiotics								
Metronidazole	6–14/7–21	7.5 mg/kg q6h	D	100%	100% **Dose for CAVH**	50%	HEMO: Dose AD CAPD: Dose for CrCl <10	Hemo clears metronidazole and its metabolites (AAC 29:235, 1986)
Sulfadiazine	17/34	1.0 gm q6h	I	q8–12h	q24h	q48–72h or avoid	HEMO/CAPD: No data	
Sulfamethoxa-zole	10/20–50	1.0 gm q8h	I	q12h	q18h **Dose for CAVH**	q24h	HEMO: 1 gm AD CAPD: 1 gm qd	
Trimethoprim	11/20–49	100–200 mg q12h	I	q12h	q18h	q24h	HEMO: Dose AD CAPD: q24h	CAVH: q18h
TMP/SMX-DS								
Treatment	As above	5 mg/kg IV q8h	D	100%	50%	Not recommended		
Prophylaxis	As above	tab 1 q24h or 3x/week po	No change	100%	100%	100%		
Vancomycin[2]	6/200–250	500 mg q6h or 1 gm q12h	D&I	500 mg q6–12h	500 mg q24–48h	500 mg q48–96h	HEMO/CAPD: 1.0 gm q1 wk	CAVH: 500 mg q24–48h

[1] Regardless of CrCl, 1st dose is 500 mg, and then adjust dose and interval

[2] Vancomycin serum levels may be overestimated in renal failure if measured by either fluorescence polarization immunoassay or radioimmunoassay; vanco breakdown products interfere. EMIT method OK.

AD = after dialysis; **CAVH** = continuous arteriovenous hemofiltration. See page 111 for other footnotes and abbreviations

TABLE 16 (3)

ANTIMICROBIAL	HALF-LIFE (NORMAL/ESRD) hr	DOSE FOR NORMAL RENAL FUNCTION[§]	METHOD* (see footnote)	ADJUSTMENT FOR RENAL FAILURE Estimated creatinine clearance (CrCl), ml/min			HEMODIALYSIS, CAPD	COMMENTS
				>50–90	10–50	<10		
ANTIFUNGAL ANTIBIOTICS								
Amphotericin B	24/unchanged	Non-lipid: 0.3–0.8 mg/kg/d ABCC:[1] 3–6 mg/kg/d ABLC:[1] 15 mg/kg/d LAB:[1] 3–5 mg/kg/d	I	q24h	q24h **Dose for CAVH**	q24–36h	HEMO: None CAPD: Dose for CrCl <10	Toxicity lessened by saline loading; risk amplified by concomitant cyclo-sporine A, aminoglycosides, or pentamidine
Fluconazole	37/100	200–400 mg q24h	D	100%	50% **Dose for CAVH**	50%	HEMO: 200 mg AD CAPD: Dose for CrCl <10	
Flucytosine[2]	3–6/75–200	37.5 mg/kg q6h	I	q12h	q16h **Dose for CAVH**	q24h	HEMO: Dose AD CAPD: 0.5–1.0 gm q24h	
Itraconazole	21/25	100–200 mg q12h	D	100%	100%	50%	HEMO/CAPD/CAVH: 100 mg q12–24h	
ANTIPARASITIC DRUGS								
Atovaquone	No data	750 mg po bid		No data in patients with renal or hepatic impairment				
Dapsone	No data	100 mg po/day		No data in patients with renal or hepatic impairment				
Pentamidine	29/118	4 mg/kg/d	I	q24h	q24–36h	q48h	HEMO/CAPD/CAVH: None	
Pyrimethamine	96/96	50–75 mg/day	No change	100%	100%	100%	HEMO/CAPD/CAVH: None	
ANTITUBERCULOUS ANTIBIOTICS *(Excellent review: Nephron 64:169, 1993)*								
Ethambutol	4/7–15	15 mg/kg q24h	I	q24h **Dose for CAVH**	q24–36h	q48h	HEMO: Dose AD CAPD: Dose for CrCl <10	25 mg/kg 4–6 hr prior to dialysis for usual 3x/week dialysis. Streptomycin recommended in lieu of ethambutol in renal failure.
Ethionamide	2.1/?	250–500 mg q12h	D	100%	100%	50%	HEMO/CAPD/CAVH: None	
Isoniazid	0.7–4/8–17	5 mg/kg/d (max. 300 mg)	D	100%	100%	50%	HEMO: Dose AD CAPD/CAVH: 50% ↓	Dose adjustment is for slow acetylators
Pyrazinamide	9/26	25 mg/kg q24h (max. dose 2.5 gm qd)	D	Avoid	Avoid	Avoid	HEMO/CAPD/CAVH: Avoid	
Rifabutin	No data	300 mg/day po		No data available				
Rifampin	1.5–5/1.8–11	600 mg/d	D	100%	50–100%	50%	HEMO: None CAPD/CAVH: Dose for CrCl <10	Biologically active metabolite
ANTIVIRAL AGENTS								
Acyclovir	2.5/20	5–12.4 mg/kg q8h	D&I	5–12.4 mg/kg q8h	5–12.4 mg/kg q12–24h	2.5–6 mg/kg q24h	HEMO: Dose AD CAPD: Dose for CrCl <10	Rapid IV infusion can cause renal failure. CAVH: 3.5 mg/kg/d

[1] **ABCC** = ampho B cholesteryl complex; **ABLC** = ampho B lipid complex; **LAB** = liposomal ampho B

[2] Concentrations <25 μg/ml should be avoided to prevent development of resistance, while >100 μg/ml avoided because of toxicity *(JAC 35:241, 1995)*

AD = after dialysis; **CAVH** = continuous arteriovenous hemofiltration. *See page 111 for other footnotes and abbreviations*

TABLE 16 (4)

ANTIVIRAL AGENTS (continued)

Cidofovir: Complicated dosing—*see package insert*

ANTIMICROBIAL	HALF-LIFE (NORMAL/ESRD) hr	DOSE FOR NORMAL RENAL FUNCTION§	METHOD* (see footnote)	ADJUSTMENT FOR RENAL FAILURE — Estimated creatinine clearance (CrCl), ml/min >50–90	ADJUSTMENT FOR RENAL FAILURE — 10–50	ADJUSTMENT FOR RENAL FAILURE — <10	HEMODIALYSIS, CAPD	COMMENTS
Induction	2.5/unknown	5 mg/kg 1x/wk for 2 wks	–	5 mg/kg 1x/wk	0.5–2 mg/kg 1x/wk	0.5 mg/kg 1x/wk	No data	Major toxicity is renal. No efficacy, safety, or pharmacokinetic data in pts with moderate/severe renal disease.
Maintenance	2.5/unknown	5 mg/kg q2wks	–	5 mg/kg q2wks	0.5–2 mg/kg q2wks	0.5 mg/kg q2wks	No data	
Didanosine tablets	0.6–1.6/4.5	125–200 mg q12h	I	q12h	q24h	q24–48h	HEMO: Dose AD CAPD/CAVH: Dose for CrCl <10	Based on incomplete data. Data are estimates.
Famciclovir	1.6–2.9/10–22	500 mg q8h	D&I	q8h	250–500 mg q12–48h	250 mg q48h	HEMO: 250 mg AD CAPD/CAVH: No data	

Foscarnet — CrCl as ml/min/kg body weight—ONLY FOR FOSCARNET

Foscarnet (CMV dosage) Dosage adjustment based on est. CrCl (ml/min) div. by pt's kg	HALF-LIFE (NORMAL/ESRD) hr	DOSE FOR NORMAL RENAL FUNCTION§	>1.4	>1.0–1.4	>0.8–1.0	>0.6–0.8	>0.5–0.6	>0.4–0.5	<0.4	COMMENTS
	Normal half-life (T½) 3 hrs with terminal T½ of 18–88 hrs. T½ very long with ESRD	Induction: 60 mg/kg q8h x2–3 wks IV	60 q8h	45 q8h	50 q12h	40 q12h	60 q24h	50 q24h	Do not use	See package insert for further details
		Maintenance: 90–120 mg/kg/d IV	120 q24h	90 q24h	65 q24h	105 q48h	80 q48h	65 q48h	Do not use	

ANTIMICROBIAL	HALF-LIFE (NORMAL/ESRD) hr	DOSE FOR NORMAL RENAL FUNCTION§	METHOD* (see footnote)	ADJUSTMENT FOR RENAL FAILURE — >50–90	ADJUSTMENT FOR RENAL FAILURE — 10–50	ADJUSTMENT FOR RENAL FAILURE — <10	HEMODIALYSIS, CAPD	COMMENTS
Ganciclovir (IV:)	2.9/30	Induction 5 mg/kg q12h IV	D&I	5 mg/kg q12h	1.25–2.5 mg/kg q24h	1.25 mg/kg 3x/wk	HEMO: Dose AD CAPD: Dose for CrCl <10	
		Maintenance 5 mg/kg q24h IV	D&I	2.5–5.0 mg/kg q24h	0.6–1.25 mg/kg q24h	0.625 mg/kg 3x/week	HEMO: 0.6 mg/kg AD CAPD: Dose for CrCl <10	
(po:)		1.0 gm tid po	D&I	0.5–1.0 gm tid	0.5–1.0 gm qd	0.5 gm 3x/week	HEMO: 0.5 gm AD	
Indinavir	1.8/No data	800 mg tid po		No data on influence of renal insufficiency. Less than 20% excreted unchanged in urine. Probably no dose reduction.				
Lamivudine	5–7/15–35	150 mg bid po	D&I	150 mg bid	100–150 mg qd	25–50 mg qd	HEMO: Dose AD; CAPD/CAVH: No data	
Nelfinavir/Nevirapine:	No data available at this time							
Ritonavir	3–5/No data	600 mg bid po		Negligible renal clearance. At present, no patient data				
Saquinavir	No data	600 mg tid po		Minimal renal excretion. No data available at this time				
Stavudine, po	1–1.4/5.5–8	30–40 mg q12h	D/I	100%	50%	50% q24h	HEMO: Dose AD CAPD/CAVH: No data	
Valacyclovir	2.5/3.3	1.0 gm q8h	D&I	1.0 gm q8h	1.0 gm q12–24h	0.5 gm q24h	HEMO: Dose AD CAPD: Dose for CrCl <10	CAVH: No data
Zalcitabine	2.0/>8	0.75 mg q8h	I	0.75 mg q8h	0.75 mg q12h	0.75 mg q24h	HEMO: Dose AD CAPD/CAVH: No data	
Zidovudine	1.1–1.4/1.4–3	200 mg q8h	D&I	200 mg q8h	200 mg q8h	100 mg q12h	HEMO: 100 mg AD CAPD: Dose for CrCl <10	CAVH: 100 mg q8h

§ Dosages are for life-threatening infections; * **D** = dosage reduction, **I** = interval extension; ** Per cent refers to % change from dose for normal renal function.
Abbreviations: **HEMO** = hemodialysis; **CAPD** = chronic ambulatory peritoneal dialysis; **ESRD** = endstage renal disease; **NUS** = not available in the U.S.

TABLE 17
DRUG/DRUG INTERACTIONS: ANTIRETROVIRAL DRUGS and DRUGS USED IN TREATMENT OF HIV-ASSOCIATED INFECTIONS AND MALIGNANCIES

This is a selected list. For drug-drug interactions of other antimicrobials, please refer to Table 19 of the SANFORD GUIDE TO ANTIMICROBIAL THERAPY. Significance/Certainty: ± = theory/anecdotal; + = of probable clinical import; ++ = of definite clinical import

ANTI-INFECTIVE AGENT (A)	OTHER DRUG (B)	EFFECT	SIGNIFICANCE/ CERTAINTY
Acyclovir (Zovirax)	Nephrotoxic drugs	Crystalluria of A may aggravate	+
Aminoglycosides— parenteral (amikacin, gentamicin, kanamycin, netilmicin, sisomicin, streptomycin, tobramycin) *NOTE: Capreomycin is an aminoglycoside, used as alternative drug to treat mycobacterial infections.*	Amphotericin B	↑ nephrotoxicity	++
	Cis platinum (Platinol)	↑ nephro & ototoxicity	+
	Cyclosporine	↑ nephrotoxicity	+
	Neuromuscular blocking agents	↑ apnea or respiratory paralysis	+
	Loop diuretics (e.g., furosemide)	↑ ototoxicity	++
	Methoxyflurane, enflurane	↑ nephrotoxicity	±
	"Noise"	↑ ototoxicity	±
	NSAIDs	↑ nephrotoxicity	+
	Non-polarizing muscle relaxants	↑ apnea	+
	Radiographic contrast	↑ nephrotoxicity	+
	Vancomycin	↑ nephrotoxicity	+
Aminoglycosides— oral (kanamycin, neomycin)	Oral anticoagulants (dicumarol, phenindione, warfarin)	↑ prothrombin time	+
Amphotericin B and ampho B lipid formulations	Antineoplastic drugs	↑ potential nephrotoxicity	+
	Corticosteroids & ACTH	May potentiate hypokalemia	+
	Digitalis	↑ toxicity of B if hypokalemia	+
	Flucytosine	Possible ↑ toxicity of A	±
	Nephrotoxic drugs: aminoglycosides, cidofovir, cyclosporin, foscarnet, pentamidine	↑ nephrotoxic potential of A	++
Atovaquone	Rifampin (perhaps rifabutin)	↓ serum levels of A; ↑ levels of B	+

Azole Antifungal Agents[1]   (**Flu** = fluconazole, **Itr** = itraconazole, **Ket** = ketoconazole, + = occurs, NRS = not reported but not studied)

Flu	Itr	Ket	OTHER DRUG (B)	EFFECT	SIGNIFICANCE/ CERTAINTY
+	NRS	NRS	Amitriptyline	↑ levels of B	+
+	+	+	Antihistaminics, non-sedating[2]	↑ levels of B (cardiac arrhythmias)	++
−	+	−	Carbamazepine	↓ levels of A	+
+	+	+	Cisapride	↑ levels of B (arrhythmias, ↑ Q-T interval)	++
+	+	+	Cyclosporine, tacrolimus	↑ levels of B, ↑ risk of nephrotoxicity	+
NRS	+	+	Didanosine	↓ absorption of A	+
−	+	+	H₂ blockers, antacids, sucralfate	↓ absorption of A	+
+	+	+	Hydantoins (phenytoin, Dilantin)	↑ levels of B, ↓ levels of A	++
−	+	+	Isoniazid	↓ levels of A	+
NRS	+	NRS	Lovastatin/simvastatin	Rhabdomyolysis reported	+
+	+	+	Midazolam/triazolam, po	↑ levels of B	++
+	+	+	Oral anticoagulants	↑ effect of B	++
+	+	NRS	Oral hypoglycemics	↑ levels of B	++
−	+	+	Proton pump inhibitors	↓ absorption of A	+
+	+	+	Rifampin/rifabutin	↑ levels of B, ↓ serum levels of A	+
		+	Tacrolimus	↑ levels of B with toxicity	++
+	NRS	+	Theophyllines	↑ levels of B	+
+	−	NRS	Zidovudine	↑ levels of B	+

ANTI-INFECTIVE AGENT (A)	OTHER DRUG (B)	EFFECT	SIGNIFICANCE/ CERTAINTY
Clindamycin (Cleocin)	Kaolin	↓ absorption of A	+
	Muscle relaxants, e.g., atracurium, baclofen, diazepam	↑ frequency/duration of respiratory paralysis	+
	Erythromycin	Mutual antagonism	+
Cycloserine	Ethanol	↑ frequency of seizures	+
	INH, ethionamide	↑ frequency of drowsiness/dizziness	+
Dapsone	Didanosine	↓ absorption of A	+
	Oral contraceptives	↓ effectiveness of B	+
	Pyrimethamine	↑ in marrow toxicity	+
	Rifampin/Rifabutin	↓ serum levels of A	+
	Trimethoprim	↑ levels of A & B (methemoglobinemia)	+
	Zidovudine	May ↑ marrow toxicity	+
Delavirdine (Rescriptor)	Alprazolam, midazolam, triazolam	↑ levels of B	++

[1] Major interactions given; unusual or minor interactions manifest as toxicity of non-azole drug due to ↑ serum levels: Caffeine (Flu), digoxin (Itr), felodipine (Itr), fluoxetine (Itr), indinavir (Ket), lovastatin/simvastatin, quinidine (Ket), tricyclics (Flu), vincristine (Itr), and ↓ effectiveness of oral contraceptives.

[2] Antihistaminics, non-sedating: astemizole, terfenadine, loratadine (less or no azole interactions)

ANTI-INFECTIVE AGENT (A)	OTHER DRUG (B)	EFFECT	SIGNIFICANCE/ CERTAINTY
Delavirdine *(con't)*	Astemizole, terfenadine	↑ levels of B	++
	Cisapride	↑ levels of B	++
	Clarithromycin	↑ levels of B	++
	Dapsone	↑ levels of B	++
	Dihydropyridine Ca++ channel blockers	↑ levels of B	++
	Ergot alkaloids	↑ levels of B	++
	Protease inhibitors	↑ levels of B	++
	Quinidine, rifamycins	↑ levels of B	++
	Warfarin	↑ levels of B	++
Didanosine (ddl) (Videx)	Cisplatin, dapsone, INH, metronidazole, nitrofurantoin, stavudine, vincristine, zalcitabine	↑ risk of peripheral neuropathy	+
	Ethanol, lamivudine, pentamidine	↑ risk of pancreatitis	+
	Fluoroquinolones	↓ absorption 2° to chelation	+
	Low pH drug solubility: dapsone, indinavir, itra/ketoconazole, pyrimethamine, rifampin, trimethoprim	↓ absorption	+
Ethambutol (Myambutol)	Aluminum salts (includes didanosine buffer	↓ absorption of A & B	+
	Verapamil	↓ levels of B	±

Fluoroquinolones (*Cipro* = ciprofloxacin; *Grepa* = grepafloxacin; *Levo* = levofloxacin; *Lome* = lomefloxacin; *Norflox* = norfloxacin; *Oflox* = ofloxacin; *Spar* = sparfloxacin; *Trova* = trovafloxacin)

Cipro	Grepa	Levo	Lome	Norflox	Oflox	Spar	Trova	OTHER DRUG (B)	EFFECT	SIGNIFICANCE/ CERTAINTY
	+					+		Antiarrhythmics	↑ Q-T interval (torsade)	++
+	+				+			Insulin, oral hypoglycemics	↑ & ↓ blood sugar	+
+	+			+			+	Caffeine	↑ levels of B	+
+			+	+	+			Cimetidine	↑ levels of A	+
+			+	+	+	+		Cyclosporine	↑ levels of B	±
+	+	+	+	+	+	+	+	Didanosine	↓ absorption of A	++
+	+	+	+	+	+	+	+	Cations: Al+++, Ca++, Fe++, Mg++, Zn++ (antacids, vitamins, dairy products), citrate/citric acid	↓ absorption of A	++
+	+	+	+	+	+	+		NSAIDs	↑ risk CNS stimulation/seizures	++
+								Phenytoin	↑ or ↓ levels of B	+
+			+	+	+			Probenecid	↓ renal clearance of A	+
+	+	+	+	+	+	+	+	Sucralfate	↓ absorption of A	++
+	+			+				Theophylline	↑ levels of B	++
+		+	+	+	+			Warfarin	↑ prothrombin time	+

ANTI-INFECTIVE AGENT (A)	OTHER DRUG (B)	EFFECT	SIGNIFICANCE/ CERTAINTY
Foscarnet (Foscavir)	Bisphosphonates	May ↑ risk of hypocalcemia	±
	Nephrotoxic drugs: aminoglycosides, ampho B, cis-platinum, cyclosporine	↑ risk of nephrotoxicity	+
	Pentamidine IV	↑ risk of severe hypocalcemia	++
Ganciclovir (Cytovene)	Didanosine	↑ serum levels of B	±
	Imipenem	↑ risk of seizures reported	+
	Probenecid	↑ levels of A	+
	Zidovudine	↓ levels of A, ↑ levels of B	+
Gentamicin	*See Aminoglycosides—parenteral*		
Indinavir	*See protease inhibitors*		
Isoniazid	Alcohol, rifampin	↑ risk of hepatic injury	+
	Aluminum salts	↓ absorption (take fasting)	+
	Carbamazepine, phenytoin	↑ levels of B with nausea, vomiting, nystagmus, ataxia	++
	Itraconazole, ketoconazole	↓ levels of B	+
	Oral hypoglycemics	↓ effects of B	+
	Warfarin	↑ effects of B	±

Macrolides (*Ery* = erythromycin, *Dir* = dirithromycin, *Azi* = azithromycin, *Clr* = clarithromycin; + = occurs, 0 = does not occur; *NRS* = not reported but not studied)

Ery	Dir	Azi	Clr	OTHER DRUG (B)	EFFECT	SIGNIFICANCE/ CERTAINTY
+		NRS	NRS	Alfentanil	↑ action of B	±
+	NRS	NRS	+	Carbamazepine	↑ serum levels of B, nystagmus, nausea, vomiting, ataxia	++ (avoid with erythro)
+			+	Cimetidine, ritonavir	↑ levels of B	+
+	NRS	NRS	+	Cisapride	↑ Q-T interval; ↑ risk arrhythmias	++
+		NRS	NRS	Clozapine	↑ serum levels of B, CNS toxicity	+

TABLE 17 (3)

ANTI-INFECTIVE AGENT (A)				OTHER DRUG (B)	EFFECT	SIGNIFICANCE/ CERTAINTY
Ery	**Dir**	**Azi**	**Clr**			
Macrolides *(continued)*						
+		NRS	NRS	Corticosteroids	↑ effects of B	+
+	+	+	+	Cyclosporine	↑ serum levels of B with toxicity	+
+	NRS	+	+	Digoxin, digitoxin	↑ serum levels of B (10% of cases)	+
+			+	Ergot alkaloids	↑ levels of B	++
+		NRS	NRS	Felodipine, fluoxetine	↑ levels of B	±
+		NRS	+	Lovastatin	Rhabdomyolysis reported	±
+		NRS		Midazolam, triazolam	↑ levels of B, ↑ sedative effects	+
+			+	Phenytoin	↑ levels of B	+
+	+	+	+	Pimozide	↑ Q-T interval	++
+			+	Rifampin, rifabutin	↓ levels of A	+
+			+	Tacrolimus	↑ levels of B	++
+	0	0	+	Terfenadine, astemizole	↑ Q-T interval; ↑ risk of arrhythmias	++
+	0	0	+	Theophyllines	↑ serum levels of B with nausea, vomiting, seizures, apnea	++
+	NRS	NRS	+	Triazolam	↑ levels of B	+
+		NRS	+	Valproic acid	↑ levels of B	+
+	NRS	0	+	Warfarin	May ↑ prothrombin time	+
NRS		0	+	Zidovudine	↓ levels of B	+

ANTI-INFECTIVE AGENT (A)	OTHER DRUG (B)	EFFECT	SIGNIFICANCE/ CERTAINTY
Mefloquine	ß-adrenergic blockers, calcium channel blockers, quinidine, quinine	↑ arrhythmias	+
	Divalproex, valproic acid	↓ level of B with seizures	++
Methenamine mandelate or hippurate	Acetazolamide, sodium bicarbonate, thiazide diuretics	↓ antibacterial effect 2° to ↑ urine pH	++
Metronidazole	Alcohol	Disulfiram-like reaction	+
	Disulfiram (Antabuse)	Acute toxic psychosis	+
	Oral anticoagulants	↑ anticoagulant effect	++
	Phenobarbital, hydantoins	↑ metabolism of A with ↓ effectiveness	+
Nelfinavir	*See protease inhibitors*		
Nevirapine (Viramune)	Oral contraceptives	↓ levels of B	±
	Protease inhibitors	↓ levels of B	±
Pentamidine, IV	Amphotericin B	↑ risk of nephrotoxicity	+
	Foscarnet	↑ risk of hypocalcemia	+
	Pancreatitis-associated drugs, e.g., alcohol, valproic acid	↑ risk of pancreatitis	+

Protease Inhibitors—Anti-HIV Drugs (**Indin** = indinavir; **Nelfin** = nelfinavir; **Riton** = ritonavir; **Saquin** = saquinavir)
Only a partial list—check package insert

Indin	**Nelfin**	**Riton**	**Saquin**	OTHER DRUG (B)	EFFECT	SIGNIFICANCE/ CERTAINTY
				Analgesics:		
		+		1. Alfentanil, fentanyl, hydrocodone, tramadol	↑ levels of B	+
		+		2. Codeine, hydromorphone, morphine	↓ levels of B	+
		+		Anti-arrhythmics: amiodarone, lidocaine, mexiletine	↑ levels of B	+
	+	+	+	Anticonvulsants: carbamazepine, clonazepam, phenytoin, phenobarbital	↓ levels of A, ↑ levels of B	++
		+		Antidepressants, all tricyclic	↑ levels of B	+
		+		Antidepressants, all other	↑ levels of B	+
		+		Antihistamine: Loratadine *(see below)*	↑ levels of B	++
				Anti-HIV protease inhibitors:		
	+			Indinavir	↑ levels of A & B	+
	+			Ritonavir	↑ levels of A	++
+	+	+		Saquinavir	↑ levels of B	++
				Anti-HIV reverse transcriptase inhibitors:		
+	+	+		Zidovudine	↑ levels of B for indin/nelfin; ↓ for riton	+
+	+		+	Nevirapine	↓ levels of A—avoid	++
+	+	+	+	Astemizole/terfenadine	↑ levels of B—do not use	++
+	+	+		Benzodiazepines	↑ levels of B—do not use	++
		+		Beta blockers: Metoprolol, pindolol, propranolol, timolol	↑ levels of B	+
		+		Calcium channel blockers (all)	↑ levels of B	++
+	+	+	+	Cisapride	↑ levels of B—do not use	++
	+	+		Contraceptives, oral	↓ levels of B	++

Protease Inhibitors—Anti-HIV Drugs (**Indin** = indinavir; **Nelfin** = nelfinavir; **Riton** = ritonavir; **Saquin** = saquinavir)
Only a partial list—check package insert (continued)

Indin	Nelfin	Riton	Saquin	OTHER DRUG (B)	EFFECT	SIGNIFICANCE/ CERTAINTY
		+	+	Corticosteroids: prednisone, dexamethasone	↓ levels of A, ↑ levels of B	+
		+		Cyclosporine	↓ levels of B	+
		+	+	Delavirdine	↑ levels of A	+
		+		Diazepam and others	↑ level of B—do not use	++
+	+	+	+	Erythromycin, clarithromycin	↑ levels of A & B	+
+	+		+	Grapefruit juice	↓ indinavir & ↑ saquinavir levels	++
+	+		+	Ketoconazole, itraconazole	↑ levels of A	+
		+		Metronidazole	Poss. disulfiram reaction, alcohol	+
+	+	+	+	Rifampin, rifabutin	↓ levels of A, ↑ levels of B	++
			+	Ritonavir	↑ levels of A	+++
		+		Theophylline	↓ levels of B	+
		+		Warfarin	↑ levels of B	+

ANTI-INFECTIVE AGENT (A)	OTHER DRUG (B)	EFFECT	SIGNIFICANCE/ CERTAINTY
Pyrazinamide	INH, rifampin	May ↑ risk of hepatotoxicity	±
Pyrimethamine	Lorazepam	↑ risk of hepatotoxicity	+
	Sulfonamides, TMP/SMX	↑ risk of marrow suppression	+
	Zidovudine	↑ risk of marrow suppression	+
Quinine	Digoxin	↑ digoxin levels; ↑ toxicity	++
	Mefloquine	↑ arrhythmias	+
	Oral anticoagulants	↑ prothrombin time	++
Rifamycins (rifampin, rifabutin) *See footnote for less severe or less common interactions*[1]	Al OH, ketoconazole, PZA	↓ levels of A	+
	Beta adrenergic blockers (metoprolol, propranolol)	↓ effect of B	+
	Clarithromycin	↑ levels of A[2]	++
	Corticosteroids	↑ replacement requirement of B	++
	Cyclosporine	↓ effect of B	++
	Delavirdine	↑ levels of A	+
	Disopyramide	↓ levels of B	++
	Fluconazole	↑ levels of A[2]	+
	Indinavir, nelfinavir, ritonavir	↑ levels of A (↓ dose of A)	+
	INH	Converts INH to toxic hydrazine	++
	Itraconazole[2], ketoconazole	↓ levels of B, ↑ levels of A[2]	++
	Methadone	↓ serum levels (withdrawal)	+
	Oral anticoagulants	Suboptimal anticoagulation	++
	Oral contraceptives	↓ effectiveness; spotting, pregnancy	+
	Phenytoin	↓ levels of B	+
	Quinidine	↓ effect of B	+
	Sulfonylureas	↓ hypoglycemic effect	+
	Tacrolimus	↓ levels of B	++
	Theophylline	↓ levels of B	+
	TMP/SMX	↑ levels of A	+
	Tocainide	↓ effect of B	+
Rimantadine	*See Amantadine*		
Ritonavir	*See protease inhibitors*		
Saquinavir	*See protease inhibitors*		
Stavudine	Dapsone, INH	May ↑ risk of peripheral neuropathy	±
Sulfonamides	Cyclosporine	↓ cyclosporine levels	+
	Methotrexate	↑ antifolate activity	+
	Monoamine oxidase inhibitors (phenelzine)	↑ toxicity of A	?
	Oral anticoagulants	↑ prothrombin time; bleeding	+
	Phenytoin	↑ levels of B; nystagmus, ataxia	+
	Sulfonylureas	↑ hypoglycemic effect	+
	Thiopental	↑ thiopental levels	±
	Phenobarbital, rifampin	↓ levels of A	+
Trimethoprim	Amantadine, dapsone, digoxin, methotrexate, procainamide, zidovudine	↑ serum levels of B	++

[1] The following is a partial list of drugs with rifampin-induced ↑ metabolism and hence lower than anticipated serum levels: ACE inhibitors, dapsone, diazepam, digoxin, diltiazem, doxycycline, fluconazole, fluvastatin, haloperidol, nifedipine, progestins, triazolam, tricyclics, zidovudine

[2] Up to 4 weeks may be required after RIF discontinued to achieve detectable serum itra levels; ↑ levels associated with uveitis or polymyolysis

TABLE 17 (5)

ANTI-INFECTIVE AGENT (A)	OTHER DRUG (B)	EFFECT	SIGNIFICANCE/ CERTAINTY
Trimethoprim *(con't)*	Potassium-sparing diuretics	↑ serum K^+	+ +
	Thiazide diuretics	↓ serum Na^+	+
Trimethoprim/Sulfa-methoxazole	Azathioprine	Reports of leucopenia	+
	Cyclosporine	↓ levels of B, ↑ serum creatinine	+
	Loperamide	↑ levels of B	+
	Methotrexate	Enhanced marrow suppression	+ +
	Oral contraceptives, pimozide, and 6-mercaptopurine	↓ effect of B	+
	Phenytoin	↑ levels of B	+
	Rifampin	↑ levels of B	+
	Warfarin	↑ activity of B	+
Vancomycin	Aminoglycosides	↑ frequency of nephrotoxicity	+ +
Zalcitabine (ddC) (HIVID)	Valproic acid, pentamidine (IV), alcohol, lamivudine	↑ pancreatitis risk	+
	Cisplatin, INH, metronidazole, vincristine, nitrofurantoin, d4T, dapsone	↑ risk of peripheral neuropathy	+
Zidovudine (ZDV) (Retrovir)	Amphotericin B, flucytosine, fos-carnet, ganciclovir, cidofovir	↑ levels of A with renal toxicity	+
	Atovaquone, fluconazole, metha-done	↑ levels of A	+
	Clarithromycin	↓ levels of A	±
	Nelfinavir	↓ levels of A	+ +
	Probenecid, TMP/SMX	↑ levels of A	+
	Rifampin/rifabutin	↓ levels of A	+ +

TABLE 18
ANTIMICROBICS IN PREGNANCY

DRUG	FDA PREGNANCY CATEGORIES*	PLACENTAL TRANSFER (%)	BREAST FEEDING	ADVERSE EFFECTS: FETUS, MOTHER
Antibacterial Agents				
Aminoglycosides:				
Amikacin	D	16	OK	Ototoxicity
Beta Lactams				
Imipenem/cilastatin	C	ND	OK	None
Clindamycin	ND	6–46	OK	None
Fluoroquinolones	C	80–90	No	Potential arthropathy
Macrolides:				
Azithromycin	B	ND	ND	None
Clarithromycin	C	ND	OK	Fetal toxicity in primates
Erythromycin	B	5–20	OK	None
Metronidazole	B	+	No	None: do not use in 1st trimester
Antifungal Agents:				
Amphotericin B	B	+	OK	None
Fluconazole	C	ND	ND	NHS
Itraconazole	C	ND	No	NHS
Ketoconazole	C	+	No 48 hrs.	NHS
Antiparasitic Agents:				
Pentamidine	C	+	No	NHS
Pyrimethamine	C	+	No	None: do not use in 1st trimester
Sulfonamides	C	70–90	No	Potential kernicterus & hem-G6PD
Trimethoprim	C	30–100	OK	None
Antimycobacterial Agents:				
Dapsone	C	+	OK	Hem-G6PD
Ethambutol	ND	30	OK	None
Isoniazid	C	100	OK	None
Pyrazinamide	C	ND	OK	None
Rifabutin	B	ND	ND	–
Rifampin	C	33	OK	Postnatal bleeding in infant
Streptomycin	D	10–40	OK	Ototoxicity (16% deafness)
Antiviral Agents:				
Acyclovir, valacyclovir	C	70	OK	None
Cidofovir	C	ND	No	–
Delavirdine	C	ND	No	Teratogenic in rats
Didanosine	B	50	ND	None
Famciclovir	B	ND	ND	–
Foscarnet	C	ND	ND	–
Ganciclovir	C	ND	No	Carcinogenic in animals, NHS
Indinavir	C	ND	No	–
Lamivudine	C	100	No	–
Nelfinavir	B	ND	No	–
Nevirapine	C	100	No	–
Ritonavir	B	15–100	No	–
Saquinavir	B	Minimal	No	–
Stavudine	C	76	No	–
Zalcitabine	C	30–50	ND	Tumors in rodents
Zidovudine	C	85	? No	None
Anabolic Agents:				
Megestrol acetate (oral)	X	ND	No	Use contraindicated

* **FDA Pregnancy Categories: A**—adequate studies in pregnant women, no risk; **B**—animal studies no risk, but human studies not adequate <u>or</u> animal toxicity but human studies no risk; **C**—animal studies show toxicity, human studies inadequate but benefit of use may exceed risk; **D**—evidence of human risk, but benefits may outweigh; **X**—fetal abnormalities in humans, risk > benefit; **ND** = no data

Abbreviations: **Hem-G6PD** = hemolysis in individuals with G6PD deficiency; **NHS** = no controlled human studies

TABLE 19
SPECTRUM AND TREATMENT OF HIV/AIDS-ASSOCIATED MALIGNANCIES*

I. **Spectrum of associated malignancies: AIDS-defining neoplasms** *(see Table 9A)*
- A. Kaposi's sarcoma and other KSHV/HHV8 related neoplasms:
  1. Primary body cavity lymphoma
  2. Multicentric Castleman's disease
  3. Possibly multiple myeloma
- B. HIV-associated lymphoma
  1. Primary CNS lymphoma
  2. Non-Hodgkin's lymphoma
- C. Cervical carcinoma
- D. Other neoplasms with increased incidence
  1. Anogenital neoplasia and squamous cell carcinoma of the anus
  2. Basal cell carcinoma of the skin
  3. Hodgkin's disease
  4. Seminoma
  5. Pediatric leiomyosarcoma

II. **Kaposi's sarcoma (KS)**
- A. **Etiology**
  1. Human herpesvirus type 8 (HHV8); also called Kaposi's sarcoma-associated herpesvirus (KSHV)
  2. HHV8/KSHV
     - a. DNA found in all KS tumors
     - b. Infection precedes KS
     - c. Seropositivity rate predicts KS rate
     - d. Latent in most cells; lytic in <5% of cells
     - e. Targets spindle cells
- B. **Diagnosis**
  1. Clinical appearance and then biopsy
  2. HHV8/KSHV serologies in development
- C. **Treatment**
  1. Immune reconstitution (improvement) with effective antiretroviral therapy of HIV infection
     - a. Reports of clearance of HHV8 from circulating cells: *Ln 349:775, 1997*
     - b. Reports of resolution, stabilization, regression of KS: *AIDS 11:261 & 1300, 1997*
  2. Therapeutic value of antiviral drugs that target HHV8/KSHV directly
     - a. Two groups report in vitro inhibition of lytic infection by cidofovir (most active), ganciclovir, and foscarnet *(AIDS 11:1327, 1997; JCI 99:2082, 1997)*
     - b. Only anecdotal clinical reports, using foscarnet *(Scand J Inf Dis 26:749, 1994)*
  3. Local therapy—often used for cosmetic purposes

Therapy	Drug/Dose	Comment
Radiation	Single dose: 800 cGy	For single/grouped lesions. Relieves facial edema.
Intralesional therapy	Vinblastine 0.01 mg in 0.1 ml sterile water Interferon alfa 1.0 million units Human chorionic gonadotropin 2000 IU per lesion *(NEJM 335:1261, 1996)*	
Cryotherapy	Liquid nitrogen	For isolated small lesions
Photodynamic (investigational)	IV photofrin 48 hrs prior to exposure to 100–300 J/cm² of 630 nM light	Partial response in 68% of lesions

  4. Systemic therapy—see next section for doses

	Stage of KS	Recommended Treatment
a.	All stages, if possible	Observe response to combination antiretroviral rx and concomitant improvement in immune status of the patient
b.	If progression despite combination antiretroviral rx or failure of antiretrovirals to substantively ↓ HIV viral burden or ↑ CD4 count:	
	(1) Slowly progressive	(a) Observe or (b) Add interferon alfa to antiretrovirals or (c) Investigational therapy 　　(i) IM human chorionic gonadotropin *(Lancet 346:118, 1995)* 　　(ii) Thalidomide *(CID 23:501, 1996)*
	(2) Rapidly progressive	Vincristine + vinblastine
	(3) Widespread, symptomatic	(a) Liposomal doxorubicin or liposomal daunorubicin (b) Doxorubicin + vincristine + bleomycin
	(4) Refractory disease	Paclitaxel (Taxol)

5. Doses, reported responses, and toxicity of drugs used for systemic therapy** of Kaposi's sarcoma*.
    References: *Med Clin No Amer 81:471, 1997; Scand J Inf Dis 29:3, 1997*

Drug(s)	Dose	Reported Response, %	Toxicity
Bleomycin (with doxorubicin & vincristine)	10 mg/M²	87	Doxorubicin: marrow suppression; G-CSF 5 µg/kg/d (usually 300 µg) may be required. Bleomycin: myocardial toxicity and heart failure with total dose of 550 mg/M² Vincristine: peripheral neuropathy (sensory loss, paresthesias)
Doxorubicin (with bleo & vincristine)	10–20 mg/M²	87	
Human chorionic gonadotropin *(investigational)*	150,000–700,000 u IM 3x/wk	?	Only pain at injection site
Interferon alfa	4–18 mill. units/day 5 d./ wk. given subcutaneously	2–20	Flu-like symptoms
Liposomal doxorubicin	20 mg/M² q2–3 wks	30–95	Neutropenia (15–25%), alopecia, nausea, back pain, flushing, chest tightness
Liposomal daunorubicin	40 mg/M² q2–3 wks	30–95	
Paclitaxel (Taxol)	100 mg/M² q2 wks	53	Severe hypersensitivity reaction in 2% pts; premedicate with steroids, diphenhydramine & H_2 antagonist; pancytopenia; many others
Thalidomide *(investigational) (CID 23:501, 1996)*	3 mg/kg/d	?	Rash, sedation, dry mouth, constipation
	For compassionate use call 1-800-801-8328		
Vinblastine	0.05–0.1 mg/kg/wk	25–30	*See vincristine, above*
Vincristine (with doxorubicin & bleo)	2 mg	87	
Vinblastine + vincristine	2 mg vincristine/wk alternating with 0.1 mg/kg vinblastine/wk	45	

*   For drugs, review package insert regarding dosage, precautions in administration and toxicities. For details, see Kaplan, LD, Northfelt, DW: Malignancies associated with AIDS, in *Medical Management of AIDS*, 5th Ed., Eds.: M.A. Sande, P.A. Volberding, W.B. Saunders & Co., 1997.

** With systemic disease, chemotherapy is palliative only, does not alter survival.

III. **Primary body cavity lymphoma**
    A. Etiology: HHV8/KSHV; some cells also positive for EBV
    B. Diagnosis: Biopsy of tumor masses in pleural space, intraabdominal cavity
    C. Treatment:
       1. No reports to date on influence of anti-HIV therapy
       2. Chemotherapy—*see non-Hodgkin's lymphoma (VI.C)*

IV. **Multicentric Castleman's disease**
    A. Rare lymphoproliferative disorder
    B. Etiology: HHV8/KSHV
    C. Clinical: Fever, lymphadenopathy, splenomegaly
    D. Treatment: Not defined

V. **Multiple myeloma**—relationship to HHV8/KSHV unclear
    A. Patients seronegative and myeloma cells negative for HHV8
    B. BUT cultured marrow stromal cells from myeloma patients positive for HHV8

VI. **HIV-associated lymphoma** *(Med Clin No Amer 81:495, 1997)*
    A. **General**
       1. Compared to immunocompetent pts, present in advanced stage
       2. HIV-associated non-Hodgkin's lymphomas virtually all of B-cell origin
       3. Viral association
          a. Systemic lymphomas—no viral association
          b. CNS lymphoma—EBV DNA present in 100%
          c. Body-cavity lymphomas—HHV8 genome present in virtually all
          (Ref.: Am J Clin Path 105:221, 1996)
    B. **Primary CNS lymphoma**
       1. Usually in patients with very low CD4 counts
       2. Treatment
          a. Whole brain irradiation
          b. Prolongs survival up to 5 months (median survival 10–18 mos.)

TABLE 19 (3)

C. **Non-Hodgkin's lymphoma**
    1. Complete response in 33–57%; relapse in 25% of complete responders within 6 mos.; median survival 4–8 mos.
    2. Treatment

Disease	Drugs/Modalities/Regimens	Comments
Non-Hodgkin's lymphoma	All patients with CD4 <200: low-dose mBACOD. With CD4 >200, consider standard-dose chemotherapy, i.e., CHOP regimen. Survival directly related to CD4 count. If CD4 <100, results are so poor that many would not recommend rx. *(Good reference: Cancer Control 2:97, 1995)*	

	Low-dose mBACOD regimen:
	  Day 1:
	    Cyclophosphamide 300 mg/M² IV
	    Doxorubicin 25 mg/M² IV
	    Vincristine 1.4 mg/M² IV (not to exceed 2.0 mg)
	  Day 15:
	    Methotrexate (MTX) 500 mg/M² with leucovorin rescue 25 mg po q6h x6 beginning 24 hrs after completion of MTX
	  CNS: Cytosine arabinoside 50 mg intrathecally on days 1, 8, 21, 28
	    Add Helmet-Field irradiation if marrow pos. 2000 cGy or if CSF pos., 4000 cGy.
	  Rx: 4–6 cycles at 28-day intervals. Start zidovudine 200 mg q4h at completion of chemotherapy.
		ACTG 142 (198 pts randomized to low-dose mBACOD with GM-CSF support): Complete response 46 vs 50%, median survival 34 vs 31 weeks. Toxicity, neutropenia, in 22% low-dose cycles, 36% of standard-dose cycles. With CNS rx, no isolated CNS relapse *(Blood 74: 897a, 1989; Rev Inf Dis 12:938, 1990; JAMA 266:84, 1991)*. Only 10% of cycles complicated by neutropenia of <500/mm³, rx with GM-CSF. Median survival 6.5 months. Infusional cyclophosphamide, doxorubicin + etoposide + G-CSF, 8/12 pts complete response *(Blood 81:2810, 1993)*.

	CHOP regimen: cyclophosphamide + doxorubicin + vincristine + prednisone. Addition of GM-CSF or G-CSF ↓ neutropenia and febrile episodes.	
	CDE regimen: cyclophosphamide + doxorubicin + etoposide—median survival 18 months in 1 study.	

VII. **Cervical carcinoma**
    A. Epidemiology
        1. More frequent, more severe
           a. As CD4 count falls
           b. If co-infection with human papillomavirus (co-infection in 66% of HIV-infected women)
        2. 25–40% Pap smears abnormal in HIV-infected women
    B. Terminology of pre-invasive cervical disease
        Following terms more or less synonymous: cervical dysplasia, cervical intraepithelial neoplasia (CIN), and squamous intraepithelial lesions (SIL)
    C. Recommendations
        1. Pap smears x2 in year one and then annually if normal
        2. More frequent Pap smears if:
           a. Previous abnormal Pap smear
           b. History of papilloma (wart) virus infection
           c. Post-treatment for CIN (SIL)
           d. Symptomatic AIDS or CD4 count <200/mm³
        3. If Pap smear shows SIL or evidence of papillomavirus, refer for colposcopy and/or biopsy.
        4. Low-grade lesions, follow closely
        5. High-grade lesions, treat by ablation (e.g., radiotherapy) or excision. Avoid cryosurgery due to high recurrence rates.

VIII. **Anal neoplasia**
    A. Epidemiology
        1. HIV-infected immunodeficient patients at increased risk of human papillomavirus (HPV)-related anal neoplasia.
        2. HPV DNA found in roughly 50% of anal cytology specimens from HIV-infected men.
    B. Recommendations for HIV-infected men with history of anal intercourse
        1. Anal Pap smear
        2. Routine anoscopy with biopsy as indicated
        3. Wide surgical resection for established neoplasia

TABLE 20
RECOMMENDATIONS FOR ROUTINE IMMUNIZATION OF HIV+ CHILDREN (ASYMPTOMATIC AND SYMPTOMATIC)[1]
(Modified from USPHS/IDSA Guidelines [*MMWR 46:34, 1997; CID 25(Suppl.3):S330, 1997*])

Vaccine ▼ / Age ►	Birth	1 mo.	2 mos.	4 mos.	6 mos.	12 mos.	15 mos.	18 mos.	24 mos.	4–6 yrs.	11-12 yrs.	14–16 yrs.
↓ Recommendations for these vaccines are the same as those for immunocompetent children ↓												
Hepatitis B[2]	Hep B-1	Hep B-1										
		Hep B-2	Hep B-2	Hep B-2	Hep B-3	Hep B-3	Hep B-3	Hep B-3			Hep B[3]	
Diphtheria, Tetanus, Pertussis[4]			DTaP or DTP	DTaP or DTP	DTaP or DTP		DTaP or DTP	DTaP or DTP		DTaP or DTP	Td	Td
Hemophilus influenzae[5] type b			Hib	Hib	Hib	Hib	Hib					
↓ Recommendations for these vaccines differ from those for immunocompetent children ↓												
Polio[6]			IPV	IPV		IPV	IPV	IPV		IPV		
Measles, Mumps, Rubella[7]						MMR	MMR	MMR	MMR	MMR		
Influenza[8]					Influenza (a dose is required every year)	Influenza (a dose is required every year)	Influenza (a dose is required every year)	Influenza (a dose is required every year)	Influenza (a dose is required every year)	Influenza (a dose is required every year)		
Streptococcus pneumoniae[9]									Pneumo-coccal			
Varicella						CONTRAINDICATED in all HIV-infected persons	CONTRAINDICATED in all HIV-infected persons	CONTRAINDICATED in all HIV-infected persons	CONTRAINDICATED in all HIV-infected persons	CONTRAINDICATED in all HIV-infected persons	CONTRAINDICATED in all HIV-infected persons	CONTRAINDICATED in all HIV-infected persons

NOTE: Modified from the immunization schedule for immunocompetent children. This schedule also applies to children born to HIV-infected mothers whose HIV infection status has not been determined. Once a child is known not to be HIV-infected, the schedule for immunocompetent children applies. This schedule indicates the recommended age for routine administration of currently licensed childhood vaccines. Some combination vaccines are available and may be used whenever administration of all components of the vaccine is indicated. Providers should consult the manufacturers' package inserts for detailed recommendations.

[1] Vaccines are listed under the routinely recommended ages. Bars ☐ indicate range of acceptable ages for vaccination. Shaded bars ▨ indicate catch-up vaccination; at 11–12 years of age, hepatitis B vaccine should be administered to children not previously vaccinated.

[2] *Infants born to HBsAg (hepatitis B surface antigen)-negative mothers* should receive 2.5 μg of Merck vaccine (Recombivax HB) or 10 μg of SmithKline Beacham (SB) vaccine (Engerix-B). The 2nd dose should be administered >1 month after the 1st dose.
Infants born to HBsAg-positive mothers should receive 0.5 ml of hepatitis B immune globulin (HBIG) within 12 hrs of birth and either 5 μg of Merck vaccine (Recombivax HB) or 10 μg of SB vaccine (Engerix-B) at a separate site. The 2nd dose is recommended at 1–2 months of age and the 3rd dose at 6 months of age.
Infants born to mothers whose HBsAg status is unknown should receive either 5 μg of Merck vaccine (Recombivax HB) or 10 μg of SB vaccine (Engerix-B) within 12 hrs of birth. The 2nd dose of vaccine is recommended at 1 month of age and the 3rd dose at 6 months of age. Blood should be drawn at the time of delivery to determine the mother's HBsAg status; if it is positive, the infant should receive HBIG as soon as possible (no later than 1 week of age). The dosage and timing of subsequent vaccine doses should be based on the mother's HBsAg status.

[3] Children and adolescents who have not been vaccinated against hepatitis B in infancy may begin the series during any childhood visit. Those who have not previously received 3 doses of hepatitis B vaccine should initiate or complete the series during the 11- to 12-year-old visit. The 2nd dose should be administered at least 1 month after the 1st dose, and the 3rd dose should be administered at least 4 months after the 1st dose and at least 2 months after the 2nd dose.

[4] DTaP (diphtheria and tetanus toxoids and acellular pertussis vaccine) is the preferred vaccine for all doses in the vaccination series, including completion of the series in children who have received >1 dose of whole-cell DTP vaccine. Whole-cell DTP is an acceptable alternative to DTaP. The 4th dose of DTaP may be administered as early as 12 months of age, provided 6 months have elapsed

TABLE 20 (2)

since the 3rd dose, and if the child is considered unlikely to return at 15–18 months of age. Td (tetanus and diphtheria toxoids, adsorbed, for adult use) is recommended at 11–12 years of age if at least 5 years have elapsed since the last dose of DTP, DTaP, or DT. Subsequent routine Td boosters are recommended every 10 years.

[5] Three H. influenzae type b (Hib) conjugate vaccines are licensed for infant use. If PRP-OMP (PedvaxHIB [Merck]) is administered at 2 and 4 months of age, a dose at 6 months is not required. After the primary series has been completed, any Hib conjugate vaccine may be used as a booster.

[6] Inactivated poliovirus vaccine (IPV) is the only polio vaccine recommended for HIV-infected persons and their household contacts. Although the 3rd dose of IPV is generally administered at 12–18 months, the 3rd dose of IPV has been approved to be administered as early as 6 months of age. Oral poliovirus vaccine (OPV) should NOT be administered to HIV-infected persons or their household contacts.

[7] MMR should not be administered to severely immunocompromised children. HIV-infected children without severe immunosuppression should routinely receive their 1st dose of MMR as soon as possible upon reaching the 1st birthday. Consideration should be given to administering the 2nd dose of MMR vaccine as soon as 1 month (i.e., minimum 28 days) after the 1st dose, rather than waiting until school entry.

[8] Influenza virus vaccine should be administered to all HIV-infected children >6 months of age each year. Children aged 6 months–8 years who are receiving influenza vaccine for the 1st time should receive 2 doses of split virus vaccine separated by at least 1 month. In subsequent years, a single dose of vaccine (split virus for persons ≤12 years of age, whole or split virus for persons >12 years of age) should be administered each year. The dose of vaccine for children aged 6–35 months is 0.25 ml; the dose for children 3 years of age and older is 0.5 ml.

[9] The 23-valent pneumococcal vaccine should be administered to HIV-infected children at 24 months of age. Revaccination should generally be offered to HIV-infected children vaccinated 3–5 years (children aged ≤10 years) or >5 years (children aged >10 years) earlier.

NOTE: BCG is not recommended in the U.S. However, in areas with a high incidence of tuberculosis, WHO recommends BCG immunization of asymptomatic HIV+ children.

TABLE 21
IMMUNIZATION OF HIV+ ADULTS (ASYMPTOMATIC AND SYMPTOMATIC)

General Principles/Guidelines:

- In HIV+ individuals, there are activated T-cells (CD25+) and quiescent T-cells (CD25–). Only activated T-cells produce virus and spread infection. In HIV+ adults, significant (2–36 fold) transient (≤6 weeks) ↑ in plasma viral RNA after pneumococcal, influenzal and tetanus immunization *(NEJM 334:1222, 1996)*. A similar phenomenon occurs with acute infections, i.e., influenza. At present, there are no data suggesting that this is clinically relevant. Concurrently, antibody responses are ↓ in HIV+ individuals. Our recommendations are presented in the following table.
- Administration of live attenuated vaccines is contraindicated in individuals with advanced HIV infection (AIDS) (MMR is an exception).
- Immunization (when indicated) with killed whole cell vaccines and/or purified antigens should be done as soon as reasonable after HIV infection diagnosed, before CD4 cells ↓ further *(JID 171:1217, 1995)*.
- Extended primary series and/or more frequent boosters often indicated.
- When specifically indicated, immune globulin (IG) and specific immune globulins can be administered.

RECOMMENDATIONS FOR ROUTINE IMMUNIZATION OF HIV+ ADULTS (United States)
(From Update on Adult Immunization, Centers for Disease Control, MMWR 40:RR-12, 1991, Nov. 15)

VACCINE/TOXOID	STAGE OF HIV INFECTION		BOOSTER DOSE	AUTHORS' RECOMMENDATIONS§ *(AIDS Clin Care 8:11, 1996)*
	ASYMPTOMATIC HIV+*	SYMPTOMATIC (AIDS)*		
Td (tetanus/diphtheria)	Yes	Yes	10 yrs	+ (if IDU)
HbCV (Haemophilus influenzae type b conjugate vaccine)	Yes	Yes	None	0
Pneumococcal	Yes	Yes	6 yrs	+
Influenza	Yes	Yes	Annual	+
HBV (Hepatitis B)	(Yes)**	(Yes)**	None	+
eIPV (polio)	(Yes)**	(Yes)**	(None)	0

Abbreviations: Td = tetanus and diphtheria toxoids, adsorbed (for adult use); **MMR** = measles, mumps and rubella vaccine; **HbCV** = Haemophilus influenzae type b conjugate vaccine; **Pneumococcal** = pneumococcal polysaccharide (23 component) vaccine; **HBV** = Hepatitis B vaccine; **eIPV** = enhanced-potency inactivated polio vaccine; **IDU** = injection drug user
* Asymptomatic—CDC category A1, A2; Symptomatic—CDC A3, B1–3, C1–3; ** See Comments; § + = benefit > risk, 0 = benefit probably < risk.

COMMENTS ON "ROUTINE" VACCINES/TOXOIDS*

VACCINE/TOXOID	COMMENTS
Td	"Injection" drug users at ↑ risk of tetanus
HbCV	Is of unproven benefit and immune responses ↓; although the risk of H. influenzae type b disease is ↑ and adverse reactions are minimal, it is no longer recommended.
Pneumococcal	Risk of bacteremia is ↑ [as high as 9.4/1000/yr (*J Inf Dis 162:1012, 1990*)]. Revaccination 6 years after 1st dose is recommended. Benefit appears > risk.
Hepatitis A	In the past several years hepatitis A has ↑ in frequency in homosexual men in the U.S., Canada and Australia (*MMWR 45:155, 1992*). Outbreaks have also been reported in injection drug users (*Am J Pub Health 79:463, 1989*). <10% U.S.-born young adults have antibody (*Mil Med 157:579, 1992*). 2 hepatitis A vaccines, inactivated, are licensed in U.S. FDA-approved indications include: persons engaged in high-risk sexual activity (homosexually active men), injection drug users. Use in high-risk HIV+ individuals is ?.
Hepatitis B	If lifestyle or occupation was risk factor for HIV it is also a risk factor for hepatitis B. Series of 3 IM injections in deltoid, using 1½-inch needle (not into the buttocks), should be given. Test for antibody to HBs Ag 1–6 months after completing series. If anti-HBs is <10 milli-international units, revaccinate with 1 or more doses.
Influenza	Annual immunization with the current vaccine is recommended regardless of age. Benefit appears > risk.
eIPV (enhanced-potency inactivated polio vaccine)	In adults ≥18 years, use only if specifically indicated: travel to developing countries (not Central or South America), prior to (~8 weeks, time for initial 2 doses) household exposure to individuals given oral polio vaccine.
OPV (oral polio vaccine)	Contraindicated
Specific immunoglobulins: Hepatitis B (HBIG), human rabies (HRIG), tetanus (TIG), vaccinia (VIG), varicella-zoster (VZIG)	Can be used for same indications, same dosage as in non-HIV infected individuals

* For further details, see Wilson, et al., *Ann Int Med 114:582, 1991*

TABLE 22A
MEASURES TO BE TAKEN BY PHYSICIANS IN PREPARING HIV+ PATIENTS AND INDIVIDUALS LIKELY TO HAVE "RISKY" BEHAVIOR FOR OVERSEAS TRAVEL*

The likelihood of developing an illness during a 3-week vacation in a tropical area is about 50%. Since illnesses are likely to be more serious and/or become chronic in the HIV+ patient, there is advice to be given and measures to be taken to minimize risks. These include:

- If the traveler is likely to engage in risky behavior during travel, ascertain the HIV antibody status before travel, especially if travel is planned to a developing country.
- If the traveler is known to be HIV+, take account of legal restrictions on travel for persons with HIV infection[2]. Assess the immune status (CD4 cell count) in infected persons.
- Review planned itinerary and activities in light of the patient's immune status and review the added risks for travel, especially to developing or tropical countries. In some instances, it may be prudent to recommend a change in itinerary or activities because of serious risks that cannot be eliminated or reduced.
- Recommend the following measures to reduce exposure to pathogens:
  Assiduously avoid food and beverages that may be contaminated, especially raw or undercooked shellfish, fish, meat, or eggs; raw, unpeeled fruits and vegetables; tap water and ice; as well as unpasteurized milk and milk products (cheese). Insist on eating only well-cooked foods and on drinking only very hot or bottled beverages.
  Reduce contact with vectors, for example, by using insect repellent and avoiding outdoor exposure at dusk or other times and places of increased insect activity.
- Urge the patient to obtain prompt evaluation of symptoms of illness and early treatment of infection. Where possible, identify a physician knowledgeable about HIV infection at the destination[3]. Arrange for continuation of medical management during travel (for example, prophylaxis for Pneumocystis carinii pneumonia).
- Use vaccine and prophylactic therapy as indicated by the planned itinerary and activities. Prescribe antimicrobial agents (with or without antimotility drugs) and counsel the patient on their use for early treatment of diarrheal disease.[4]

[1] The most up-to-date source is: Health Information for the International Traveler, 1995. HHS Publication (CDC) No. 93-8280. Available from U.S. Government Printing Office, Washington, DC 20402.
[2] Duckett M., Orkin AJ: AIDS-related migration and travel policies and restrictions: a global survey. AIDS 3:(Suppl 1) S231-252, 1989.
[3] For a list of English-speaking doctors abroad and health information: International Association for Medical Assistance to Travelers (IAMAT), 417 Center St., Lewiston, NY 14092.
[4] For suggestions regarding a medical kit and advice (for all travelers): Sanford JP: Self-help for the traveler who becomes ill. *Inf Dis Clin NA 6:405, 1992.*
* *Reproduced with permission from Wilson ME, von Reyn CF, Fineberg HV: Infections in HIV-infected travelers: risks and prevention (Table 2). Ann Int Med 114:582, 1991. USPHS/IDSA Guidelines CID 21(Suppl. 1):520, 1995.*

TABLE 22B

IMMUNIZATION OF HIV+ ADULTS TRAVELING TO DEVELOPING COUNTRIES*

VACCINE/TOXOID/ AGENT	HIV STATUS**		COMMENTS
	ASYMPTOMATIC	**SYMPTOMATIC**	
"Routine" for All Developing Countries			
eIPV	Yes	Yes	*See above.* OPV contraindicated
Typhoid Vi polysaccharide vaccine (Connaught)	Yes	Yes	Boosters recommended q2 yrs. Live attenuated typhoid vaccine contraindicated
Immune globulin (IG)	Yes	Yes	For 2-3 months travel, 0.02 ml/kg IM single dose
"Special" Depending on Itinerary: Country and Activity			
Cholera (inactivated vaccine)	*See Comments*	*See Comments*	Vaccine does not prevent transmission, efficacy ~50%, risk to U.S. travelers very low. WHO does not recommend, but some countries require (check with Health Dept.). If required, have vaccination completed, signed, dated and validated to avoid risk of revaccination and quarantine.
Rabies (pre-exposure) (inactivated vaccine)	Yes, if indicated (Animal handlers, travelers spending 1 month or more in country where rabies is a constant threat)	Yes, if indicated	Course: Three 1.0 ml of HDCV or RVA IM on days 0, 7, 28. Test serum for antibodies 2 weeks after 3rd dose.
Meningococcal (polysaccharide vaccine)	Yes, if traveling to area where meningococcal disease is epidemic or endemic (sub Sahara Africa)		
Yellow Fever (live attenuated)	Yes (±); offer choice if potential exposure unavoidable	No (contraindicated)	
Japanese Encephalitis	Yes, if indicated: travel to Asia, in monsoon (summer) months, staying in rural areas		Requires 3 injections: day 0, 7, and 30. An abbreviated schedule at days 0, 7, 14 can be used but less effective *(MMWR 42:RR-1, 1993)*.
Plague (inactivated)	Yes, if indicated: to areas of endemic plague, especially if staying in rural areas, not in tourist hotels		
BCG (Bacillus Calmette-Guerin) vaccine	No	No	Is live attenuated vaccine

*   All travelers should have current routine immunizations, *Table 21, pages 122–123*

**   Asymptomatic—CDC category A1, A2; Symptomatic—CDC A3, B1-3, C1-3 *(Table 3, page 9)*.

TABLE 23
INFECTION CONTROL FOR HIV

I. General. 1996 Hospital Infection Control Practices Advisory Committee, CDC Guidelines, Revised; *Am J Inf Cont 24:24, 1996)*
  A. The revised guidelines contain two tiers of precautions:
      1. "Standard Precautions": all hospitalized patients, regardless of diagnosis
      2. "Transmission-based Precautions": patients suspected or known to be infected
  B. Standard Precautions **(use with all patients)**
      1. Wash hands between patient contacts, after contact with blood, body fluids, secretions, excretions, and equipment contaminated by them.
      2. Wear gloves (barrier protection) when touching blood, etc., as in (1). Change gloves between patients. Wash hands after removing gloves.
  C. Transmission-Based Precautions

Type Precaution	Requirements
Airborne	• Private room, negative air pressure, ≥6 exchanges per hour, discharge air to outside or filter air
	• Respiratory protection (i.e., N95 particulate respirator, 3M—still requires fit-testing) for all persons entering room
Droplet	• Private room if possible
	• Masks if working within 3 feet of patient
Contact	• Glove when entering room, change after contact (B.2)
	• Gown for substantial contact with patient or environmental surfaces

  D. Precautions by Clinical Syndrome, emphasis on HIV-associated infections

Syndrome	Potential Pathogens	Type Precautions
Diarrhea	See Table 9, pages 50 & 51	Contact
Respiratory (cough, sputum production, ± fever)		
Until TB excluded*	M. tuberculosis	Airborne
TB excluded	Strep. pneumoniae, H. influenzae, influenza virus	Droplet
Above excluded	P. carinii, fungal, Kaposi's	Standard
Skin (maculopapular, vesicular, excoriated, ulcerative lesions)	H. simplex, VZV, Staph. aureus, Group A strep, syphilis, scabies	Contact
Abscess, draining wounds, decubiti	H. simplex, Staph. aureus, enterobacteria-ceae, pseudomonas	Contact

  * Until results of AFB stains on 3 specimens negative or until 2 weeks of treatment with clinical response

II. Prevention of Needle Injuries
      Dispose at site of use in puncture-proof container (not plastic bags)
      Do NOT resheath, snip, or perform other post-use manipulation
      If using new "safety" needles, ensure adequate training/practice prior to use
      With blunted suture needles, risk is ~0.
      Double-gloving: blood-hand contact ↓ from 71 to 32/100 procedures.

III. Tuberculosis Prevention and Control
  A. Screening
      1. Recommendations for tuberculin testing (with purified protein derivative):
          • HIV-infected persons
          • Injection drug users
          • Prison/jail inmates
          • Homeless persons
          • Immunosuppressed persons
          • Health care workers. OSHA TB Compliance Directive (2.106, Feb. 9, 1996) requires a "two-step baseline for new employees who had initially negative PPD and who had not had a documented negative TB skin test result during preceding 12 months." *See A.2 below.*
          • Upon admission to nursing homes, residential care facilities, hospices
      2. Procedure and interpretation
          Tuberculin test (abbreviation TBnT). The standard is the Mantoux test, 5 TU PPD in 0.1 ml diluent stabilized with Tween 80. Read at 48–72 hours measuring maximum diameter of induration.
              • ≥5 mm is **positive** in the following: + HIV or risk factors, recent close case contacts, chest x-ray consistent with healed tuberculosis.
              • ≥10 mm is **positive** in the following: foreign-born in countries of high prevalence, IV drug users, low income populations, nursing home residents, patients with medical conditions which ↑ risk.
              • ≥15 mm is **positive** in all individuals *(Am Rev Resp Dis 142:725, 1990).*
          Two-stage TBnT: use in individuals to be tested regularly, i.e., health care workers. TBn reactivity may ↓ over time but boosted by skin testing. If unrecognized, individual may be incorrectly diagnosed as recent converter. If 1st TBnT is reactive but <10 mm, repeat 5 TU in 1 week, if then ≥10 mm = +, not recent conversion *(Am Rev Resp Dis 119:587, 1979).*

          (Regardless of BCG immunization status; prior BCG does not contraindicate PPD testing unless documented history of an accelerated reaction.)

3. Anergy testing indicated only if results affect clinical care *[MMWR 46(RR-15):1, 1997]*. Application of 1 of the following intradermally:
   - Mumps antigen
   - Candida antigen
   - Tetanus antigen

   Any reactivity is considered positive by most experts.

B. INH prophylaxis for PPD positives if no or inadequate prior treatment
   1. Not HIV-infected: 9 months INH
      a. All persons with positive PPD <35 years of age. [Recent model suggests that INH prophylaxis with careful monitoring of liver function tests may be beneficial in patients >35 years of age as well *(Ann Int Med 127:1051, 1997).*]
      b. All recent (within 2 years) PPD converters (after active disease excluded)
   2. HIV-infected persons
      a. INH for 12 months
      b. Rifampin plus pyrazinamide for 2 months (under investigation)
      c. Study in Uganda suggests 3 regimens effective for prophylaxis in PPD+, HIV+ patients: INH for 6 months, INH + RIF for 3 months, INH + PZA for 3 months *(NEJM 337:801, 1997)*.
   3. Multiply drug resistant TB contacts *(contact CDC for advice)*

C. Active disease (institute airborne isolation, *I.C above*)
   Maintain a high index of suspicion! Nearly all outbreaks of nosocomial tuberculosis related to **failure to identify infected patients**. Once isolation implemented, transmission ceases *(CID 22:597, 1996)*.

IV. Invasive (Surgical or Other) Procedures
   Procedure-specific
      Barrier precaution for high-risk exposure: double or triple glove, plastic apron, double sleeves, water-resistant shoe covers, face shield
      "Sharps" precautions: avoid hand-to-hand passage of sharps (use Mayo tray or emesis basin), "no touch" surgery, minimize needles in the field, coordinate surgical team
      Alternative techniques: blunt needles, staples, Bovie cautery

V. Sterilization and Disinfection: It is imperative that the risk of disease transmission by instruments be negligible. This requires standardized procedures. Following are several guidelines: *[for details: 1. Disinfection, Sterilization and Preservation, 4th Ed., editor S.S. Block, Lea & Febiger, Philadelphia, 1991; 2. Am J Inf Cont 22:19, 1994]*

Levels of resistance of microorganisms to germicidal chemicals (level of disinfection required: high, intermediate, low):
   Most resistant: bacterial spores (high) > mycobacteria (intermediate) > non-lipid viruses (polio, rhino) (low) > fungi (candida, crypto) (low) > vegetative bacteria (pseudomonas, staph) (low) > lipid viruses (HSV, CMV, hepatitis B, HIV) (low); least resistant

Activity levels of selected procedures/liquid germicides:
Sterilization: steam autoclaving
                glutaraldehyde
Disinfection: glutaraldehyde (high to intermediate)
                hydrogen peroxide (high to intermediate)
                chlorine compounds, 500-1000 mg/L free chlorine (household bleach is excellent, inexpensive) (intermediate)
                alcohols, 70% isopropyl (intermediate)
                phenolic compounds (intermediate-low)
                iodophor compounds (intermediate-low)
                quaternary ammonium compounds, 0.1-0.2% (low)

Instrument-related risks of disease transmission/level of sterilization/disinfection required/comments:
Critical instruments: routinely penetrate skin or mucous membranes during use, e.g., needles, scalpel blades: require sterilization
Semicritical instruments: come in contact with intact mucous membranes during use, e.g., flexible fiberoptic endoscopes, laryngoscopes, vaginal specula: require high level disinfection
Noncritical instruments: normally come in contact with intact skin, e.g., blood pressure cuffs, stethoscopes, ECG electrodes: sterilization/disinfection between use is not critical, clean if soiled (household bleach)

Environmental surfaces: If soiled: clean, low-level disinfectant, chlorine compounds (household bleach) very active against HIV. Skin antiseptics are NOT appropriate for disinfecting inanimate surfaces!

APIC Guideline for Infection Prevention and control in flexible endoscopy (Am J Inf Cont 22:19, 1994):
   Mechanical cleansing (most important step): carry out immediately before secretions dry, alcohol and aldehyde compounds not to be used for mechanical cleaning (coagulate protein):
   - When endoscope removed from patient, flush air/water channel for 10-15 seconds. Aspirate detergent through biopsy/suction channel for 10-15 seconds
   - External cleansing. Totally immerse in warm water and detergent
   - Brush through suction biopsy channel
   - Flush each internal channel
   - Rinse
   Disinfection:
   - Totally immerse in 2% glutaraldehyde or other disinfectant of similar potency for not less than 5 min.
   - Rinse with water, then dry
   Storage:
   - After disinfection, rinse each channel with 70% alcohol, dry with compressed air
   - Store in hanging position (not coiled in box)

TABLE 24
ALTERNATIVE THERAPIES FOR HIV*

- Early unorthodox treatments included megadose vitamin C, AL-721 (a mixture of lipids extracted from egg yolks with acetone), dinitrochlorobenzene (DNCB) (a topical sensitizer), ribavirin (an antiviral agent effective against respiratory syncytial virus, Hantaan and several arenaviruses) and dextran sulfate.
- Extent of usage of alternative therapies varies but is in the range of 30–70% of patients with HIV. Hence, care providers at least must be aware of such agents.
- With the current abundance of available antiretroviral agents, alternative therapies are sought for conditions without truly effective interventions, e.g., immune suppression, wasting syndrome.
- There are many alternative agents; this is a list of ones in common, current use.

AGENT	NATURE OF AGENT	ADVERSE EFFECTS/COMMENTS
Antioxidants		
Vitamin C (large doses)	Proposed activity against oxygen free radicals resulting in less CD4 lymphocyte destruction	Diarrhea
Beta-carotene		3 studies now confirm higher death rates with drug rx from cancer, heart disease and stroke *(NEJM 330:1029, 1994)*.
Cysteine precursors (N-acetyl cysteine, NAC)	Cysteine precursor, used for mucolytic rx in bronchitis and systemically for acetaminophen poisoning	Minimal toxicity. Phase I NIAID study shows minimal oral bioavailability; no change in CD4, p24 antigen, plasma viremia or cysteine levels.
SPV-30	An extract of boxwood evergreen tree with "purported anti-HIV activity"	French pilot study found ↑ CD4 counts without significant side-effects. Larger controlled trial and "trial by mail" showed no surrogate benefits.
Chinese herbs	Numerous preparations utilized for control of various HIV-related symptoms	No measurable clinical or surrogate marker effect with a 31-herb mixture given for 12 weeks in placebo-controlled trial *(J AIDS 12:386, 1996)*.
Acupuncture	Traditional Chinese medicine approach to anesthesia and pain management	Studied vs amitriptyline vs placebo for peripheral neuropathy in CPCRA study and found to be ineffective.
Marijuana	Leaves and flowering tops of a number of Cannabis species; anti-emetic and appetite stimulant properties	Widespread use in the absence of clinical trials; active component (delta-9 THC) licensed drug; impact unknown on immune system, lungs (? aspergillus) and possibly drugs metabolized by liver.
DHEA (dehydroepiandrosterone)	Naturally occurring adrenal steroid with purported immune modulating and antiviral activity	Phase I trial showed no surrogate benefits, few adverse effects. Possible virilization (voice, hirsutism) in women. Widely used to ↑ body mass *(J AIDS 6:459, 1993)*.
Nandrolone (Deca-Durabolin)	Injectable anabolic steroid	Ongoing trials to evaluate effects in wasting syndrome in both men and women. Impact on immune system unknown at present.
Tea Tree Oil (Malalcuca)	Australian bush plant extract with in vitro activity vs candida isolates	Microbiologic and clinical efficacy of 15 cc mouthwash qid in refractory thrush reported *(XI Intl Conf. 2:109, WeB 3305, 1996)*; blisters possible, nausea if swallowed.
Allicin	A high-dose garlic concentrate from China used for refractory diarrhea	Community trial of 30 mg bid in pts with cryptosporidiosis reported improved stool consistency, ↓ frequency, and some clearing of organism
Cat's claw (Una de Gato)	Peruvian highlands herb with "panacea" properties; utilized as immune stimulant and antioxidant	No efficacy data available, but agent reportedly has low toxicity even at high doses; taken as a tea preparation.

TABLE 25
AIDS INFORMATION AND REFERRAL SERVICES

- AIDS/HIV Clinical Trials conducted by National Institutes of Health and FDA-approved efficacy trials: 1-800-874-2572
- For a wide variety of AIDS/HIV information, resources, publications, call the National AIDS Clearinghouse: 1-800-458-5231
- To find out about AIDS resources in your area, call the National AIDS Hotline: 1-800-342-2437
- The AIDS/HIV Treatment Directory is published by the American Federation for AIDS Research (AmFAR) and is updated semi-annually; 733 Third Ave., 12th Floor, New York, NY 10017-3204. Telephone: 1-800-392-6327
- The HIV/AIDS Treatment Information Service (Public Health Coordinating Group): 1-800-HIV-0440

TABLE 26
LIST OF GENERIC AND COMMON TRADE NAMES

GENERIC NAME	TRADE NAME	GENERIC NAME	TRADE NAME	GENERIC NAME	TRADE NAME
Acyclovir	Zovirax	Ethionamide	Trecator	PAS	Paser
Amikacin	Amikin	Etoposide	VePesid	Pentamidine	Pentam 300
Amphotericin B	Fungizone	Famciclovir	Famvir	Pentamidine aerosol	NebuPent
Ampho B cholesteryl complex	Amphotec	Filgrastim (G-CSF)	Neupogen	Primaquine	Primaquine
Ampho B lipid complex	Abelcet	Fluconazole	Diflucan	Pyrazinamide	Pyrazinamide
Ampho B liposomal	AmBisome[NUS]	Flucytosine	Ancobon	Pyrimethamine	Daraprim
Atovaquone	Mepron	Foscarnet	Foscavir	Ribavirin	Virazole
Azithromycin	Zithromax	Ganciclovir	Cytovene	Rifabutin	Mycobutin
Bleomycin	Blenoxane	Human growth hormone (rHGH)	Serostim	Rifampin	Rifadin
Capreomycin	Capastat			Ritonavir	Norvir
Cidofovir	Vistide	Imipenem	Primaxin	Saquinavir	Invirase
Ciprofloxacin	Cipro	Indinavir	Crixivan	Sargramostim (GM-CSF)	Leukine, Prokine
Clarithromycin	Biaxin	Interferon alfa	Roferon-A, Intron A	Stavudine (d4T)	Zerit
Clindamycin	Cleocin	Iodoquinol	Yodoxin	Thiacetazone	Tibione
Clofazimine	Lamprene	Isoniazid	INH, Laniazid, Tubizid	Trimethoprim	Proloprim, Trimpex
Cycloserine	Seromycin	Itraconazole	Sporanox	Trimethoprim/ Sulfamethoxazole	Bactrim, Septra
Daunorubicin-liposome	DaunoXome	Ketoconazole	Nizoral		
Delavirdine	Rescriptor	Lamivudine (3TC)	Epivir	Trimetrexate	Neutrexin
Didanosine (ddl)	Videx	Megestrol	Megace	Valacyclovir	Valtrex
Doxorubicin	Adriamycin	Nelfinavir	Viracept	Vidarabine	Vira-A
Doxorubicin-liposome	Doxil	Nevirapine	Viramune	Vinblastine	Velban
Dronabinol	Marinol	Norfloxacin	Noroxin	Vincristine	Oncovin
Erythropoietin	Epogen, Procrit	Ofloxacin	Floxin	VP16	VePesid
Ethambutol	Myambutol	Paclitaxel	Taxol	Zalcitabine (ddC)	HIVID
		Paromomycin	Humatin	Zidovudine (ZDV)	Retrovir

TRADE NAME	GENERIC NAME	TRADE NAME	GENERIC NAME	TRADE NAME	GENERIC NAME
Abelcet	Ampho B lipid emulsion	HIVID	Zalcitabine (ddC)	Retrovir	Zidovudine
		Humatin	Paromomycin	Rifadin	Rifampin
Adriamycin	Doxorubicin	Intron A	Interferon alfa	Rimactane	Rifampin
AmBisome[NUS]	Ampho B liposomal	Invirase	Saquinavir	Roferon-A	Interferon alfa
Amikin	Amikacin	Lamprene	Clofazimine	Septra	TMP/SMX
Amphotec	Ampho B cholesteryl complex	Leukine	Sargramostim (GM-CSF)	Seromycin	Cycloserine
Ancobon	Flucytosine			Serostim	Human growth hormone [HGH(m)]
Bactrim	TMP/SMX	Marinol	Dronabinol		
Biaxin	Clarithromycin	Megace	Megestrol	Sporanox	Itraconazole
Blenoxane	Bleomycin	Mepron	Atovaquone	Taxol	Paclitaxel
Capastat	Capreomycin	Myambutol	Ethambutol	Tibione	Thiacetazone
Cleocin	Clindamycin	Mycobutin	Rifabutin	Trecator	Ethionamide
Cipro	Ciprofloxacin	NebuPent	Pentamidine aerosol	Trimpex	Trimethoprim
Crixivan	Indinavir	Neupogen	Filgrastim (CSF)	Valtrex	Valacyclovir
Cytovene	Ganciclovir	Neutrexin	Trimetrexate	Velban	Vinblastine
Daraprim	Pyrimethamine	Noroxin	Norfloxacin	VePesid	Etoposide (VP16)
DaunoXome	Daunorubicin-liposome	Norvir	Ritonavir	Videx	Didanosine (ddl)
		Oncovin	Vincristine	Viracept	Nelfinavir
Diflucan	Fluconazole	Paser	PAS	Viramune	Nevirapine
Doxil	Doxorubicin-liposome	Pentam 300	Pentamidine	Virazole	Ribavirin
		Primaxin	Imipenem + cilastatin	Vistide	Cidofovir
Epivir	Lamivudine			Yodoxin	Iodoquinol
Epogen	Erythropoietin	Procrit	Erythropoietin	Zerit	Stavudine (d4T)
Famvir	Famciclovir	Prokine	Sargramostim (GM-CSF)	Zithromax	Azithromycin
Floxin	Ofloxacin			Zovirax	Acyclovir
Foscavir	Foscarnet	Proloprim	Trimethoprim		
Fungizone	Amphotericin B	Rescriptor	Delavirdine		

TABLE 27

COSTS OF COMMONLY USED AGENTS AND LABORATORY TESTS FOR AN HIV-INFECTED ADULT[*]

AGENT OR TEST	TRADE NAME	COMMON REGIMEN	COST/YR ($)
Antiretroviral treatment			
Zidovudine (AZT, ZDV)	Retrovir	200 mg orally 3x/day	3,490
Didanosine (ddI)	Videx	200 mg orally 2x/day	2,160
Zalcitabine (ddC)	HIVID	0.75 mg orally 3x/day	2,520
Stavudine (d4T)	Zerit	20 mg orally 2x/day	2,730
Lamivudine (3TC)	Epivir	150 mg orally 2x/day	2,800
Saquinavir	Invirase	600 mg orally 3x/day	7,080
Ritonavir	Norvir	600 mg orally 2x/day	8,120
Indinavir	Crixivan	800 mg orally q8h	6,020
Nevirapine	Viramune	200 mg orally 2x/day	3,020
Prophylaxis against Pneumocystis carinii pneumonia or toxoplasmosis			
TMP/SMX	Bactrim DS	160 mg TMP and 800 mg SMX orally 3x/wk	30
Dapsone		100 mg orally daily	70
Atovaquone	Mepron	750 mg orally 2x/day	8,190
Prophylaxis against Mycobacterium avium complex			
Rifabutin	Mycobutin	300 mg orally daily	1,890
Clarithromycin	Biaxin	500 mg orally 2x/day	2,380
Azithromycin	Zithromax	1200 mg orally every week	1,510
Antifungal prophylaxis or treatment			
Clotrimazole troche	Mycelex	10 mg orally 5x/day	1,360
Nystatin suspension	Mycostatin	5 ml orally 4x/day	2,660
Fluconazole	Diflucan	100 mg orally daily	2,510
Ketoconazole	Nizoral	200 mg orally daily	1,070
Itraconazole	Sporanox	200 mg orally daily	4,260
Prophylaxis against cytomegalovirus			
Ganciclovir, oral	Cytovene	1 gm orally 3x/day	17,080
Herpes simplex treatment			
Acyclovir	Zovirax	400 mg orally 2x/day	1,610
Nutritional maintenance			
Food supplement	Ensure	1 8-oz. can orally 3x/day	1,610
	Ensure Plus	1 8-oz. can orally 3x/day	1,970
Dronabinol	Marinol	2.5 mg orally 2x/day	1,820
Megestrol acetate	Megace	800 mg orally daily	3,290
Laboratory monitoring			
Complete blood count and chemistry profile[†]		4x/year	200
CD4 cell count		4x/year	400
HIV viral load measurement		4x/year	800

Adapted from Feder and Milch, NEJM 336:954, 1997

* Costs are based on average wholesale prices, rounded to the nearest $10, with prices for generic products used when available. TMP/SMX denotes trimethoprim/sulfamethoxazole.

† The chemistry profile includes measurements of electrolytes and renal and liver function tests.

TABLE 28

INDUCED SPUTUM FOR IDENTIFICATION OF PULMONARY PATHOGENS, SPUTUM COLLECTION
(Ng et al., Arch Path Lab Med 113:488, 1989)

(1) No solid food for 8 hours

(2) Immediately before induction: vigorously brush teeth, gingival margins, tongue and buccal surfaces with water or saline. Rinse thoroughly. Gargle several times with water.

(3) Inhale aerosol solution of 3% saline generated by ultrasonic nebulizer (DeVilbiss Model 35B or UltraNeb-100) for 20 minutes (3 to 7 ml/minute)

(4) Expectorate one specimen during the first few minutes of inhalation and the second during the remainder of the procedure. Label each. The second is more likely to be representative of distal respiratory tract secretions. Examine the first only if the second is non-diagnostic.

INDEX TO MAJOR ENTITIES

Bold numbers indicate
    • *Major description of syndrome, disease or infection & rx*
    • *Drug dosage, side-effects, & modification in renal/hepatic insufficiency*

Bold numbers indicate
- *Major description of syndrome, disease or infection & rx*
- *Drug dosage, side-effects, & modification in renal/hepatic insufficiency*

Bold numbers indicate
- *Major description of syndrome, disease or infection & rx*
- *Drug dosage, side-effects, & modification in renal/hepatic insufficiency*

Bold numbers indicate
- *Major description of syndrome, disease or infection & rx*
- *Drug dosage, side-effects, & modification in renal/hepatic insufficiency*

NOTES

NOTES

NOTES

NOTES

NOTES

NOTES